ABBREVIA

H&P	Histc
HPF	High-power field (microscopy)
HPV	Human papillomavirus
HSIL	High-grade squamous intraepithelial lesions
HSV	Herpes simplex virus
IAS	Internal anal sphincter
IBD	Inflammatory bowel disease (Crohn disease, ulcerative colitis, indeterminate colitis)
IBS	Irritable bowel syndrome
ICU	Intensive care unit
I&D	Incision and drainage (abscess)
IMA	Inferior mesenteric artery
IMRT	Intensity-modulated radiation therapy
IMV	Inferior mesenteric vein
IPAA	Ileal J-pouch anal anastomosis
IPS	Irritable pouch syndrome
IRA	Ileorectal anastomosis
LAR	Low anterior resection
LBO	Large bowel obstruction
LGV	Lymphogranuloma venereum
LIS	Lateral internal sphincterotomy
LLQ	Left lower quadrant
LSIL	Low-grade squamous intraepithelial lesions
LUQ	Left upper quadrant
LV	Leucovorin
MACE	Malone antegrade colonic enema
MAP	*MYH*-associated polyposis
MELD	Model for end-stage liver disease
MRCP	Magnetic resonance cholangiopancreatography
MRI	Magnetic resonance imaging
MRSA	Methicillin-resistant *Staphylococcus aureus*
MSI	Microsatellite instability
MSM	Men who have sex with men
MSS	Microsatellite stability
NGT	Nasogastric tube
NPO	Nothing by mouth (*nulla per os*)
NSAID	Nonsteroidal anti-inflammatory drug

McGraw-Hill Manual

Colorectal Surgery

To my wife Petra,
and my sons Benjamin, Linus, and Julian

McGraw-Hill Manual
Colorectal Surgery

Andreas M. Kaiser
Associate Professor of Clinical Colorectal Surgery
USC Department of Colorectal Surgery
Keck School of Medicine, University of
Southern California
Los Angeles, California

Mc Graw Hill **Medical** 2009

New York Chicago San Francisco Lisbon London Madrid Mexico City
New Delhi San Juan Seoul Singapore Sydney Toronto

The *McGraw-Hill* Companies

McGraw-Hill Manual Colorectal Surgery

1 2 3 4 5 6 7 8 9 0   CTP/CTP   0 9 8

ISBN 978-0-07-159070-9
MHID 0-07-159070-6

This book was set in Times by International Typesetting and Composition.
The editors were Marsha Loeb and Harriet Lebowitz.
The production supervisor was Sherri Souffrance.
The illustration manager was Armen Ovsepyan.
Project management was provided by Preeti Longia Sinha, International
Typesetting and Composition.
The designer was Eve Siegel; the cover designer was Thomas De Pierro.
Cover photo: Surgical laser used in treating colon cancer. Jan
Halaska/Photo Researchers, Inc.
China Printing & Translation Services, Ltd., was printer and binder.

This book is printed on acid-free paper.

Library of Congress Cataloging-in-Publication Data

Kaiser, Andreas M.
      McGraw-Hill manual. Colorectal surgery / Andreas M. Kaiser.
         p. ; cm.
      ISBN 978-0-07-159070-9 (pbk. : alk. paper)   1. Colon (Anatomy)—
Surgery—Handbooks, manuals, etc.   2. Rectum—Surgery—Handbooks,
manuals, etc.   3. Colon (Anatomy)—Diseases—Handbooks, manuals,
etc.   4. Rectum—Diseases—Handbooks, manuals, etc.   I. Title.
II. Title: Colorectal surgery.
      [DNLM: 1. Colonic Diseases—diagnosis—Handbooks.   2. Colonic
Diseases—therapy—Handbooks.   3. Colorectal Surgery—methods—
Handbooks.   4. Rectal Diseases—diagnosis—Handbooks.   5. Rectal
Diseases—therapy—Handbooks. WI 39 K13m 2009]
      RD544.K37 2009
      617.5'547—dc22

                                                              2008023059

CONTENTS

ACKNOWLEDGMENTS

I am deeply indebted to my wife, Petra Lott, for her unrestricted constant support in whatever new adventure I take on—despite the numerous obligations she has to deal with in her own professional and academic life. Furthermore I am most grateful to the professors and academic mentors that were key to my professional career development, in particular to Felix Largiader (University of Zurich, Switzerland), Michael L. Steer (Harvard University), and Robert W. Beart Jr (University of Southern California). Last but not least, it is no secret that a big token of appreciation goes to my professional colleagues for their daily support and efforts to maintain a stimulating academic and practice environment, as well as to an uncounted number of students, residents, and fellows I had the privilege to teach, challenge, and interact with.

PREFACE

Healthcare with its high degree of specialization, the rapid and dynamic technical revolution, and fast-pace day-to-day activities has become increasingly complex and demanding at all levels of providers. Colorectal Surgery—as the historically first subspecialty within the realm of surgery to establish its own training programs and board certification—is no exception. Margins for making mistakes have decreased, while the daily pressure continues to increase with shortened hospitalizations and more rapid patient turnovers. Doing the right thing in a particular situation means knowing about possible strategies and alternatives with their likely outcomes.

There are numerous excellent, very comprehensive textbooks on colorectal surgery which remain the backbone of in-depth study and knowledge acquisition. For a rapid "double-check review" of the evidence, the amount of available data and information from these and other heavy-weight sources tends to be overwhelming. The role of a short and concise handbook is never designed to replace the standard textbooks but to complement them and to provide a handy, quick, and well organized "on-the-move" reference when there is no time to halt.

The McGraw-Hill Manual in Colorectal Surgery is intended to serve as this quick, highly structured notes-style source of information about colorectal diseases and their management. The book is written for established colorectal surgeons, general surgeons, and other specialists likewise, as well as for students, residents, and fellows in those areas, who deal with patients, prepare/study for an operation or presentation, or need a rapid refresher text for the boards or maintenance of certification (MOC) exams. The content was chosen such that the major areas of the colorectal core curriculum are covered according to national and professional guidelines. The central focus and point of view is the one of colorectal surgery, whereas covering every possible detail and common general surgery principles would have been beyond the scope of this manual.

The text is divided in seven chapters plus two appendices:

- Symptoms and Differential Diagnosis
- Evaluation Tools
- Anatomy and Physiology
- Diseases and Problems
- Operative Techniques
- Nonsurgical Management

- Perioperative Management
- Appendix I Medications
- Appendix II Diagnostic Guides

Topics in each of these chapters are written in notes-style format. To avoid lengthy sentences, the arrow symbol ($\rightarrow$) is liberally used as a logical *downstream linker* to indicate *what follows*—logically, medically, anatomically, in pathogenesis, or with regards to the management. Common abbreviations used throughout the text are explained in the appendix.

The text follows a predictable structure to allow the reader to focus on all aspects of a particular topic or just the parts relevant to their momentary needs. The content covers the majority and all relevant aspects outlined in the curriculum for colorectal residencies, defines the standard of care according to published guidelines, and highlights ongoing controversies within colorectal surgery. Furthermore, it provides a description of the most common surgical procedures of the specialty in a step-by-step fashion. Where applicable, ICD-9 codes have been added to the topic headings. In addition to the table of contents, cross references to chapters with related topics are placed at the bottom of each topic in order to facilitate navigation within the text and book. Illustrations are not the main focus of this guide, but are incorporated for selected key aspects that benefit from the visual support.

The author and the publisher are equally aware of the changing preferences and interpersonal variability in the way information is carried around and accessed these days. The traditional print edition in pocket-size format will therefore be supplemented with alternate e-media formats (eg, AccessSurgery)—(a) to follow an increasing demand, and (b) with the intent to maintain accuracy of the information by timely updates and revisions. Regardless of the chosen medium, the readers are advised to consult more extensive information where needed to gain adequate detail in specific areas. Recommendations for selection and dosing of medications can only serve as a general idea, but will always need to be verified before being applied to an individual patient's care.

Andreas M. Kaiser, MD FACS

Los Angeles, California

March 2008

Chapter 1

Symptoms and Differential Diagnosis

ABDOMINAL DISTENTION

Highlights of the Symptom

- Localization/point of origin: peritoneal cavity (ascites, bowel dilation), abdominal wall (hernia, obesity).
- Associated symptoms: nausea, vomiting, abdominal pain and cramping, altered bowel function, bleeding?
- Symptom evolution: acute/progressive, intermittent, recurrent, chronic.
- Appearance: diffuse, focal area.
- Grading: mild, severe.
- Underlying systemic disease: congenital malformation, malignancy, cardiovascular disease, IBD, history of previous surgeries.
- Probability of being sign of serious disease (liability issue): high.

Pathogenesis-Oriented Differential Diagnosis

1. Malformation
   - acquired: obesity, organomegaly (liver, spleen)
   - cystic fibrosis (mucoviscidosis) with fecal impaction in the small bowel
   - megacolon (Hirschsprung disease)
   - colonic malrotation
   - intestinal atresia
2. Vascular
   - ischemia-related bowel obstruction (ischemic stricture)
3. Inflammatory
   - inflammatory process with bowel obstruction (diverticulitis, Crohn disease)
   - toxic megacolon
4. Tumor
   - tumor-related bowel obstruction (neoplasm, endometriosis)
   - carcinomatosis
   - pseudomyxoma peritonei
5. Degenerative/functional
   - adhesion-related bowel obstruction
   - Ogilvie syndrome
   - hernia
   - pseudohernia from denervation of abdominal wall musculature

  – fecal impaction

  – ascites (eg, liver cirrhosis)

6. Traumatic/posttraumatic

  – hematoma

Top of the List

1. Constitutional: obesity.

2. Bowel obstruction (SBO, LBO).

3. Hernia.

4. Megacolon/pseudoobstruction.

5. Ascites.

Keys to Diagnosis

• Patient's surgical/medical history: habitus, symptom progression, previous abdominal surgeries, tumor, etc.

• Clinical examination: patient's general condition and habitus, presence/absence of (tympanitic) bowel sounds, focal/diffuse tenderness to palpation, organomegaly, peritoneal signs, stool in rectal vault.

• Imaging:

  – Abdominal x-ray series, chest x-ray: evidence of bowel obstruction (SBO vs LBO), free air, distended loops of bowel, air/fluid levels, gastric dilation, transition point, presence of air in distal colon, calcifications, pneumobilia.

  – CT scan (if possible with oral and IV contrast): ascites, hernia, small or large bowel dilation, transition point, extensive mucosal thickening, intestinal pneumatosis, pneumobilia, portal vein gas, suspicion of closed loop, intraabdominal/retroperitoneal mass, extent and location of tumor burden, etc.

  – Ultrasound: ascites, tumor.

Cross-reference

BLEEDING PER RECTUM

Highlights of the Symptom

- Localization/point of origin: upper GI, mid-GI, lower GI, anorectal.
- Associated symptoms: pain, pruritus, prolapse, altered bowel habits, constipation, diarrhea, dizziness, weakness, weight loss?
- Time factor: onset, constant, certain times, certain activity, link to menstrual cycle?
- Symptom evolution: continuous, intermittent, worsening, one-time, self-limited.
- Appearance: BRBPR, dark blood, melena, invisible/occult bleeding, false positive (nonhematogenous red color).
- Severity: acute/massive, acute/moderate, sporadic, occult, anemia.
- Underlying systemic disease: hematologic, liver disease, medications (ASA, warfarin).
- Probability of being sign of serious disease (liability issue): high.

Pathogenesis-Oriented Differential Diagnosis

1. Malformation
   - AV malformations, angiodysplasia, Osler disease
   - Meckel diverticulum
   - congenital aneurysms
2. Vascular
   - ischemic colitis
   - mesenteric ischemia
   - vasculitis
   - Osler disease
   - rectal varices
   - hemorrhoids
   - anorectal Dieulafoy lesion
   - acquired (pseudo-)aneurysms
   - radiation injury
   - esophageal varices
3. Inflammatory
   - colitis (infectious, idiopathic, postradiation)
   - SRUS

- – fissure
- – perianal dermatitis
- – peptic ulcer disease, Mallory-Weiss syndrome

4. Tumor
    - – epithelial: cancer, adenomatous polyps
    - – mesenchymal: lymphoma, leiomyoma, GIST, etc
    - – neurogenic: melanoma
    - – endometriosis

5. Degenerative/functional
    - – diverticulosis
    - – stercoral ulcers
    - – prolapse
    - – intussusception
    - – Mallory-Weiss syndrome

6. Traumatic/posttraumatic
    - – blunt/penetrating trauma
    - – anal intercourse, autoeroticism, foreign body
    - – iatrogenic
    - – paraplegia with need for manual stimulation

Top of the List

Local bleeding source

1. Fissure.

2. Hemorrhoids.

3. Neoplasm.

4. Prolapse.

5. Trauma.

Higher bleeding source

1. Diverticulosis (distal > proximal).

2. Tumor.

3. Colonic AV malformation (proximal > distal).

4. IBD.

5. Ischemia.

6. Bleeding proximal to ileocecal valve (Meckel, Crohn, varices, Mallory-Weiss, peptic ulcer, etc).

Children:

1. Anal fissure

2. Intussusception

3. Meckel diverticulum

4. Polyps

Keys to Diagnosis

- Clinical examination: general condition, abdominal exam, rectal exam, anoscopy/rigid sigmoidoscopy.
- Blood work: CBC, PT, PTT → rule out coagulopathy.
- Colonoscopy: limited by poor visibility (unprepped colon, strong light absorption of blood that results in darkness); distribution of blood in the colon has only limited value in localization of bleeding source.
- Tagged red blood cell scan: > 0.5 mL bleeding, particularly the first 15–30 min are meaningful for localization.
- Angiography: > 1 mL/min bleeding.
- Bleeding proximal to ileocecal valve: NGT insertion, EGD, capsule endoscopy.

Cross-reference

Topic	*Chapter*
Colonoscopy	2 (p 71)
Angiography	2 (p 128)
Nuclear scintigraphy	2 (p 131)
Anal fissure	4 (p 161)
Hemorrhoids	4 (p 167)
Colorectal cancer	4 (pp 252–265)
Lower GI bleeding	4 (p 391)

COLITIS OR PROCTITIS

Highlights of the Symptom

- Definition: visible inflammatory changes in colon or rectum (edema, ulcerations, friability).
- Localization/point of origin: begin at the dentate line? Most distal segment disease-free or with limited disease (caveat: distal begin of disease potentially masked by previous local therapy!).
- Associated symptoms: altered bowel habits, diarrhea, bleeding, mucous discharge, urgency, tenesmus, weight loss, pelvic or abdominal pain, abdominal distention, fever, toxic signs, urinary tract infections? Extraintestinal manifestations?
- Time factor: sudden onset, gradual onset, relapsing, one-time, continuous.
- Symptom evolution: gradual worsening, on/off relapsing.
- Appearance: diffuse involvement of affected segment, patchy/discontinuous involvement, very localized.
- Severity: extent of involvement, chronic/acute/fulminant/toxic.
- Underlying systemic disease: known IBD, status postcancer treatment (radiation, chemotherapy, bone marrow transplantation, etc).
- Probability of being sign of serious disease (liability issue): high.

Pathogenesis-Oriented Differential Diagnosis

1. Malformation

  – cavernous hemangioma ($\rightarrow$ no true inflammation)

2. Vascular

  – ischemic colitis (peripheral vascular disease, embolic disease, vasculitis)

  – radiation injury

3. Inflammatory

  – IBD: ulcerative colitis, Crohn disease

  – *C difficile* colitis, diverticulitis

  – infectious colitis (amebic, shigella, enterohemorrhagic *E coli,* tuberculosis, cytomegalovirus, etc)

  – STD proctitis: lymphogranuloma venereum, gonorrhea, etc

  – side effect: bowel cleansing (aphthoid ulcers or diffuse), NSAIDs, etc

  – eosinophilic colitis

4. Tumor

  – colorectal cancer (eg, signet cell cancer results in diffuse infiltration with lack of mass effect)

  – extraintestinal cancer

  – lymphoma, Kaposi sarcoma

  – endometriosis

5. Degenerative/functional

  – SRUS

  – stercoral ulcerations (fecal impaction)

6. Traumatic/posttraumatic

  – anal intercourse, autoeroticism, foreign body

  – iatrogenic

Top of the List

1. IBD

2. Specific proctitis/colitis (*C difficile,* infectious, STD).

3. Ischemic colitis (caveat: ischemic proctitis unlikely!).

4. Radiation proctitis/colitis.

Keys to Diagnosis

- History: narration with specific details, identification of risk factors (family, travel, radiation, cardiovascular surgery, anoreceptive intercourse, etc).
- Clinical examination: anoscopy/rigid sigmoidoscopy or partial/full colonoscopy, endoscopic picture, and biopsies.
- Histology: type of inflammation, granulomatous disease.
- Stool analysis: cultures, *C difficile* toxin, ova and parasites, possible fecal WBCs.
- Serum analysis: possible serum titers for viral/amebic pathogens.
- Possible imaging studies, eg, small bowel follow-through or CT enterography: small bowel involvement?

Cross-reference

CONSTIPATION

Highlights of the Symptom

- Appearance: decreased frequency of bowel movements, increased consistency of the stools, change in shape (pencil-/pellet-like bowel movements), need for straining or manual support, incomplete evacuation; multiple/repetitive small bowel movements.
- Localization/point of origin: intestinal transport, evacuation.
- Associated symptoms: bleeding, weight loss, fever, dehydration (primary/secondary), vaginal bulging, etc.
- Time factor: acute vs chronic.
- Symptom evolution: one-time, gradually worsening, lifelong.
- Underlying systemic disease: tumor, cardiopulmonary disease, diabetes, renal disease, etc.
- Probability of being sign of serious disease (liability issue): age-dependent.

Pathogenesis-Oriented Differential Diagnosis

1. Malformation
   - atresia
   - Hirschsprung disease
2. Vascular
   - ischemic stricture
3. Inflammatory
   - Crohn diseaes with stricture
   - chronic diverticulitis with stricture
   - anastomotic stricture
4. Tumor
   - tumor-related obstruction
5. Degenerative/functional
   - dietary
   - social (poor habits)
   - drug-induced
   - immobility
   - endocrine/metabolic: hypothyroidism, diabetes, hyperparathyroidism
   - psychiatric/neurologic (Parkinson disease, multiple sclerosis, etc)
   - constipation-predominant IBS

- slow transit constipation (colonic inertia)
- pelvic floor dysfunction: functional outlet obstruction, intussusception, prolapse, rectocele
- Chagas disease
- pregnancy (pelvic/abdominal lack of space, endocrine-induced decrease of motility, insufficient fluid intake)

6. Traumatic/posttraumatic
   - spinal injury, paraplegia
   - retroperitoneal/spinal pathology (hematoma, fracture, etc)

Top of the List

1. Habits.
2. Drug-induced.
3. Functional (IBS, slow transit constipation).
4. Morphologic obstruction (tumor, stricture etc).
5. Pelvic floor dysfunction.

Keys to Diagnosis

- Patient's surgical/medical history: habits, daily routine (diary), alarm symptoms, previous abdominal surgeries, tumor, systemic disease, etc. Previous colonic evaluations?
- Clinical examination: patient's general condition, abdominal distention, palpable mass, tenderness to palpation? Digital rectal exam: perineal descent, stool in rectal vault, stool quality, rectocele, sphincter and puborectalis muscle tone, etc?
- Based on evidence from H&P, the likelihood of a morphologic problem has to be determined in order to decide on further tests:
  - Colonic evaluation.
  - Colonic function tests: colonic transit time, defecation proctogram.
  - CT scan.
  - Contrast studies.

Cross-reference

DIARRHEA

Highlights of the Symptom

- Localization/point of origin: intestinal, colonic, systemic.
- Associated symptoms: nausea, vomiting, abdominal pain and cramping, abdominal distention, high ileostomy output of watery (tealike) quality, bleeding, altered bowel habits, diarrhea, urinary tract infections?
- Time factor: acute vs chronic.
- Symptom evolution: single episode (self-limited).
- Appearance: increased frequency, decreased consistency (loose, watery, etc), added components (blood, mucus), etc.
- Severity: decompensated → dehydration; compensated → preserved hydration and organ function.
- Underlying systemic disease: IBD, celiac disease, history of previous abdominal surgeries, antibiotic use, etc.
- Probability of being sign of serious disease (liability issue): moderate.

Pathogenesis-Oriented Differential Diagnosis

1. Malformation
    - short bowel syndrome (postresection)
    - internal fistula (eg, gastrocolic, enterocolonic, enteroenteric fistula)
2. Vascular
    - acute mesenteric ischemia (first stage)
    - chronic intestinal ischemia
    - massive GI bleeding
3. Inflammatory
    - infectious enteritis/enterocolitis (viral, bacterial, parasites, fungal, STDs, etc)
    - toxic colitis (eg, *C difficile* colitis, chemotherapy)
    - collagenous colitis (abortive form of ulcerative colitis?)
    - microscopic colitis (abortive form of ulcerative colitis?)
    - IBD (ulcerative colitis, Crohn disease)
    - pouchitis
    - radiation enteritis
    - celiac disease

4. Tumor
  – neuroendocrine tumor (eg, VIPoma)
5. Degenerative/functional
  – contrast-induced
  – IBS (diarrhea predominant)
  – dietary (eg, artificial sweeteners, enteral tube feeding)
  – drug-induced (eg, laxatives, bowel cleansing, HAART, chemotherapy, etc)
  – bile acid–induced (eg, postileal resection, Crohn disease)
  – malabsorption
  – pancreatic insufficiency
  – stress-induced
  – paradoxical diarrhea (in fecal impaction)
6. Traumatic/posttraumatic
  – loss of bowel

Top of the List

Acute diarrhea
1. Infectious enterocolitis (including traveler's diarrhea).
2. Iatrogenic (contrast-induced, drugs, cleansing).
3. Antibiotic-associated diarrhea.
4. IBD.

Chronic diarrhea
1. IBS.
2. IBD.
3. Malabsorption.
4. Collagenous/microscopic colitis.

Keys to Diagnosis

- Patient's surgical/medical history: exposure (travel, foods, oral–anal intercourse, etc)? Other family members affected? Previous endoscopies? Previous abdominal surgeries, tumor, antibiotic treatment, immunosuppression (HIV, drug-induced), current medications, etc.
- Clinical examination: patient's general condition (hydration, hemodynamic status), abdominal distention, hyperactive bowel sounds, focal/diffuse tenderness to palpation, peritoneal signs, stool in rectal vault (fecal impaction?), etc.

• Further testing (typically not needed for acute self-limited diarrhea):
  – Stool analysis: cultures, toxins, O&P, 24-hour fat content.
  – Blood/urine tests: celiac disease, 5-HIAA, etc.
  – Endoscopy:
    • Colonoscopy with biopsies (even if macroscopically normal → assess for collagenous or microscopic colitis).
    • EGD → consider small bowel biopsy to rule out celiac disease?
    • Capsule endoscopy?
  – Imaging:
    • Contrast studies: small bowel follow-through, CT enterography.
• Response to empirical treatment (antidiarrheals, cholestyramine, etc).

Cross-reference

Topic	*Chapter*
HIV-associated diseases	4 (p 206)
STDs	4 (p 210)
Carcinoid tumor	4 (p 287)
Infectious colitis	4 (p 315)
IBD	4 (pp 320–327)
IBS	4 (p 434)

DISCHARGE
Highlights of the Symptom

- Localization/point of origin: per rectum, perianal, per vagina?
- Associated symptoms: perianal/perineal moisture ($\rightarrow$ skin irritation), odor, bleeding, pain, itching, tenesmus, urgency, prolapse, altered bowel habits, diarrhea, weight loss, pulmonary symptoms?
- Time factor: onset, constant, cyclic, certain time, certain activity?
- Symptom evolution: continuous, intermittent, worsening, one-time, self-limited.
- Appearance: aqueous; clear, colorless mucus; brownish; feculent; purulent.
- Underlying systemic disease: fistula-in-ano, fecal incontinence/soiling, rectovaginal fistula, IBD (ulcerative colitis, Crohn disease), HIV, STDs, tuberculosis.
- Probability of being sign of serious disease (liability issue): moderate.

Pathogenesis-Oriented Differential Diagnosis

1. Malformation
  – ectropion (eg, post–Whitehead hemorrhoidectomy)

2. Vascular
  – prolapsing internal hemorrhoids
  – radiation proctitis

3. Inflammatory
  – proctitis/colitis (infectious, idiopathic, postradiation)
  – SRUS
  – abscess
  – fistula-in-ano
  – anastomotic leak
  – dermatitis (eczema, contact allergy, etc)

4. Tumor
  – large adenoma (particularly villous adenoma)
  – anorectal tumors (cancer, Paget disease, Bowen disease)

5. Degenerative/functional
  – IBS
  – rectal prolapse/intussusception
  – fecal incontinence

    – transpiration
    – inadequate local hygiene
6. Traumatic/posttraumatic
    – anal intercourse, autoeroticism, foreign body
    – rectourinary fistula

Top of the List

1. Abscess/fistula.

2. Incontinence/transpiration.

3. Prolapse (rectal, hemorrhoidal).

4. Villous adenoma.

5. IBS.

6. Neoplasm.

7. Proctitis.

8. Trauma.

Keys to Diagnosis

• Patient history: precipitating/risk factors, characterization of symptoms.
• Clinical examination: careful anorectal exam including inspection, palpation, anoscopy/rigid sigmoidoscopy.
• Colonoscopy: (a) for diagnostic purposes if diagnosis not clear from local exam; (b) colonic evaluation per guidelines.
• Functional studies: anophysiology testing, defecating proctogram, etc.

Cross-reference

Topic	*Chapter*
Hemorrhoids	4 (p 167)
Perianal/-rectal fistula	4 (p 178)
Fecal incontinence	4 (p 189)
STDs	4 (p 210)
Colorectal cancer	4 (pp 252–265)
Rectal prolapse	4 (p 423)

EXTRALUMINAL AIR

Highlights of the Symptom

- Radiologic finding: conventional x-ray, CT scan.
- Associated abdominal symptoms: nausea, vomiting, abdominal pain and cramping, distention, GI dysfunction, tissue crepitans?
- Evolution: primary progression/regression, temporary resolution (eg, postoperative) with secondary recurrence?
- Location: peritoneal, retroperitoneal, mediastinal, abdominal wall/soft tissue.
- Probability of being sign of serious disease (liability issue): high.

Pathogenesis-Oriented Differential Diagnosis

1. Malformation
   – Chilaiditi syndrome, situs inversus: pseudo–free air
2. Vascular
   – portal vein gas: sign of ischemic bowel necrosis
3. Inflammatory
   – perforated viscus (colon, peptic ulcer, appendicitis, etc): → confined or free perforation
   – anastomotic leak → confined or free perforation
   – abscess → small pocket of extraluminal air
   – appendicitis: rarely leading to pneumoperitoneum
   – emphysematous cholecystitis
   – necrotizing soft tissue infection
4. Tumor
   – perforated tumor → confined or free perforation
5. Degenerative/functional
   – spontaneous pneumoperitoneum without peritonitis: aspiration of air, eg, through vagina and tubes
   – peritoneal dialysis
6. Traumatic/postsurgical
   – postoperative pneumoperitoneum: normal resolution expected within 7 days, sporadically taking up to $2^1/_2$ –3 weeks (however, worsening not compatible with delayed absorption → new pathology has to be suspected)
   – postoperative while nonvacuum drains still in place

– postcolonoscopy: small amounts of gas possible even without perforation

– colonoscopic/endoscopic perforation → generally massive pneumoperitoneum and/or retroperitoneal air (due to insufflation of pressured gas)

– post–transanal endoscopic microsurgery (TEM): extensive retroperitoneal gas expected.

– postcardiopulmonary resuscitation: air leak from pressured ventilation → pneumomediastinum/pneumothorax with abdominal extension; rib fractures → sharp injury to lung/diaphragm

– pneumobilia: status post-ERCP/sphincterotomy, status post-hepaticojejunostomy

Top of the List

1. Perforated viscus.

2. Normal postoperative.

3. Anastomotic leak.

4. Abscess.

Keys to Diagnosis

• Patient's immediate surgical/medical history: type and time frame of previous abdominal surgeries or procedures, prodromal symptoms (eg, epigastric or LLQ pain, etc).

• Clinical examination: patient's general condition, vital signs, abdominal distention, tenderness to percussion/palpation, peritoneal signs (involuntary guarding, rebound tenderness), bowel sounds, drains, etc.

• Context synthesis: combination of radiologic data with information from H&P.

• Additional imaging: eg, water-soluble contrast study.

Cross-reference

FISTULA

Highlights of the Symptom

- Localization/point of origin (primary opening): stomach, small bowel, colon, rectum, anal canal.
- Localization of secondary openings: abdominal skin, small bowel, colon, rectum, vagina/uterus, bladder/urethra, perirectal skin.
- Associated symptoms: drainage (stool, pus, gas, urine), incontinence, fever, sepsis, abscess, abdominal or perirectal pain, bleeding, skin irritation, change in bowel habits (eg, diarrhea), malnutrition, weight loss.
- Time factor: onset with acute presentation, onset without memorable episode of acute event, associated with preceding event (abdominal/perianal) or procedure.
- Symptom evolution: worsening, improving, one-time episode with complete/incomplete resolution, high-/low-output or alternating, recurrent, sporadic cyclic.
- Appearance: diameter, length, visible mucosa, perifocal induration/erythema, tenderness.
- Severity: severe (with sepsis, malnutrition), moderately symptomatic (manageable, not manageable), asymptomatic except for abnormal passage, completely asymptomatic.
- Underlying systemic disease: Crohn disease, cancer, radiation enteropathy, adhesions, preceding surgery, systemic infection (tuberculosis, actinomycosis, etc), hidradenitis suppurativa, chronic LGV.
- Probability of being sign of serious disease (liability issue): low to high.

Pathogenesis-Oriented Differential Diagnosis

1. Malformation
   - pilonidal cyst
   - congenital anogenital malformations
   - urachus fistula
2. Vascular
   - radiation injury (acute, chronic)
   - incarcerated hernia
3. Inflammatory
   - Crohn disease (intestinal)
   - diverticulitis
   - massive adhesions

  – cryptoglandular disease

  – hidradenitis suppurativa

  – burrowing fissure

  – tuberculosis

  – actinomycosis

  – chronic LGV

4. Tumor

  – advanced neoplasm (cancer, lymphoma, etc)

5. Degenerative/functional

  – diverticulosis

  – giant hernia with loss of domain

6. Traumatic/posttraumatic

  – Iatrogenic: eg, postsurgical leak, stapler injury, enterotomies, instrument perforation, implant, etc

  – blunt/penetrating trauma (eg, impalement)

  – anal intercourse, autoeroticism, foreign body

  – obstetric injury

  – iatrogenic (postsurgery, instrument perforation, enterotomies, etc)

Top of the List

Anal/perirectal

1. Cryptoglandular fistula.

2. Hidradenitis suppurativa.

3. Crohn disease.

4. Posttraumatic/postsurgical.

Abdominal

1. Diverticulitis.

2. Cancer.

3. Crohn disease.

4. Postsurgical (eg, enterotomy, leak, infected implant).

Keys to Diagnosis

• Patient history: events/interventions preceding onset, exact description of symptoms and severity, underlying diseases, evidence for FRIEND (foreign body, radiation, infection, epithelialization, neoplasm, distal obstruction)?

- Clinical examination: anorectal exam including anoscopy/sigmoidoscopy, vaginal exam if needed, abdominal exam, general condition, and nutritional status.
- Further testing:
  - Anorectal: assessment in clinic as tolerated, complete during surgery, imaging only under selected circumstances.
  - Abdomen: CT abdomen/pelvis, colonoscopy vs barium enema, small bowel follow-through, fistulogram, assessment of nutritional status → ultimately surgical exploration to give best assessment of the problems.

Cross-reference

INCONTINENCE

Highlights of the Symptom

- Quality of incontinence: stool, gas, urine.
- Location: anal, vaginal, urethra.
- Warning symptoms: urgency ("reduced time to bathroom"), inappercept episodes.
- Descriptive severity: staining < soilage < seepage < accidents.
- Grading of severity and impact: scoring systems: eg, CCF/Wexner fecal incontinence score (frequency of five parameters), Fecal Incontinence Quality of Life (FIQL) score.
- Associated symptoms: bleeding, prolapse (rectal, vaginal, bladder), altered bowel habits, diarrhea/constipation, urinary incontinence, urinary tract infections, abdominal discomfort?
- Evolution: acute-limited, progressive, sporadic, persistent.
- Timing: interval since original injury?
- Underlying systemic disease: IBD, IBS, malignancy, history of previous surgeries, diabetes, neurologic including spinal disease, history of chemoradiation?
- Probability of being sign of serious disease (liability issue): low.

Pathogenesis-Oriented Differential Diagnosis

1. Malformation
    - meningomyelocele → neurogenic incontinence
    - imperforate anus (postreconstructive pull-through procedure)
    - cloaca-like deformity (acquired, congenital)
    - keyhole deformity (acquired)
2. Vascular
    - radiation injury with stricture formation
3. Inflammatory
    - IBD
    - fistula-in-ano
4. Tumor
    - anorectal cancer
5. Degenerative/functional
    - age-related
    - idiopathic sphincter dysfunction

  – rectal/hemorrhoidal prolapse
  – pelvic floor dysfunction
  – pelvic organ prolapse syndrome
  – neuropathy (eg, diabetes, drug-induced)
  – functional fecal incontinence (normal sphincter and nerve function)

6. Traumatic/posttraumatic
  – obstetric injury
  – surgical injury (hemorrhoidectomy, fistulotomy, sphincterotomy)
  – post-sphincter–salvaging coloanal or ileoanal reconstruction
  – spinal injury
  – brain injury

Top of the List

1. Obstetric injury (10% known at time of delivery, 30% occult).
2. Anorectal surgeries (hemorrhoidectomy, fistulotomy, sphincterotomy).
3. Altered bowel habits (IBS, IBD, diet intolerance, constipation with over-flow incontinence).
4. Status post colo-/ileoanal reconstruction.

Keys to Diagnosis

• Patient's surgical/medical history: gravity/parity, obstetric injuries, previous anorectal, vaginal or abdominal surgeries, malignancy, radiation treatment; underlying diseases, bowel function.
• Clinical examination: anal configuration, sphincter function (sphincter complex, auxiliary muscles), evidence for morphologic changes (inflammation, mass, stricture, etc).
• Investigations:
  – Anophysiology studies including endorectal ultrasound: sphincter defect, manometry, neuropathy, anorectal sensation, rectal compliance.
  – Endoscopy.

Cross-reference

INTESTINAL STRICTURE

Highlights of the Symptom

- Localization/point of origin: proximal/mid/distal small bowel, large bowel.
- Associated symptoms: nausea, vomiting, abdominal pain and cramping, abdominal distension, high ileostomy output of watery (tealike) quality, bleeding, altered bowel habits, diarrhea, urinary tract infections? Dehydration, hemodynamic instability, sepsis?
- Symptom evolution: asymptomatic, acute, intermittent/recurrent, chronic.
- Appearance: endoscopic, radiologic, during surgery.
- Severity: no functional impact, causing mild/moderate/severe symptoms (partial SBO/LBO, complete SBO/LBO).
- Underlying systemic disease: Crohn disease, malignancy, history of previous surgeries.
- Probability of being sign of serious disease (liability issue): moderate to high.

Pathogenesis-Oriented Differential Diagnosis

1. Malformation
   - atresia
   - anastomotic stricture

2. Vascular
   - mesenteric ischemia (peripheral vascular disease, embolic disease, vasculitis)
   - portal vein thrombosis
   - radiation injury with stricture formation

3. Inflammatory
   - peritoneal adhesions
   - Crohn disease
   - diverticulitis/appendicitis with inflammatory encasement of small bowel loop(s)
   - pancreatitis (mixture of direct inflammation and mid-colic ischemia)

4. Tumor
   - peritoneal carcinomatosis (various primary tumors)
   - desmoid
   - lymphoma, mesenchymal tumors
   - endometriosis
   - primary small bowel cancer: rare

5. Degenerative/functional
   – ileus (postoperative)
   – internal wrapping of small bowel around ileostomy-bearing small bowel segment
   – volvulus
   – intussusception
   – fecoliths/fecal impaction in small bowel of patients with cystic fibrosis
   – gallstone ileus
6. Traumatic/posttraumatic
   – blunt abdominal trauma
   – abdominal compartment syndrome (post-trauma, post–burn injury, etc)
   – retroperitoneal/spinal pathology (hematoma, fracture, etc)

Top of the List

Small bowel
1. Crohn disease.
2. Adhesions.
3. Small bowel cancer (primary, carcinomatosis).

Large bowel
1. Cancer.
2. Diverticulitis.
3. Crohn disease.
4. Ischemia.

Keys to Diagnosis

• Patient's surgical/medical history: previous abdominal surgeries, tumor, etc.
• Clinical examination: patient's general condition, abdominal distention (may be absent if very proximal obstruction), presence/absence of (tympanitic) bowel sounds, focal/diffuse tenderness to palpation, peritoneal signs, stool in rectal vault.
• Imaging:
   – Abdominal x-ray series, chest x-ray: SBO vs LBO, free air, air/fluid levels, gastric dilation, small bowel dilation (> 2.5 cm) with plicae circulares, transition point, presence of air in the distal colon, distended loops of bowel, calcifications, pneumobilia.

– CT scan (if possible with oral and IV contrast): small bowel dilation, transition point, extensive mucosal thickening, intestinal pneumatosis, pneumobilia, portal vein gas, suspicion of closed loop, tumor burden, etc.

– Contrast studies: small bowel follow-through: (a) with barium if chronic partial SBO, (b) diatrizoate meglumine (Gastrografin) or 50%/50% Gastrografin/barium if more acute partial SBO.

Cross-reference

Topic	*Chapter*
Contrast enema	2 (p 99)
SBFT	2 (p 107)
Colorectal cancer	4 (pp 252–265)
IBD—Crohn disease	4 (p 327)
LBO	4 (p 355)
Diverticular disease	4 (p 368)

LARGE BOWEL OBSTRUCTION *(LBO)*

Highlights of the Symptom

- Grading: partial LBO, complete LBO.
- Localization: anal canal, rectum, left-sided, right-sided.
- Associated symptoms: time of last bowel activity, abdominal distention, abdominal pain and cramping, nausea, vomiting (miserere: feculent vomiting), bleeding, altered bowel habits, urinary tract infections? Dehydration, hemodynamic instability, sepsis?
- Evolution: acute, intermittent, recurrent, chronic.
- Underlying systemic disease: Crohn disease, malignancy, cardiovascular disease, history of previous surgeries.
- Probability of being sign of serious disease (liability issue): high.

Pathogenesis-Oriented Differential Diagnosis

1. Malformation
   - anorectal malformation: imperforate anus/atresia
   - Hirschsprung disease
2. Vascular
   - ischemic colonic stricture (peripheral vascular disease, embolic disease, vasculitis)
   - radiation injury with stricture formation
   - ischemic anastomotic stricture
3. Inflammatory
   - Crohn disease
   - chronic diverticulitis with stricture formation
   - inflammatory anastomotic stricture (eg, leak)
   - anal stenosis (postsurgical, chronic diarrhea, Crohn disease, etc)
4. Tumor
   - colorectal cancer, anal cancer
   - peritoneal carcinomatosis (various primary tumors)
   - desmoid
   - lymphoma, mesenchymal tumors
   - endometriosis

5. Degenerative/functional
   – ileus (postoperative)
   – internal wrapping of small bowel around ostomy-bearing large bowel segment.
   – intussusception
   – hernia (inguinal/ventral/internal)
   – colonic pseudoobstruction (Ogilvie syndrome)
6. Traumatic/posttraumatic
   – blunt abdominal trauma
   – abdominal compartment syndrome (post-trauma, post–burn injury, etc)
   – retroperitoneal/pelvic/spinal pathology (hematoma, fracture, etc)

Top of the List

1. Neoplasm.
2. Chronic diverticulitis.
3. Pelvic radiation injury with stricture formation.
4. Anastomotic stricture.
5. Herniation (external, internal).
6. Crohn disease.

Keys to Diagnosis

• Patient's surgical/medical history: symptom characterization, previous abdominal/pelvic/anorectal surgeries, tumor, radiation treatment, etc.
• Clinical examination: patient's general condition, abdominal distention, presence of incarcerated hernia, presence/absence of (tympanitic) bowel sounds, focal/diffuse tenderness to palpation, peritoneal signs, stool in rectal vault.
• Imaging:
   – Abdominal x-ray series, chest x-ray: SBO vs LBO, free air, small bowel dilation and air/fluid levels (sign of incompetent ileocecal valve), large bowel dilatation (> 6 cm in transverse, >12 cm in cecum), transition point, air in the distal colon, calcifications, pneumobilia.
   – CT scan (if possible with oral and IV contrast): large bowel dilation, tumor burden, transition point, extensive mucosal thickening, intestinal pneumatosis, portal vein gas, nondistended small bowel ($\rightarrow$ suspicion of closed loop), etc.
   – Contrast studies: water-soluble contrast enema: point of obstruction vs pseudoobstruction?

Cross-reference

LUMP OR MASS

Highlights of the Symptom

- Localization/point of origin: perianal, rectal, presacral, rectovaginal, abdominal, lymph nodes.
- Associated symptoms: obstruction, presence/absence of pain, discharge, incontinence, fever, weight loss, night sweats, etc.
- Time factor: rapid onset, slow progression, on-off, related to menstrual cycle.
- Symptom evolution: unchanged, worsening, sporadic, constant, improving.
- Appearance: visible lump, preserved epithelial cover, ulceration, erythema, discharge, tenderness.
- Severity: benign, malignant.
- Underlying systemic disease: known malignancy, IBD, endometriosis, etc.
- Probability of being sign of serious disease (liability issue): high.

Pathogenesis-Oriented Differential Diagnosis

1. Malformation
   - cyst
   - skin tag
2. Vascular
   - cavernous hemangioma
   - external hemorrhoid
   - thrombosed hemorrhoid
3. Inflammatory
   - sentinel skin tag (from chronic anal fissure)
   - abscess/fistula opening
   - actinomycosis
   - gumma
   - inflammatory mass (diverticulitis, Crohn disease, appendicitis, etc)
   - reactive lymphadenopathy
4. Tumor
   - hypertrophied anal papilla
   - cancer (including regional/distant metastases)
   - desmoid
   - lymphoma, sarcoma, GIST, other malignant mesenchymal tumors

– benign mesenchymal tumors

– endometriosis

– condyloma, giant condyloma (Buschke-Lowenstein)

5. Degenerative/functional

– hernia

– rectocele/cystocele/vaginal prolapse

6. Traumatic/posttraumatic

– hematoma

Top of the List

Anorectal

1. Thrombosed hemorrhoid.

2. Sentinel skin tag.

3. Abscess.

4. Condylomata.

5. Neoplasm.

Abdominal

1. Neoplasm.

2. Hernia.

3. Inflammatory mass (diverticulitis, Crohn disease, appendicitis, etc).

Keys to Diagnosis

Anorectal mass/lump

• Patient's surgical/medical history: location of the mass, previous surgeries, symptom descriptors, risk factors, risk behavior.

• Clinical examination: exact location, palpation (including inguinal lymph nodes), visualization (including anoscopy, sigmoidoscopy).

• Surgical intervention or biopsy.

• Rarely imaging needed: endorectal ultrasound, CT abdomen/pelvis, MRI, etc.

Abdominal mass/lump

• Patient's surgical/medical history: location of the mass, previous surgeries, previous colonic evaluations, symptom descriptors, risk factors.

• Clinical examination: patient's general condition, abdominal scars, ostomy, hernia, tenderness to palpation, peritoneal signs, stool in rectal vault, palpable mass, organomegaly.

• Imaging: CT scan, abdominal ultrasound.

Cross-reference

MEGACOLON

Highlights of the Symptom

- Setting: patient's age at presentation, inpatient vs outpatient.
- Symptom evolution: acute, chronic progressive, intermittent, recurrent.
- Signs of toxicity: fever/sepsis, tachycardia, elevated WBC.
- Associated symptoms: abdominal pain and cramping, GI dysfunction (diarrhea, ileus, constipation), mental status change.
- Underlying colonic disease: IBD, *C difficile* colitis, intestinal ischemia, amebic or other infectious colitis, Ogilvie syndrome (colonic pseudoobstruction), Hirschsprung disease, Chagas disease.
- Comorbidities: immunosuppression, cardiovascular disease, embolic disease, retroperitoneal/mediastinal pathology, spinal disease.
- Probability of being sign of serious disease (liability issue): high.

Pathogenesis-Oriented Differential Diagnosis

1. Malformation
- – Hirschsprung disease

2. Vascular
- – ischemic colitis

3. Inflammatory
- – IBD (ulcerative colitis, Crohn colitis)
- – *C difficile* colitis
- – other infectious colitis

4. Tumor
- – tumor-related LBO

5. Degenerative/functional
- – Ogilvie syndrome
- – Chagas disease
- – volvulus

6. Traumatic/posttraumatic
- – blunt colon trauma
- – new spinal cord injury with acute colonic distention
- – retroperitoneal/spinal pathology (hematoma, fracture, etc)

Top of the List

Acute/toxic megacolon

1. Ulcerative colitis.

2. *C difficile* colitis.

3. Any other acute colitis (infectious, ischemic).

4. Volvulus.

Chronic/nontoxic megacolon

1. Ogilvie syndrome.

2. Chagas disease (endemic countries).

3. Hirschsprung disease.

Keys to Diagnosis

- Patient's surgical/medical history: age at presentation, endemic country, current/recent bowel function, known history of IBD, recent antibiotic use, previous surgeries (abdominal, cardiovascular, spinal), tumor, etc.
- Clinical examination: patient's general condition, hemodynamic stability, extent of abdominal distention, peritoneal signs.
- Imaging:
  - Abdominal x-ray series: colonic diameter > 6 cm ($1^1/_2$ vertebral heights) in transverse colon, > 12 cm in cecum.
  - CT scan: colonic diameter, colonic wall thickening, mucosal enhancement, pneumatosis, portal vein gas?
  - Contrast studies: contraindicated under acute circumstances.

Cross-reference

Topic	Chapter
C difficile colitis	4 (p 308)
IBD—ulcerative colitis	4 (p 320)
Hirschsprung disease	4 (p 450)
Total abdominal colectomy	5 (p 557)

PAIN, ABDOMINAL

Highlights of the Symptom

- Localization/point of origin: upper abdomen, periumbilical, lower abdomen, migrating pain, referred pain location.
- Associated symptoms: nausea, vomiting, diffuse distention, local bulging, hypotension, respiratory distress, bleeding (coffee ground, melena), mass/lump, altered bowel habits, constipation, diarrhea, drainage, fevers/chills.
- Timing: onset, constant, certain times, certain activity, waking up at night.
- Evolution: increasing, decreasing, intermittent, certain time/activity.
- Duration of episode: minutes, hours, days, weeks, or more.
- Appearance: dull, sharp, on-off.
- Maximum: acute, relief through bowel activity, paroxysmal, sporadic.
- Underlying systemic disease: tumor, chemotherapy/immunosuppression, radiation, atrial fibrillation, peptic ulcer disease, kidney stones, etc.
- Probability of being sign of serious disease (liability issue): moderate to high.

Pathogenesis-Oriented Differential Diagnosis

1. Malformation
    – paraesophageal hernia, upside-down stomach
    – ectopic pregnancy
    – SBO
    – Meckel diverticulum
    – pancreas divisum
2. Vascular
    – mesenteric ischemia
    – myocardial infarction, pulmonary embolism
    – ruptured aortic aneurysm
    – incarcerated hernia
    – splenic infarction
3. Inflammatory
    – appendicitis, diverticulitis, pancreatitis, cholecystitis, pyelonephritis
    – perforated viscus (peptic ulcer, diverticulitis, etc)
    – GYN pathology (adnexal, pelvic inflammatory disease, Fitz-Hugh-Curtis, etc)
    – primary bacterial peritonitis

4. Neoplastic
   – advanced tumor → bowel perforation, strangulation, necrosis, obstruction, etc
5. Degenerative/functional
   – urinary retention
   – volvulus
   – intermittent hernia
   – IBS
   – urolithiasis
   – spinal origin
   – diabetic pseudoperitonitis, Mediterranean fever, porphyries
   – Munchausen syndrome
6. Traumatic/posttraumatic
   – blunt/penetrating trauma
   – autoeroticism, foreign body
   – splenic rupture
   – anastomotic leak

Top of the List

Acute diffuse pain
1. Perforated viscus.
2. Pancreatitis.
3. Urinary retention.
4. Primary bacterial peritonitis.
5. Mediterranean fever, porphyries, hemascos, etc.

Acute localized pain
1. RLQ: appendicitis, Crohn disease, lymphadenitis mesenterica, urolithiasis, Meckel diverticulum, GYN pathology, hernia.
2. LLQ: diverticulitis, GYN pathology, LBO, urolithiasis, neoplasm, hernia.
3. RUQ: cholecystitis, urolithiasis, peptic ulcer, pyelonephritis, pancreatitis.
4. LUQ: pancreatitis, peptic ulcer disease, paraesophageal hernia, Boerhaave syndrome, splenic rupture, incarcerated diaphragmatic hernia.
5. Central: incisional pain, hernia, early appendicitis, SBO.
6. Flanks: urolithiasis, pyelonephritis, hydronephrosis, ruptured aortic aneurysm, aortitis, spinal.

Chronic pain
1. IBS/constipation.
2. Adhesions.
3. Chronic diverticulitis.
4. Recurrent (sub-)volvulus or intussusception.

Keys to Diagnosis

• Patient history: circumstances of the pain, evolution, associated symptoms? Precursor symptoms? Underlying diseases? Bowel function? Previous interventions/tests?
• Clinical examination: hemodynamic and cardiopulmonary stability, femoral pulses, presence of incarcerated hernia, diffuse/localized tenderness to palpation, peritoneal signs, involuntary guarding, bowel sounds, etc.
• Monitoring: ECG, urine output, etc.
• Imaging:
  – Upright chest x-ray or left lateral decubitus: evidence of free air?
  – Cross-sectional imaging (eg, abdominal ultrasound, CT): evidence of organ pathology?
  – Contrast imaging: road map of the pathology.
• GI evaluation: EGD, colonoscopy, SBFT, etc.
• Surgical exploration?

Cross-reference

PAIN, PERIRECTAL

Highlights of the Symptom

- Localization/point of origin: outside, inside, tailbone, perineum, lateral, radiating.
- Associated symptoms: swelling, lump, bleeding, prolapse, altered bowel habits, constipation, diarrhea, drainage, fevers/chills.
- Timing: onset, constant, certain time, certain activity, waking up at night.
- Evolution: increasing, decreasing, intermittent, certain time/activity.
- Duration of episode: minutes, hours, days, weeks, or more.
- Appearance: dull, sharp, on-off.
- Maximum: acute, related to bowel activity (during/after), paroxysmal, sporadic.
- Underlying systemic disease: tumor, chemotherapy/immunosuppression, radiation.
- Probability of being sign of serious disease (liability issue): low.

Pathogenesis-Oriented Differential Diagnosis

1. Malformation
   - lymphangioma, hemangioma
2. Vascular
   - thrombosed external hemorrhoid
3. Inflammatory
   - anal fissure
   - perirectal abscess
   - horseshoe abscess
   - prostatitis
   - herpes simplex infection
   - HIV-associated anal ulcer
   - proctitis
   - perianal dermatitis, exulcerations
4. Neoplastic
   - epithelial: anal SCC, rectal cancer (with muscle or bone infiltration)
   - mesenchymal: GIST, etc
   - neurogenic: melanoma

5. Degenerative/functional

  – levator ani syndrome

  – anismus

  – proctalgia fugax

  – rectocele

  – intussusception

  – spinal pathology with radicular pain

6. Traumatic/posttraumatic

  – blunt/penetrating trauma

  – autoeroticism, foreign body

  – iatrogenic: eg, postsurgery, post–digital rectal exam

  – coccygodynia

Top of the List

1. Anal fissure.

2. Thrombosed external hemorrhoid.

3. Abscess.

Keys to Diagnosis

• Patient history: association with defecation? Steadily increasing? Associated symptoms? Bowel function? Level of activity? Previous interventions/tests?

• Clinical examination:

  – External inspection: asymmetric appearance, erythema = abscess? bluish lump = thrombosed external hemorrhoid?

  – External palpation: exact pain localization, tissue induration?

  – Lateral traction on buttocks: fissure visible?

  – Only if diagnosis not yet made and exam tolerable to patient: → digital rectal exam (eg, tenderness/induration in postanal space, palpation of prostate, levator muscles, etc), anoscopy/proctoscopy.

Cross-reference

PROLAPSE

Highlights of the Symptom

- Grading: extent of prolapse, spontaneous reduction, need for manual reduction, nonreducible, or immediately reprolapsing.
- Localization: anorectal, vaginal.
- Associated symptoms: bleeding, pain, underlying bowel function (diarrhea/constipation), change in bowel habits, incontinence (stool, gas, urine), weight loss.
- Symptom evolution: acute, sporadic, recurrent, chronic.
- Underlying systemic disease: wasting, malnutrition, tuberculosis, liver disease, neurologic disease (cerebral, spinal), malignancy, cystic fibrosis, history of previous surgeries.
- Probability of being sign of serious disease (liability issue): low.

Pathogenesis-Oriented Differential Diagnosis

1. Malformation/predisposition
   - cystic fibrosis (mucoviscidosis)
   - external skin tags/hemorrhoids
2. Vascular
   - internal hemorrhoids
3. Inflammatory
   - solitary rectal ulcer syndrome
4. Tumor
   - rectal neoplasm: may be lead point for intussusception/prolapse (Figure 1–1)
   - anorectal neoplasm: true prolapse vs pseudoprolapse (fungating mass)
   - large hypertrophic anal papilla
   - external skin proliferation (condyloma, neoplasm, etc)
5. Degenerative/functional
   - rectal mucosal prolapse
   - full-thickness rectal prolapse
   - vaginal prolapse
   - cystocele
   - rectocele
6. Traumatic/posttraumatic
   - ectropion

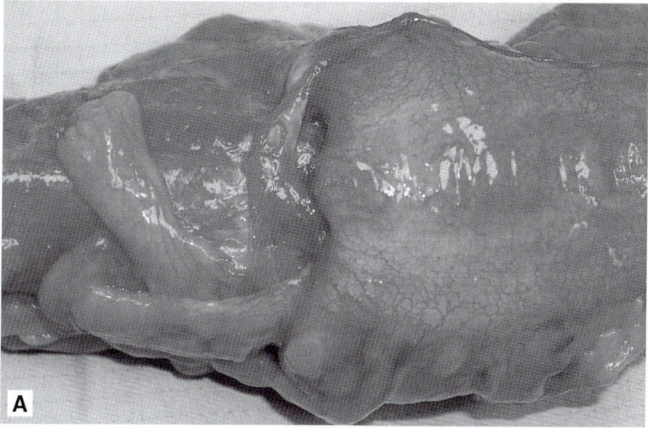

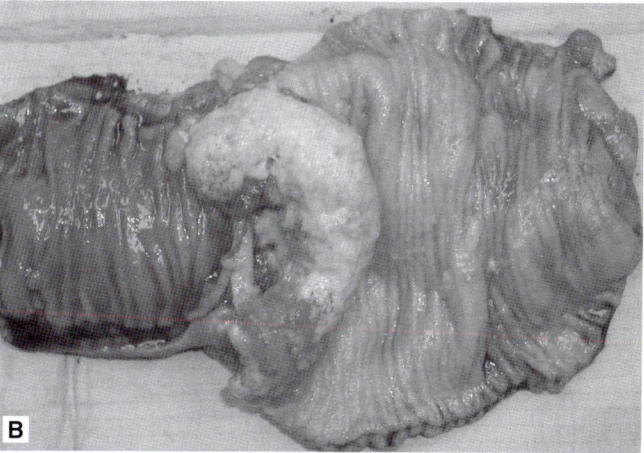

Figure 1–1. Intussusception with cancer as lead point.

Top of the List

1. Skin tags.
2. Hemorrhoidal prolapse.
3. Rectal prolapse.
4. Tumor.

Keys to Diagnosis

- Patient's history: obstetric history (parity, etc), previous abdominal or spinal surgeries (hysterectomy, tumor, spinal disc, etc), underlying bowel function (constipation/ diarrhea).
- Clinical examination:
  - Patient's age and general condition (cachexia)?
  - Anal configuration (tags, patulousness, pelvic floor descent, sphincter tone)? Presence/absence of complications (incarceration, necrosis, ulceration, active bleeding)? Rectocele/cystocele?
  - Visible prolapse? If no prolapse visible → patient instructed to perform Valsalva maneuver on the toilet to try to trigger the prolapse:
    - Prolapse with radial pattern = hemorrhoidal prolapse.
    - Prolapse with concentric pattern = rectal prolapse.
  - Anoscopy/proctoscopy: tumor (lead point), hemorrhoids, ulcerations and thickening (solitary rectal ulcer syndrome).
- Imaging:
  - Defecating proctogram: only needed if diagnosis in doubt or co-pathology suspected.
  - Dynamic MRI: assessment of coexisting pelvic floor dysfunction.

Cross-reference

SMALL BOWEL OBSTRUCTION *(SBO)*

Highlights of the Symptom

- Grading: partial SBO, complete SBO.
- Localization: proximal jejunum, mid-small bowel, ileum.
- Associated symptoms: time of last bowel activity, nausea, vomiting, abdominal pain and cramping, abdominal distention, high ileostomy output of watery (tealike) quality, bleeding, altered bowel habits, diarrhea, urinary tract infections?
- Evolution: acute, intermittent, recurrent, chronic.
- Underlying systemic disease: Crohn disease, malignancy, cardiovascular disease, history of previous surgeries.
- Probability of being sign of serious disease (liability issue): moderate to high.

Pathogenesis-Oriented Differential Diagnosis

1. Malformation
- atresia

2. Vascular
- mesenteric ischemia (peripheral vascular disease, embolic disease, vasculitis)
- portal vein thrombosis
- radiation injury with stricture formation

3. Inflammatory
- peritoneal adhesions
- Crohn disease
- diverticulitis/appendicitis with inflammatory encasement of small bowel loop(s)

4. Tumor
- peritoneal carcinomatosis (various primary tumors)
- desmoid
- lymphoma, mesenchymal tumors
- endometriosis
- primary small bowel cancer: rare

5. Degenerative/functional
- ileus (postoperative)
- internal wrapping of small bowel around ostomy-bearing bowel segment

– intussusception
– fecoliths/fecal impaction in small bowel of patients with cystic fibrosis
– gallstone ileus
– hernia (external, internal)

6. Traumatic/posttraumatic
– blunt abdominal trauma
– abdominal compartment syndrome (post-trauma, post–burn injury, etc)
– retroperitoneal/spinal pathology (hematoma, fracture, etc)

Top of the List

1. Adhesions.

2. Herniation (external, internal).

3. Tumor (eg, carcinomatosis).

4. Crohn disease.

Keys to Diagnosis

• Patient's surgical/medical history: symptom characterization, previous abdominal surgeries, tumor, history of previous SBOs.

• Clinical examination: patient's general condition, abdominal distention (may be absent if very proximal obstruction), presence of incarcerated hernia, presence/absence of (tympanitic) bowel sounds, focal/diffuse tenderness to palpation, peritoneal signs, stool in rectal vault.

• Imaging:
– Abdominal x-ray series, chest x-ray: SBO vs LBO, free air, air/fluid levels, gastric dilation, small bowel dilation (> 2.5 cm) with plicae circulares, transition point, presence of air in the distal colon, calcifications, pneumobilia.
– CT scan (if possible with oral and IV contrast): small bowel dilation, transition point, extensive mucosal thickening, intestinal pneumatosis, pneumobilia, portal vein gas, suspicion of closed loop, tumor burden, etc.
– Contrast studies: small bowel follow-through: (a) with barium if chronic partial SBO, (b) Gastrografin or 50%/50% Gastrografin/barium if more acute partial SBO.

Cross-reference

SEPSIS

Highlights of the Symptom

- Grading: subfebrile vs febrile, hemodynamically stable/unstable.
- With/without sepsis-like symptoms: tachycardia, decrease of peripheral vascular resistance, hypotension, high cardiac output, thrombocytopenia, hypophosphatemia, coagulopathy/DIC.
- Organ dysfunction: pulmonary, cardiovascular, renal, neurologic, hepatic, bone marrow, GI.
- Associated abdominal symptoms: nausea, vomiting, abdominal pain and cramping, distention, wound infection, wound discharge, altered drain output, GI dysfunction?
- Postoperative timing:
  - 1–3 days: atelectasis/pulmonary.
  - 3–6 days: wound infection/fascial dehiscence.
  - 5–7 days: anastomotic leak.
- Evolution: acute, fulminant, persistent/smoldering.
- Underlying systemic disease: immunosuppression, malignancy, other systemic disease, single- or multiorgan dysfunction, coagulopathy.
- Probability of being sign of serious disease (liability issue): high.

Pathogenesis-Oriented Differential Diagnosis

1. Malformation
  - valvular heart disease (bicuspid aortic valve, mitral valve prolapse) → bacterial endocarditis
  - atrial myxoma
2. Vascular
  - ischemic necrosis
  - thromboembolic
  - herniation, strangulation
  - line sepsis
3. Inflammatory
  - anastomotic leak
  - abscess: pelvic, paracolonic, interloop, subhepatic, subdiaphragmatic, etc
  - wound infection
  - fascial dehiscence/evisceration

– superimposed infection: cholecystitis, pancreatitis, *C difficile* colitis, diverticulitis, appendicitis, line sepsis
– pneumonia (including malinspiration, aspiration, ARDS)
– urinary tract infection
– endocarditis, septic thrombus

4. Tumor
   – extensive tumor load (with tumor necrosis)
   – hematologic and lymphatic proliferations
   – treatment- or tumor-induced neutropenia

5. Degenerative/functional
   – atelectasis
   – ileus (postoperative)
   – sacral decubitus (with/without osteomyelitis)
   – factitious fever

6. Traumatic/posttraumatic
   – sepsis-like syndrome
   – fat embolism

Top of the List

1. Infection: surgery-related > pulmonary > non–surgery-related.
2. Neoplasm.
3. Autoimmune disease.

Keys to Diagnosis

• Patient's surgical/medical history: type and time frame of previous abdominal surgeries (particularly contaminated/dirty), aspiration, central lines, tumor extent, etc; recovery progress, ie, bowel function, respiratory function, pain control, urination, etc.

• General clinical examination: patient's general condition, vital signs, arrhythmias, respiratory excursions, oxygenation, abdominal distention, wound appearance, excessive amber drainage (ie, sign of fascial dehiscence), bowel sounds, focal/diffuse tenderness to careful percussion, peritoneal signs, appearance of drains.

• Gentle digital rectal exam (if anastomosis in reach): obvious or subtle evidence for leak?

• Cultures: blood, sputum, urine, wounds/drains.

- Imaging:
  - Abdominal x-ray series, chest x-ray: persistent or recurrent free air, air/fluid levels, gastric dilation.
  - Chest x-ray: atelectasis, pulmonary consolidations, effusions.
  - Ultrasound or CT scan (abdomen/pelvis, or inclusion of chest) with possible CT-guided drainage: evidence for abscess, leak, free air, etc.
  - Water-soluble contrast studies, particularly if relatively distal anastomosis: evidence for anastomotic leak.

Cross-reference

SKIN RASH

Highlights of the Symptom

- Localization/distribution pattern: perianal, groin, diffuse.
- Associated symptoms: itching, pain, bleeding, fever/chills, edema, moisture, incontinence, drainage, prolapse, etc.
- Time factor: constant, one-time, recurrent.
- Symptom evolution: progressive, worsening, on/off, triggered by certain treatment/activity.
- Appearance: symmetric, asymmetric, circumscribed with sharp demarcation, border enhancement, dry/wet, elevation/lump, underlying induration.
- Underlying skin disease: atopic eczema, psoriasis, lichen, lupus erythematosus.
- Probability of being sign of serious disease (liability issue): low.

Pathogenesis-Oriented Differential Diagnosis

1. Malformation
   - acanthosis nigricans
2. Vascular
   - radiation injury (acute, chronic)
3. Inflammatory
   - unspecific perianal skin irritation
   - fungal infection
   - erythrasma
   - allergic contact dermatitis
   - irritant contact dermatitis
   - atopic dermatitis
   - erythema (phlegmon)
   - perirectal abscess
   - lichen sclerosus
   - psoriasis
4. Tumor
   - Paget disease
   - Bowen disease
   - eczematoid squamous cell carcinoma
   - lentigo, melanoma

5. Degenerative/functional

– chronic steroid abuse

– pseudorash: change in pigmentation (hyperpigmented scar, vitiligo, pityriasis versicolor, etc)

6. Traumatic/posttraumatic

– scratch-induced (eg, scratch excoriations)

– hematoma

Top of the List

1. Unspecific perianal dermatitis.

2. Fungal infection.

3. Allergic or toxic contact dermatitis.

4. Systemic skin disease (eg, psoriasis).

Keys to Diagnosis

• Patient history: symptom characterization, previous anorectal surgeries, tumor treatment (eg, radiation treatment), current bowel function (diarrhea?), incontinence, antibiotic use, current perianal skin management (creams, ointments, hygiene, aggressive washing), etc.

• Clinical examination: patient's general condition, symmetric vs asymmetric rash, excoriations, exact localization (perianal, groins, intertriginous areas, etc), underlying induration, digital rectal exam (reduced sphincter tone?).

• Biopsy (with/without cultures): all asymmetric or otherwise suspicious lesions, symmetric lesions without complete resolution after limited period of empirical treatment.

Cross-reference

ULCERATION

Highlights of the Symptom

- Localization/point of origin: anal verge, rectum, colon.
- Appearance: solitary area, multifocal, diffuse.
- Associated symptoms: rectal pain (with/without bowel movements), abdominal pain, urgency, tenesmus, and cramping, abdominal distention, bleeding, altered bowel habits, diarrhea?
- Time factor: relapsing, progressing, self-limited.
- Symptom evolution: acute, intermittent, recurrent, chronic.
- Severity: resulting in local symptoms only vs in general morbidity.
- Underlying systemic disease: IBD (ulcerative colitis, Crohn disease), immunosuppression, HIV infection, cytomegalovirus (CMV) infection/ flare-up, constipation, NSAID use, malignancy, history of previous surgeries, anastomosis, implantation of foreign body (eg, mesh).
- Probability of being sign of serious disease (liability issue): high.

Pathogenesis-Oriented Differential Diagnosis

1. Malformation
   - congenital fistula opening
2. Vascular
   - mesenteric ischemia (peripheral vascular disease, embolic disease, vasculitis)
   - radiation injury with focal ulceration (caveat: don't biopsy anteriorly: risk to create rectovaginal fistula)
3. Inflammatory
   - solitary rectal ulcer
   - HIV-associated anal ulcer
   - CMV colitis
   - herpes colitis
   - ulcerative colitis/Crohn disease
   - caustic colitis (eg, result of bowel prep)
   - around foreign body (eg, erosion, residual suture material, staples)
   - STDs: lymphogranuloma venereum, herpes simplex, gonorrhea, syphilis, chancroid, granuloma inguinale
   - tuberculosis
   - Behçet disease

4. Tumor
   – primary anorectal or colorectal malignancy (cancer, lymphoma, etc)
   – secondary involvement by extraintestinal cancer
5. Degenerative/functional
   – stercoral ulcer
   – solitary rectal ulcer syndrome
6. Traumatic/posttraumatic
   – anoreceptive intercourse, foreign body, automanipulation
   – iatrogenic injury (eg, instrumentation, biopsy)

Top of the List

Anorectal ulceration
1. Anal fissure.
2. Fistula opening.
3. HIV-associated anal ulcer: idiopathic or specific infection (STDs).
4. Solitary rectal ulcer syndrome.
5. Anorectal neoplasia: anal cancer, lymphoma, Kaposi sarcoma.

Colonic or rectal ulceration
1. IBD: ulcerative colitis, Crohn disease.
2. Neoplasia: rectal cancer (eg scirrhous subform).
3. CMV colitis.
4. Stercoral ulcerations.
5. Solitary rectal ulcer syndrome.

Keys to Diagnosis

• Patient's surgical/medical history: personal/family history of IBD, underlying tumor diagnosis and treatments (radiation, chemotherapy), immunosuppression (drug-induced, HIV)? Nature of anorectal symptoms?

• Clinical examination: patient's general condition, descriptive parameters of ulcerations, eg,
   – Painless anorectal ulcers: neoplasia, syphilis (= painless, indurated, clean-based ulcer/chancre), granuloma inguinale.
   – Painful anorectal ulcers: neoplasia, chancroid (= painful inguinal lymphadenopathy), HSV (= multiple tender shallow ulcers/vesicular changes).
   – Colonic/rectal ulcers: associated with mass, solitary vs multiple, condition of surrounding bowel, etc.

- Biopsy: histopathology, special stains if necessary.
- Endoscopy: defining the proximal extent of disease?

Cross-reference

VAGINAL AIR AND/OR STOOL PASSAGE

Highlights of the Symptom

- Appearance: passage of gas, passage of stool through vagina, quality of material.
- Evolution: continuous, intermittent, worsening, one-time, self-limited.
- Associated symptoms: pelvic or abdominal pain, bleeding, altered bowel habits, diarrhea, urinary tract infections?
- Time of occurrence: recent child birth or anorectal surgery? History of abdominal pain or change in bowel habits?
- Underlying systemic disease: Crohn disease, malignancy, history of radiation treatment, history of previous surgeries (anorectal, bowel resection, hysterectomy, other GYN).
- Localization: high, mid-level, low rectovaginal fistula.
- Probability of being sign of serious disease (liability issue): high.

Pathogenesis-Oriented Differential Diagnosis

1. Malformation
   - congenital rectovaginal fistulae (eg, in conjunction with imperforate anus)
2. Vascular
   - radiation injury
3. Inflammatory
   - Crohn disease
   - perirectal abscess
   - Bartholin abscess
   - specific infections: tuberculosis, LGV, actinomycosis
   - diverticulitis
   - intra-abdominal/pelvic abscess postanastomotic leak (LAR, bowel resection)
   - endometritis, vaginitis (without fistula)
4. Tumor
   - pelvic (anorectal or GYN) or abdominal tumor
   - endometriosis
5. Degenerative/functional
   - pseudofistula: passage of vaginal air without true intestinal communication

6. Traumatic/posttraumatic
   – obstetric injury
   – penetrating trauma
   – anal intercourse, autoeroticism, foreign body
   – iatrogenic (instrumentation, surgeries: eg, hemorrhoidectomy, recto-
     cele repair, LAR, hysterectomy, enterotomy, etc)

Top of the List

Colovaginal (or enterovaginal) fistula
1. Diverticulitis.

2. Cancer.

3. Crohn disease.

4. Postsurgical (eg, anastomotic leak, enterotomy).

Rectovaginal fistula
1. Obstetric injury.

2. Perirectal or Bartholin abscess.

3. Crohn disease.

4. Anorectal surgery.

5. Malignancy.

6. Radiation injury.

Keys to Diagnosis

• Patient's narration: believe her even if fistula not immediately visible.

• History: previous diseases, previous surgeries, timing.

• Clinical examination: rectovaginal exam, anoscopy/rigid sigmoidoscopy,
  colposcopy, air-water test, tampon test.

• Possible imaging studies: barium enema, colpography, CT scan.

Cross-reference

..

Chapter 2

Evaluation Tools

Evaluation Tools

LIABILITY IN COLORECTAL SURGERY

Overview

Practice of colorectal surgery opens numerous vulnerabilities for lawsuits:

- Failure to timely diagnose disease: eg, colorectal cancer is the second most common type of cancer cited in malpractice lawsuits.
- Sphincter injury with fecal incontinence after anorectal surgery or midline episiotomy.
- Failure to offer continence-preserving procedure.
- Iatrogenic medical complications/death during diagnosis or treatment.
- Sponges/instruments left in the patient.
- Iatrogenic organ injury of nontarget structures (eg, colon, small bowel, ureter, major vessels, spleen, vagina).
- Lack of informed consent regarding extent or risks of procedures/endoscopies.

Specific challenges to physicians cited in malpractice cases arise from:

- Type or sequence of diagnostic procedures, eg, failure to recommend colonoscopy.
- Missing or insufficient documentation for medical rationale to recommended treatment, patient education, follow-up.
- Lack of follow-up on test results, initiation of follow-up tests (eg, after incomplete colonoscopy).
- Lack of communication.

Risk of lawsuit can never be completely eliminated but can be dramatically reduced, if the outlook of success for the plaintiff is lower, due to the fact that systematic preventive steps are undertaken:

1. To reduce misconceptions, miscommunications.
2. To follow recommended medical guidelines.
3. To adhere to excellent documentation in the chart, informed consenting process, and documentation of refusal to undergo recommended test/procedure.

Key Elements

Delays to prompt diagnostic evaluation in patients with symptoms

- Routine screening not recommended.
- Routine screening recommended but not scheduled.
- Diagnostic test recommended but not scheduled.

• Diagnostic test scheduled but not performed.
• Ordering or follow-up of screening or diagnostic procedures not documented.

Narrow diagnostic focus
• Inadequate evaluation of abnormal findings.
• Failure to convey to patient the importance of keeping test and follow-up appointments.

Lack of communication
• Multiple providers for the same patient fail to properly communicate important information.
• Patient not notified of test results.

Poor documentation
• Informed refusal not documented.
• Important clinical information missing from clinical note.

Documentation

Baseline documentation
• Adequate documentation of current history elements; clarification of patient's vague terminology (eg, "occasional," "frequent") → reduce misinterpretation of self-reported symptoms.
• Key statements must be documented by selected outside medical records, eg, pathology report (cancer, IBD), colonoscopy report (clearance of rest of the colon), operative notes (definition of anatomy, problems/adhesions during previous surgeries), medical clearance.
• Amendments to existing chart/medical record: if an addendum is absolutely necessary, it should be made after the last entry, noting current date and time, with both entries cross-referenced. Inappropriately amended medical records render a case indefensible if plaintiff's attorneys demonstrate in court that the note was written or typed after the fact. No addendum in anticipation of claim or legal action.
• Medical record: "what is not documented has not happened" → record should reflect in appropriate detail what was done for patient and demonstrate quality of care given → provide defense against allegations of inadequate care.

Interactions with patient or family
• Document all phone conversations, including those in which compliance issues are stressed.

Patient compliance and noncompliance

- To ensure that screening tests are performed: schedule before patient leaves office, or at least document discussion with patient of the recommendation for the test.
- Document all follow-up efforts to reach patient or to reschedule a test/procedure.
- Document discussions/conversations with patient and witnesses about recommended action, risks and benefits of proposed testing, as well as alternatives.
- Document patient's refusal to undergo recommended test or lifesaving procedure, preferably on a specific informed refusal form signed by patient.
- Make it a routine for high-risk patients who fail to keep appointments or when responding to phone calls to reschedule:
  – To use a form for tracking details.
  – To contact them by registered mail (with return receipt).

Cross-reference

PATIENT HISTORY

Overview

Obtaining the patient's accurate and detailed history is the most important tool to direct the subsequent examination, to create a list of possible differential diagnoses, and eventually to establish the final diagnosis without wasting valuable resources. It is further crucial in tailoring the best choice among various treatment options to the patient's individual situation. Preferably, the history is taken from the patient, often from accompanying individuals (family, translators, referring physicians): risk of "loss in translation."

Particularly in colorectal surgery, it is a high art to take a patient's history in an unprejudiced, sensitive, but nonetheless thorough manner. Efficient questioning consists of a problem-oriented focus and systematic expansion of areas, depending on the responses. It is advantageous to start by letting the patient describe the key symptoms in an open end–type narration, which is subsequently complemented with specific problem-oriented questions. Even in "simple" cases, a systematic checklist of relevant background information should be followed to ensure a complete context and hence avoid legal glitches.

Key Elements

Symptoms
- Rectal bleeding: amount, color (bright red vs dark red), onset, pattern, mixed into the stool, triggering factors, etc.
- Discharge: quality, associated symptoms, etc.
- Pain: location, onset, pattern, triggering factors, etc.
- Itching: hygiene habits, incontinence, discharge, medications applied, etc.
- Prolapse: what, how much, where? Spontaneous or manual reduction, nonreducible?
- Lump/mass: always there or protruding with bowel movements, pain?
- Bowel movements: stool quality, sudden change in bowel habits, complete/incomplete evacuation, necessary counterpressure/digital maneuvers.
- Incontinence: stool, gas, urine.
- Nausea/vomiting, weight loss, fevers/chills.
- Associated symptoms.

Past medical/surgical history
- Baseline bowel and anorectal function (prior to onset of presenting symptom).
- History of IBD, IBS, cancer (abdominal/extraabdominal), etc.

- Previous abdominal surgeries.
- Previous anorectal/pelvic surgeries or radiation treatment.
- Previous vaginal deliveries, obstetric injuries.
- Previous colonic evaluations (colonoscopy, etc).
- HIV status (if relevant for disease).
- General medical history: cardiopulmonary, vascular, diabetes, cancer, liver, neurologic, kidney.

When intervention is planned
- Documentation of preexisting symptoms (incontinence to stool/gas, sexual dysfunction, rectovaginal fistula, etc).

Family history
- Particularly risk of polyps/cancer and IBD.

General history
- Medications (current and recent past).
- Allergies.
- Review of systems.
- Profession/disability, socioeconomic environment, habits, caregivers.

Documentation

Adequate documentation of current history elements is absolutely necessary. Key statements in a patient's history must be documented by selected outside medical records, eg, pathology report (cancer, IBD), colonoscopy report (clearance of rest of the colon), operative notes (definition of anatomy, problems/adhesions during previous surgeries), medical clearance.

Cross-reference

Topic	*Chapter*
Liability in colorectal surgery	2 (p 56)
Clinical examination	2 (p 61)

CLINICAL EXAMINATION
Overview

The clinical examination is the cornerstone and the most distinguishing skill for the initial and follow-up assessments of an overwhelming part of colorectal patients, particularly patients with anorectal problems. Nothing should be taken for granted even if there are respective statements in outside records. It is an art and special privilege to examine a patient in the most intimate area of the body and requires an unprejudiced, sensitive, but nonetheless thorough manner. To optimize the exam, it is important in the short time between the history taking and the actual exam to digest the information and prepare a working array of possible, likely or unlikely findings.

Key Findings
General exam
- Habitus including weight and height → calculation of body mass index as weight (in kg) divided by square height (in m).
- Vital signs: heart rate, blood pressure, respiratory rate, temperature.
- Mobility and performance status.
- Mental/intellectual status: eg, inquisitive vs passive vs manipulative nature; anxiety, mood.
- Nutritional and hydration status.

Anorectum
- Inspection:
  - Presence/absence of external/internal stool, blood, mucus, secretions (eg, pus).
  - Anal configuration: appearance/location/asymmetries of anus, perineal body, vagina. Circumferential presence of radial folding, or absence in area of sphincter defect?
  - Perianal skin: intact, irritation (symmetric, asymmetric), erythema, discoloration, focal pathology.
  - Visible evidence of pelvic floor dysfunction: perineal descent, flattened anal verge, patulous anus, gapping of anus to lateral traction.
  - Spreading of buttocks to the anal verge: search for visible pathologic openings, eg, fistula, fissure, ulcer.
  - Visible "tissue addition": lumps, bumps, prolapse (posterior vs anterior/vaginal).
  - Visible "tissue diminution": weakened/absent perineal body.

Evaluation Tools

- Palpation, including digital rectal exam:
  - Focal external tenderness to palpation.
  - Bidigital palpation (index finger inside, external counterpressure with thumb): focal induration, eg, perirectal or ischioanal fat, deep postanal space.
  - Focal tenderness: exact location, including coccyx, prostate, levator muscles, cervical motion.
  - Sacrum palpable: if not → suspect presacral mass/abscess/hematoma/scar!
  - Palpable mass (endorectal, prostate, extraluminal).
  - Sphincter tone at rest/squeeze, intersphincteric groove, focal defects, use of auxiliary muscles for squeezing.
  - Length of anal canal.
  - Anastomosis, anastomotic leak.
  - Stricture, stenosis: length, angulation, passable?
  - Presence/absence of stool, assessment of stool quality.
  - Palpable defect (eg, rectovaginal fistula).
- Vaginal exam:
  - Palpable defect or mass.
  - Assessment of strength of rectovaginal septum.
- Anoscopy:
  - Evaluation of anal canal: internal hemorrhoids, dentate line, distal defect or mass.
- Rigid sigmoidoscopy:
  - Evaluation of distal rectum and anal canal.
  - Characterization of visible stool.

Abdomen
- Abdominal shape: scaphoid, flat, distended, obese.
- Pannus, including location of body folds.
- Distention: soft, tympanitic, mass, organomegaly.
- Presence/absence of defects, wounds, ostomy, skin abnormality.
- Presence/absence of fresh surgical wounds (incisions).
- Presence/absence and location of scars.
- Hernias: groin, umbilical, incisional hernias.
- Tenderness to palpation: location, severity.
- Peritoneal signs: guarding (involuntary), rebound tenderness, percussion tenderness.
- Bowel sounds: normo-active, hyperactive, tympanitic, absent.

Other body regions
• Lymph node regions: particularly groin, but also supraclavicular, axillary.
• Hernia: former incisions, groin.

Limitations
Access to internal pathology is limited.

Cross-reference

Topic	*Chapter*
Liability in colorectal surgery	2 (p 56)
Patient history	2 (p 59)
Evaluation tools	2 (pp 64–134)

COLORECTAL CANCER SCREENING/SURVEILLANCE

Overview

Symptoms are not reliable for early detection of colorectal cancer (CRC). There is therefore a need for risk-adjusted screening programs for asymptomatic individuals to start no later than age 50, earlier in increased or high-risk individuals. No definite guidance available about criteria to discontinue screening.

Effective screening has to be:

• Based on understanding of the adenoma-carcinoma sequence: it takes 5–10 years from the first molecular change to a clinically manifest cancer (caveat: shorter sequence in HNPCC).

• Based on individual's genetic, disease- or age-dependent risk for the development of CRC.

• Highly sensitive.

• Practical, easy to do, cost-effective.

The term *screening* is only applicable to asymptomatic people; a test in the presence of symptoms should not be called "screening" but instead, "diagnostic" evaluation.

Epidemiology

Prevalence of polyps: 20–30% in average-risk persons ≥ 50 years of age.

First colonoscopy responsible for largest benefit of polypectomy; risk for subsequent CRC in patients with small adenoma is not greater than average risk.

Current screening rates among average-risk population are unacceptably low: 20–50%. Contrast: > 50% of gastroenterologists and colorectal surgeons perform colonoscopy at intervals shorter than recommended by the guidelines → not cost-effective and diverting resources from higher yielding primary screening.

Differential Risk Assessment

• Low or average risk (65–75%): no risk factors, no CRC in any first-degree relatives.

• Moderate risk (20–30%): CRC in one first-degree relative with age ≤ 60 years or ≥ two first-degree relatives of any ages, personal history of curative resection of colorectal malignancy or large polyp (> 1 cm) or multiple colorectal polyps of any size.

• High risk (6–8%): FAP, HNPCC, IBD.

Screening Tools

Fecal occult blood test (FOBT)

- Pros: noninvasive, easy, convenient, safe.
- Cons: colon not visualized, low to moderate sensitivity/specificity, positive tests require colonoscopy and other testing. Lack of specificity: only 2% of patients with positive FOBT have a CRC, ie, 50 colonoscopies needed to identify 1 patient with CRC, 100 colonoscopies needed to save 1 patient.
- Precautions: should be repeated annually, dietary restrictions (no red meat, horseradish, vitamin C, etc).
- Data: annual FOBT associated with decrease in CRC mortality of 20–33%; sensitivity for advanced adenomas or CRC only 24%.

Flexible sigmoidoscopy

- Pros: safer than colonoscopy, more convenient, no bowel prep, most commonly no need for sedation.
- Cons: does not visualize entire colon, positive findings require full colonoscopy.
- Precautions: should be repeated every 5 years.
- Data: decrease in CRC mortality = 60% overall, 70% distal CRC; 2% of patients with normal flexible sigmoidoscopy have a significant lesion proximal to splenic flexure.

Combination of FOBT and flexible sigmoidoscopy

Data: even though offering a theoretical advantage, the benefit of combining the 2 tests remains uncertain: higher detection rate, but no proven incremental decrease in CRC mortality compared to flexible sigmoidoscopy alone (see above).

Colonoscopy

- Pros: gold standard with full colonic visualization, therapeutic capability.
- Cons: higher risk than flexible sigmoidoscopy, need for bowel prep, need for sedation.
- Precautions: should be repeated every 10 years.
- Data: National Polyp Study found 76–90% decreased CRC incidence with colonoscopy and removal of all visualized polyps compared with historical controls.

Barium enema

- Pros: full colonic visualization even in presence of nearly obstructing lesion, no need for sedation, better tolerated.
- Cons: no therapeutic capability, lower sensitivity than colonoscopy, positive or uncertain findings need colonoscopic evaluation, still needs bowel prep.

Evaluation Tools

- Precautions: should be repeated every 5 years.
- Data: sensitivity 80–85% for colorectal cancer and 50% for large polyps (> 1 cm).

CT colonography
- Pros: full colonic visualization, no need for sedation.
- Cons: no therapeutic capability, still needs bowel prep, higher discomfort (insufflation of air, no sedation given), unnecessary evaluations/surgeries for incidental findings.
- Precautions: interpretation and recommendations not clarified.
- Data: awaiting further confirmation. Current data controversial with reports of similar sensitivity vs only moderate sensitivity/specificity for larger lesions compared to colonoscopy. Sensitivity for smaller polyps definitely lower.

Fecal DNA
- Pros: noninvasive, convenient, safe.
- Cons: colon not visualized, low to moderate sensitivity/specificity, positive tests require colonoscopy and other testing.
- Precautions: should be repeated every year.
- Data: Sensitivity better than FOBT; 50% for detecting invasive CRC, 15–20% for significant adenomas.

Guidelines

Baseline screening (if normal)
Goal: Detection and elimination of precursor lesions, identification of patients at risk to stratify for frequency of future screening/surveillance.

1. Average-risk individuals, asymptomatic, non–African-American → start at age 50:
   a. Colonoscopy every 10 years (method of choice).
   b. Annual FOBT; if positive → colonoscopy.
   c. Screening sigmoidoscopy every 5 years.
   d. Double-contrast barium enema every 5 years.
2. Increased or high-risk individuals → specific guidelines:
   a. African-American ethnicity: start screening at age of 45.
   b. Positive family history (increased risk group): start at age of 40 or 10–15 years before youngest family member (whichever comes first).
   c. Ulcerative colitis: start 7 years post onset: (bi-)annual colonoscopy with multiple biopsies.

   d. FAP: start in early/mid teens (vs genetic testing).

   e. HNPCC: start around age of 25 (vs genetic testing); thereafter repeat colonoscopy every 1–3 years because of shorter adenoma-carcinoma sequence!

Repeat colonoscopy after polypectomy

Goal: Detect and remove adenomata missed on the initial exam (miss rate: 10–20% of polyps = 6 mm); assess patient's tendency to form new adenomas with advanced pathologic features.

1. Short interval (based on clinical judgment):

   a. Numerous adenomata.

   b. Malignant adenoma (cancerous polyp).

   c. Large sessile polyp.

   d. Incomplete colonoscopy or incomplete removal.

2. Three-year interval:

   a. Advanced or multiple polyps (≥ 3).

3. Five-year interval:

   a. One to two small polyps (tubular adenoma).

4. No surveillance needed:

   a. Hyperplastic polyps (exception: patients with hyperplastic polyposis syndrome).

Repeat colonoscopy after sporadic CRC (not HNPCC/Attenuated FAP)

Goals: rule out synchronous/metachronous CRC; rule out true anastomotic recurrence (< 2% risk); detect and remove adenomata missed on the initial examination; assess patient's tendency to form new adenomas with advanced pathologic stage.

1. Around time of resection ± 6 months:

   a. Full colonoscopy before resection.

   b. If colon perforated/obstructed and cannot be evaluated at the time of the resection → full colonoscopy to be performed within 6 months.

2. One-year interval:

   a. After the resection.

3. Three-year interval:

   a. If perioperative or first postoperative colonoscopy negative.

4. Five-year interval:

   a. Thereafter if normal.

HNPCC/AFAP: annual surveillance of residual colorectum.

Evaluation Tools

Follow-up

Pathology results.

Clinical side effects of polypectomy: postpolypectomy syndrome, perforation, bleeding.

Surgery for larger polyps or cancer. Prophylactic surgery?

Secondary prophylaxis?

Cross-reference

Topic	*Chapter*
Bleeding per rectum	1 (p 4)
Constipation	1 (p 9)
LBO	1 (p 27)
Flexible sigmoidoscopy	2 (p 69)
Colonoscopy	2 (p 71)
Contrast enema	2 (p 99)
CT colonography	2 (p 120)
Carcinogenesis	3 (p 156)
Tumors	4 (pp 236–265)
Chemoprevention	6 (p 636)

FLEXIBLE SIGMOIDOSCOPY

Overview

Limited colonic evaluation: justification dependent on patient's young age (< 40 years), lack of individual risk factors for colorectal cancer, status post complete colonoscopy within acceptable interval, status post subtotal colectomy.

One to two working ports allow for intervention, manipulation, suction/irrigation. Cold biopsy: using forceps. Hot biopsies are generally contraindicated because of inadequate gas elimination with enemas which carries a risk of explosion!

Sedation and analgesia are commonly not needed as major flexures do not have to be passed. Success and detection rate depend on the endoscopist's skill, time spent thoroughly inspecting the colon, and adequacy of cleansing enemas.

Alternatives

Rigid sigmoidoscopy.

Full colonoscopy.

Colonic imaging (contrast enema, CT colonography).

Indications

Diagnostic evaluation of symptomatic low-risk individuals (< 40 years old, negative personal/family history) with symptoms of likely distal origin, eg, bright red blood per rectum.

Intervention: biopsy, polypectomy, stenting, tattooing, to stop bleeding, for focal decompression.

Screening: in conjunction with Hemoccult test.

Surveillance of residual colon and rectum after total or subtotal colectomy.

Preparation

Two Fleet enemas right before test.

Office procedure: commonly no sedation needed.

Caveat: enemas insufficient to remove explosive gases → snare/cautery contraindicated!

Advantages

Combination of evaluation, biopsy, and (limited) intervention.

No lengthy preparation needed.

Evaluation Tools

Limitations and Risks

- Pathologic lesion not in reach of flexible sigmoidoscope (eg, proximal polyps and neoplasms, 20% of *C difficile* colitis, etc).
- Miss rate: up to 20–25% for polyps up to 1 cm.
- Perforation: low risk for diagnostic endoscopy, higher in interventional endoscopy and/or preexisting bowel weakness, eg, acute diverticulitis.
- Bleeding: depending on pathology/intervention, minimal for diagnostic endoscopy.
- Explosion of intestinal gas (hydrogen, methane): use of cautery in inadequately prepped colon contraindicated in flexible sigmoidoscopy.
- Size of lesions generally overestimated (magnification) → need to correlate size of lesion with diameter of inserted instruments.
- Exact orientation difficult/impossible; only absolute landmark is dentate line; if location needs specification (eg, for later surgery): tattooing of the area with India ink (1 mL in 3 separate areas on the circumference).

Characteristic Features

Pathology: melanosis coli, friability, ulcerations, edema (disappearance of vascular pattern), granular reflections ("star sky"), polyps (diminutive, sessile, pedunculated, extramucosal), mass (mucosal/extramucosal), lipoma (extramucosal, soft impressibility: pillow sign), diverticula, stricture, fistula, hemorrhoids.

Cross-reference

COLONOSCOPY

Overview

Complete evaluation of entire colon (and terminal ileum) with option of biopsy and intervention. Intended extent of examination is dependent on individual circumstances (eg, previous surgeries), expected findings, patient's age, etc.

One to two working ports allow for intervention, manipulation, suction/irrigation. Cold biopsy: using forceps. Hot biopsies: using snare and electrocautery (contraindicated with inadequate cleansing, eg, enemas only).

As the instrument has to be negotiated around angles and flexures, monitored IV sedation and analgesia are commonly administered (even though not mandatory). Success and detection rate depend on endoscopist's skills, time spent thoroughly inspecting the colon (withdrawal time > 6 minutes), and adequacy of bowel cleansing.

Advanced techniques:

- High-resolution colonoscopy with chromoendoscopy (spraying of colon with 0.4% indigo carmine dye) is associated with a higher detection rate for polyps and flat adenomas.
- Combination with endoscopic ultrasound.

Alternatives

Limited colonic evaluation: flexible sigmoidoscopy.

Single-column contrast enema: gives a road map but does not allow biopsy, intervention.

Double-contrast enema: if colon is clean and good radiologic technique is used → similar screening sensitivity as colonoscopy.

CT colonography ("virtual colonoscopy"): also needs bowel prep. Typically done without sedation → discomfort. Findings inside/outside colon precipitate further (unnecessary?) interventions.

Indications

Screening and surveillance per guidelines (asymptomatic individuals), clearing rest of colon before segmental intervention.

Diagnostic evaluation of specific symptoms (bleeding, distention, altered bowel habits, etc) in patient > 40 years of age or presence of additional risk factors. Evaluation of patients with altered bowel habits and suspicion for Crohn disease (→ intubation of ileocecal valve).

Intervention: biopsy, polypectomy, stenting, tattooing, to stop bleeding, for detorsion or decompression.

Contraindication: suspected perforation, acute diverticulitis (< 4–6 weeks after onset), fulminant colitis, unstable patient.

Preparation

Colonoscopy: full bowel cleansing the day before.

Conscious sedation and monitoring.

If intervention anticipated: discontinuation of anticoagulation (if possible) or switch to heparin with perioperative short-term pausing; discontinuation of ASA/NSAIDs not mandatory but recommended if possible.

Advantages

Combination of evaluation, biopsy, treatment, and intervention (gold standard).

Better tolerability under sedation.

Limitations and Risks

- Ten percent incomplete colonoscopy: inability to reach cecum due to technical, anatomic, or patient-related issues (pain tolerance), equipment failure: → barium enema: safe on same day unless biopsy or polypectomy performed → wait 5–7 days.
- Miss rate: 20–25% for polyps < 1 cm, 6–12% for polyps > 1 cm: more likely in insufficient prep, spastic colon.
- Bleeding: 0.1–0.5% (diagnostic), 1–2.5% (polypectomy).
- Colon perforation: 0.1% in diagnostic endoscopy, up to 1–3% in interventional endoscopy, particularly in preexisting bowel wall weakness; perforation requires surgical intervention unless very favorable conditions allow for conservative management; 4 perforation mechanisms:
  - With the instrument tip → often relatively small perforation.
  - Bowing injury from instrument looping and overstretching of colon wall → commonly very large tears.
  - Diffuse overinsufflation in weakened colon wall (eg, diverticulum).
  - As result of intervention (biopsy, snare, stent).
- Postpolypectomy syndrome: caused by cautery injury to colon wall → pain, abdominal tenderness, often starting 1–3 days after procedure; most commonly manageable with antibiotics but perforation needs to be ruled out.
- Explosion of intestinal gases (hydrogen, methane): use of cautery in inadequately prepped colon, high risk with mannitol cleansing (sugar degradation through bacteria → increased intestinal gas production).

- Size of lesions generally overestimated (magnification): → need to correlate size of lesion with diameter of inserted instruments.
- Exact orientation difficult/impossible; only absolute landmarks are dentate line, terminal ileum.

Characteristic Features

Normal structures: ileum with carpet-like mucosa (small bowel villi), Peyer plaques. Appendiceal orifice. Ileocecal valve. Cecum/ascending colon: often less clean despite otherwise good cleansing. Hepatic flexure with transparency of bluish liver. Transverse colon (triangular shape typical but not specific. Descending/sigmoid colon. Rectum with reticular vascular pattern. Retroflex view for distal rectum and hemorrhoids.

Most common pathologies:

- Degenerative: melanosis coli, diverticula, hemorrhoids, dolichocolon (too long, tortuous), megacolon (too wide), volvulus.
- Inflammation: edema (disappearance of vascular pattern), granular reflections ("star sky"), friability, ulcerations (diffuse vs skip and bear claw), cobblestoning, pseudomembranes, mucosal necrosis.
- Growth: polyps (diminutive, sessile, pedunculated, extramucosal), mass (mucosal/extramucosal), lipoma (extramucosal, soft impressibility: pillow sign.
- Anastomosis, stricture, fistula.

Cross-reference

Topic	*Chapter*
Colorectal cancer screening	2 (p 64)
Contrast enema	2 (p 99)
CT colonography	2 (p 120)
Polyps	4 (p 236)
Polyposis syndromes	4 (p 240)
Colorectal cancer	4 (p 252)
Bowel preparation/cleansing	7 (p 700)

Evaluation Tools

POUCHOSCOPY
Overview
Instrumentation (rigid or flexible) of existing pouch (ileoanal pouch, continent ileostomy) for evaluation or treatment (eg, dilation of stricture, decompression, tube insertion, etc).

Indication based on symptoms (ie, pouch dysfunction, pouchitis) or for routine surveillance of pouch and ATZ for dysplasia, polyps, or cancer (particularly in FAP).

Circumstances dictate whether flexible or rigid instrument preferable. Sedation and analgesia are commonly not needed but occasionally preferable in very sensitive patient (eg, traumatized perianal skin, etc).

Alternatives
Pouchogram: contrast x-ray.

Indications
- IBD: every 1–3 years or when symptomatic and not responding to conservative treatment, surveillance of ATZ cuff every 1–3 years.
- FAP: every year.

Preparation
Diagnostic: possibly 1 Fleet enema right before test (if poor visibility).
Therapeutic: none.

Advantages
Combination of evaluation, biopsy, and (limited) intervention.
No lengthy preparation needed.

Limitations and Risks
- Pathology missed (inadequate visibility, pocket).
- Perforation: low risk.
- Bleeding: depending on pathology/intervention, minimal for diagnostic.
- Exact orientation difficult/impossible.

Characteristic Features
Pathology: pouchitis, lymphoid hyperplasia (Peyer plaques), dysplasia, formation of polyps/tumor, mass (more likely in posterior area), acute and chronic inflammation, ulcerations (→ suggestive of Crohn disease if ulcerations in

afferent limb), length of efferent limb (eg, S-pouch), friability of ATZ, length and configuration of valve segment (continent ileostomy), fistula opening.

Cross-reference

CAPSULE ENDOSCOPY

Overview

Although the colon and upper GI tract are accessible for direct endoscopy, the small bowel in between is not. Overall, the small bowel only rarely is the primary site of disease. Concern that the test is often overused, eg, missing indication or low yield indication.

Alternatives

Small bowel follow-through.

CT enterography.

Ileoscopy.

Indications

- Obscure bleeding while EGD and colonoscopy negative.
- Evaluation of small bowel Crohn disease.
- Suspicion for small bowel tumor.
- Relative contraindication: stricture (particularly first-generation device may get trapped; newer development: biodegradable capsules).

Preparation

Overnight fasting.

Potentially small bowel follow-through to rule out stricture.

Advantages

Direct visualization of small bowel mucosa.

Limitations and Risks

- Pathology missed (inadequate visibility).
- Obstruction.
- Technique is time-consuming, expensive, and not universally available.

Characteristic Features

Pathology: varices, portal hypertension, erosions, areas of Crohn disease, small bowel tumors/polyps.

Cross-reference

Evaluation Tools

ANOPHYSIOLOGY STUDIES

Overview

Series of elective tests to assess the function and morphology of the anorectum. Common indications are workup of fecal incontinence, obstructed defecation, complex perianal fistulae, assessment and staging, as well as surveillance of anorectal tumors. Test results are not absolute, but always require correlation with patient's individual history, severity of complaints, clinical findings, and unrelated test results.

Typical test combinations:

- Fecal incontinence: "triple studies"—PNTML, manometry/anorectal sensation, ultrasound.
- Obstructed defecation: EMG, manometry/anorectal sensation, balloon expulsion test.
- Anal/rectal tumor: ultrasound, potentially with ultrasound-guided biopsy; rarely triple studies are needed if anorectal function is an important parameter for decision-making.
- Ruling out Hirschsprung disease: RAIR.

Expected Benefits

Obtain objective and reproducible evaluation of anorectal function for assessment and documentation (liability) of patient's symptoms, patient counseling, assessment of treatment effect.

Limitations

Patient cooperation required → false pathologic results possible.

Lack of 1:1 correlation of test results and symptoms → test interpretation and correlation within context of other elements of information necessary.

Latex allergy.

Preparation

Fleet enema right before testing.

Questionnaires: CCFIS (Wexner score) and FIQL.

1. Test Element: Pudendal Nerve Terminal Motor Latency (PNTML)

Purpose

Assessment of transmission time within pudendal nerve from site of stimulus to site of sphincter contraction.

Indication

Evaluation of fecal incontinence: evidence for neuromuscular component of sphincter dysfunction?

Evaluation of possible preexisting autonomic nerve damage prior to pelvic or sphincter-reconstructive surgery.

Equipment and technique

Medtronic Duet Encompass (or comparable) machine with integrated/compatible software component. St. Marks Electrode.

A grounding probe is attached to the patient's leg, and the test electrode connected and attached to the gloved finger. Insertion into posterolateral quadrants. Sequential stimulation with 50 mA until an adequate curve is reproducible.

Risks

Discomfort from electrical stimulus.

Electrical shock if improper setup (eg, too high mA, lack of grounding).

Reference values

Normal PNTML ≤ 2.5 ms (Figure 2–1A).

Interpretation

Prolonged PNTML (if reading and stimulation curve adequate) is evidence of pudendal neuropathy.

Normal PNTML: can either be true normal, or false normal if significant nerve damage present is masked by sufficient number of intact and transmitting nerve fibers.

Absent PNTML reading: either related to complete absence of pudendal nerve function, or false negative (see below).

Pitfalls

False negative: related to inadequate technique or stimulation, scar tissue, extraluminal pathology.

False positive: direct electrical stimulation of the sphincter muscle.

Comment

Majority of patients with idiopathic fecal incontinence have prolonged PNTML.

Controversy in literature about value of PNTML in predicting success of overlapping sphincteroplasty: half the reports show correlation and the other half, no relationship. Nonetheless, PNTML test is recommended prior to sphincteroplasty to protect surgeon in case of insufficient success or recurrent incontinence.

Evaluation Tools

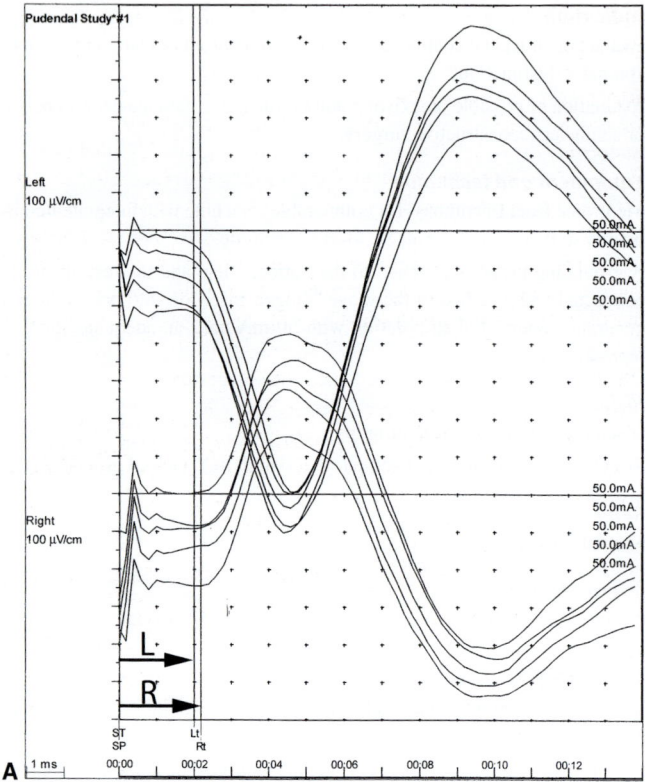

Figure 2–1A. Anophysiology—PNTML.

2. Test Element: Anal Manometry

Purpose

Objective (reproducible?) assessment of sphincter strength and sphincter tone at rest and squeeze (ie, obtain numbers for subjective impression on digital rectal exam). Definition of high-pressure zone.

Indication

Evaluation of fecal incontinence, pelvic floor and levator ani spasms, outlet obstruction, rarely in setting of anal fissure (before/after sphincterotomy).

Objective evaluation of treatment success after nonsurgical and surgical management.

Equipment and technique
Medtronic Duet Encompass (or comparable) machine with integrated/compatible data recording and analysis software. Multichannel catheter with a defined and oriented number of water-perfused channels. Pressure-sensitive pizo-electrodes are arranged around a central channel which is connected to the balloon at the catheter's end. These pressure sensors measure the pressure needed to overcome the outflow resistance. Calibration of catheter to room air pressure with probe held externally at the level of the anus. Correct orientation of the catheter with separate recording of 4–8 positional pressures: anterior, posterior, R lateral, L lateral.

- Stationary pull-through method: sequential recording of alternating 10 second periods of resting/squeeze at 6 static levels of 1-cm intervals.
- Continuous pull-through method: motor-driven extraction of the probe and continuous pressure recording: two separate drive-throughs with one at rest and one during maximal squeeze.

Risks
Discomfort from probe/balloon placement.

Reference values
Variation of normal anal canal pressures according to gender, age, measurement technique.

Interpretation
- Radial pressures: more commonly reported pressure values, recorded with circumferential measuring ports: resting pressure 50–100 mm Hg, squeeze pressure 100–350 mm Hg.
- Axial pressures: less frequently reported pressure values, recorded along longitudinal spiral of the catheter lumina.
- Volume manometry:
  - High-pressure zone: length and maximal amplitude, defining the physiologic anal canal.
  - Area under the curve: integration of pressure values of the pressure profile over the length of the anal canal; better summative information of the total outlet resistance than just a single maximal resting and squeeze pressure.

Pitfalls
False normal pressures (despite sphincter weakness): compensatory use of gluteal muscles → this pitfall can be avoided/reduced by repeat testing after

Evaluation Tools

period of lasting gluteal contraction: while skeletal muscles become tired, sphincter muscle function is relatively resistant to fatigue.

Comment

Ongoing controversy about value and best interpretation of manometry in predicting severity of fecal incontinence. Single values likely are insufficient; pressure profile potentially is more meaningful. Continued lack of an incontinence score that incorporates physiologic data.

3. Test Element: Rectoanal Inhibitory Reflex (RAIR)

Purpose

The RAIR is a physiologic relaxation of the internal sphincter muscle upon sudden distention of the rectum. Believed to play a role in anorectal sampling. Reflex may be absent in Hirschsprung disease, Chagas disease, 50% of ileoanal or coloanal anastomoses (ie, RAIR can recover in up to 50% after colo-anal or ileo-anal pullthrough procedure). Presence of RAIR reliably rules out Hirschsprung disease.

Indication

Evaluation of fecal incontinence: neurogenic component?

Evaluation of constipation → rule out Hirschsprung disease.

Equipment and technique

Same as before → continuation after previous test.

Catheter advanced such that pressure sensors in anal canal and balloon in the rectum. Await steady state pressure undulations > 0. Short insufflation of 15–40 mL of room air.

Risks

Discomfort, otherwise negligible.

Reference values

RAIR present at 15–40 mL insufflation (Figure 2–1B).

Interpretation

RAIR present: normal → high negative predictive value, ie, if RAIR present → Hirschsprung disease ruled out.

RAIR absent: consistent with Hirschsprung disease, Chagas disease, 50% of ileoanal or coloanal anastomoses → further evaluation depending on context.

Pitfalls

RAIR falsely absent: due to inadequate technique, large rectocele, megarectum, or underlying neuromuscular disease.

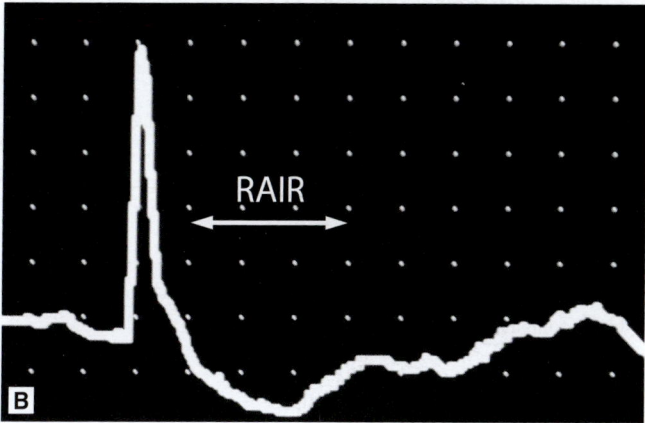

Figure 2–1B. Anophysiology—RAIR.

4. Test Element: Anorectal Sensation and Rectal Compliance

Purpose

Evaluation of somatic and visceral anorectal sensation.

Indication

Evaluation of fecal incontinence.

Evaluation of IBS.

Evaluation of constipation.

Equipment and technique

• Somatic sensation: perianal wiping with Q-tip to assess sensation (symmetry?) and to trigger anocutaneous reflex, ie, reflectory sphincter contraction.

• Visceral sensation: manometry equipment as before, but exchange of balloon into one with high material compliance: catheter advanced into rectum, followed by slow instillation of body-temperature water (maximum 450 mL) with continuous pressure measurement → recording of the following steps:

  – First sensation: patient feels balloon in the rectum (not just at the anal verge).

  – First urge: patient notices first urge to move bowels.

– Maximally tolerable volume: patient starts to feel discomfort/pain.

– Rectal compliance = Δvolume/Δpressure.

Risks

Discomfort, balloon rupture, internal balloon loss (→ always secure balloon edge externally).

Reference values

• First sensation: 10–50 mL.

• First urge: 50–100 mL.

• Maximally tolerable volume: 140–320 mL (F), 170–440 mL (M).

• Rectal compliance: 2–6 mL/mm Hg.

Interpretation

• Normal: normal sensation and compliance.

• IBS: reduced volume tolerance, normal compliance.

• IBD or rectal stricture: reduced volume tolerance, reduced compliance.

• Neurologic dysfunction: reduced sensation, increased volume tolerance, normal (or increased) compliance.

Pitfalls

Patient cooperation needed. False normal compliance if balloon distends more axially (lower resistance) than radially (high resistance). External loss of balloon (incontinence) before meaningful volume instilled.

5. Test Element: EMG

Purpose

Evaluation of neuromuscular integrity and coordination.

Indication

Evaluation of pelvic floor dyssynergia or anismus (nonrelaxing puborectalis muscle).

Occasionally for evaluation of fecal incontinence: loss of muscular contractile capacity?

Equipment and technique

Surface anal electromyography: bilateral placement of electrodes at anal verge plus additional grounding electrode → recording of summative electric sphincter muscle activity at rest, at squeeze, at straining, and during coughing.

Needle EMG: insertion of concentric needle electrode into the muscle (→ discomfort!).

Risks

Surface EMG: no risks.

Needle EMG: discomfort, infection, bleeding.

Reference values

Potential > 100 mV, fiber density.

Interpretation

Normal sequence: normal pattern at rest, followed by adequate increase during squeeze and coughing, but decrease during straining.

Dyssynergia: normal or increased pattern at rest, increase during squeeze, coughing, but also during straining.

Pitfalls

Surface EMG is relatively inaccurate as it represents summation potential of all fibers and is buffered by skin and subcutaneous tissue.

6. Test Element: Balloon Expulsion Test

Purpose

Simple screening evaluation to rule out pelvic floor dyssynergia: ability to expel balloon is a complex activity that requires proper coordination of the rectum, pelvic floor, and anal sphincter muscle.

Indication

Constipation, obstructed defecation, pelvic floor dyssynergia (anismus, paradoxical puborectalis contraction).

Equipment and technique

Balloon is inserted into rectum and insufflated with 100–200 mL of water → patient is asked to expel balloon: (1) on examination table; (2) if not possible in lateral decubitus position, transfer to restroom and attempt in sitting position.

Variation of the test: addition of defined external weight.

Risks

Discomfort, balloon rupture, internal balloon loss (→ always secure balloon edge externally).

Reference values

Normal: balloon expelled (any position).

Abnormal: balloon cannot be expelled (not even in sitting position).

Evaluation Tools

Interpretation

Normal test: no evidence for pelvic floor dyssynergia → further tests not needed.

Abnormal test: false pathologic (patient not cooperating) vs true dyssynergia → further tests (eg, defecating proctogram).

Pitfalls

Test dependent on patient cooperation.

7. Test Element: Balloon Retention Test

Purpose

Simple screening evaluation to assess functional and coordinative ability to prevent fecal accident: ability to retain balloon against external traction force is a complex activity that requires proper coordination of the rectum, pelvic floor, and anal sphincter muscle.

Indication

Fecal incontinence.

Equipment and technique

Balloon is inserted into rectum and insufflated with 100 mL of water → patient is asked to retain balloon while examiner exerts increasing external traction. Recording of extraction force.

Risks

Discomfort, balloon rupture, internal balloon loss (→ always secure balloon edge externally).

Reference values

Normal: balloon can be retained against significant external traction (> 0.5 kg).

Abnormal: balloon lost under minimal to moderate external traction (< 0.5 kg).

Interpretation

- Normal balloon retention capacity: pseudo-incontinence vs seepage due to anal disconfiguration (eg, keyhole deformity).
- Abnormal balloon retention capacity: true morphologic-functional neuromuscular incontinence

Pitfalls

Test dependent on patient cooperation.

8. Test Element: Endoanal Ultrasound (see also next section on ERUS)

Purpose
Evaluation of structural integrity and pathology in the anal canal and the rectum.

Indication
Evaluation of fecal incontinence: sphincter defect, sphincter attenuation?

Anorectal tumors: evaluation and staging.

Extraluminal pathology: ultrasound-guided biopsy.

Fistula/abscess: location, course.

Equipment and technique
Ultrasound machine with rotating 10 (7) MHz probe.

Risks
Direct trauma during insertion of probe, discomfort (balloon distention); biopsy → risk of bleeding, infection, rectourethral fistula.

Reference values
Anal canal: IAS = hypoechogenic (black) ring, EAS = hyperechogenic (white) ring, puborectalis muscle = hyperechogenic (white) parabolic muscle.

Rectum: 5-layer model of rectal wall (Figure 2–2A), prostate and seminal vesicles, rectovaginal septum.

Interpretation
Sphincter defect (IAS, EAS).

Anorectal tumor: → staging (size, penetration, invasion, lymph nodes).

Other pathology: fistula showing as hypoechogenic tract that become hyperechogenic upon injection of peroxide into external fistula opening.

Abscess: hypoechogenic pocket.

Pitfalls
Artefacts, rectocele/short anal canal mistaken for anterior sphincter defect.

Further Steps
Defecating proctogram vs dynamic MRI.

Colonic transit studies (Sitzmark study).

Cross-reference

ENDORECTAL ULTRASOUND *(ERUS)*

Overview

Use of ultrasound waves (2–15 MHz) for imaging of extraluminal structures. Ultrasound pulses are emitted from a transducer. Reflection/refraction/transmission of the signal depends on tissue composition/impedance and presence/absence of interfaces: the signals returning to the probe are recorded. The reflected beams are processed to obtain an electronic reconstruction of the tissue.

Tissue penetration depth is related inversely, and resolution directly, to frequency:

- Transcutaneous (eg, abdominal) ultrasound: 3–7 MHz.
- Endoluminal ultrasound: 7–10 MHz.

Image optimization also is dependent on:

- Focal range (too close → need to interpose water-filled layer; too far → need to lower frequency).
- Artefacts: edge effect, mirror image, interference/reverberation, shadowing, posterior enhancement, refraction, side lobe.
- Adjustment of time gain compensation.

Expected benefits

Visualization of extraluminal anatomy and pathology.

Limitations

Lesion not in reach of probe, or probe cannot be passed through lesion (eg, obstructing cancer, stricture, etc).

Procedure not tolerated (→ alternative: ERUS under anesthesia/sedation).

Operator-dependent examination!

Accuracy/sensitivity/specificity not perfect → clinical and pathologic correlation needed:

- Distinction between normal vs scar vs tumor not always possible.
- False positive (ie, reactive, noncancerous) lymph node enlargement after recent biopsy.

Preparation

Fleet enema immediately before testing.

Cancer: rigid sigmoidoscopy.

Incontinence: anophysiology studies (see earlier discussion), questionnaires.

1. Test Element: Endorectal Ultrasound (ERUS)

Purpose

Evaluation and staging of rectal cancer.

Evaluation and staging of anal cancer?

Indication

Anorectal tumors: pretreatment evaluation and staging.

Anorectal tumors: post-treatment reassessment, surveillance.

Equipment and technique

Ultrasound machine with rotating 10 (7) MHz probe, equipped with water-filled balloon.

Risks

Direct trauma during insertion of probe, discomfort (balloon distention), perforation.

Reference values

Rectum: 5 layers of rectal wall (Figure 2–2A and 2–2B).

Landmarks: prostate, seminal vesicles, rectovaginal septum, puborectalis muscle/sphincter complex.

Interpretation

• Primary lesion: distortion of the rectal wall; depth, axial and circumferential size:

    – Noninvasive polyp or T1 cancer: thickening of black-2, intact of white-2.

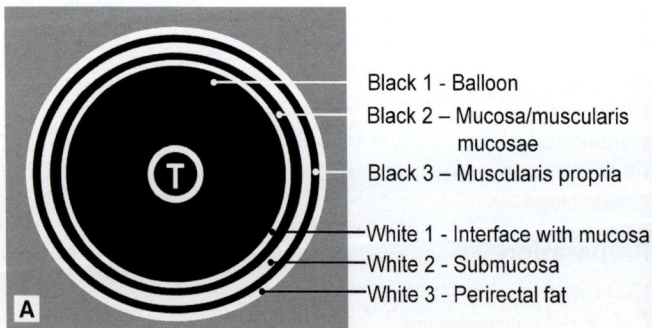

Black 1 - Balloon
Black 2 – Mucosa/muscularis mucosae
Black 3 – Muscularis propria
White 1 - Interface with mucosa
White 2 - Submucosa
White 3 - Perirectal fat

Figure 2–2A. ERUS—5-layer model of rectal wall.

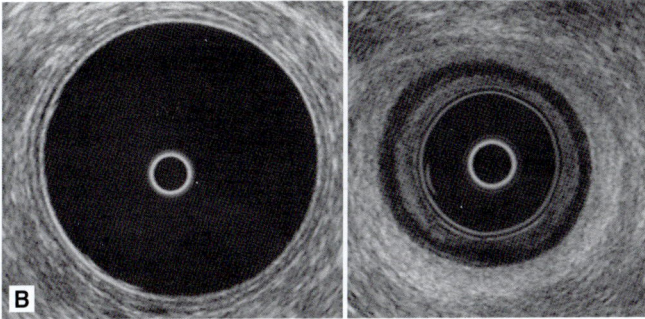

Figure 2–2B. ERUS—normal rectum (left) and anal canal (right).

- T2 cancer: interruption of white-2, no indentation into white-3.
- T3 cancer: interruption of white-2, indentation of tumor fingers into white-3.
- T4 cancer: blurring of the plane toward prostate, distortion of sphincter complex.

• Extraluminal structures:

- Lymphadenopathy: reproducible round/oval, nonbranching hypoechogenic extraluminal structures with measured diameter of 3–20 mm (sometimes even more).
- Recurrent tumor: asymmetric hypoechogenic tissue distortion, often only distinguishable from scar through observation of interval change on serial exams.
- Blood vessels: branching, can be followed over longer course, occasionally visible pulsations.
- Seminal vesicles: continuation to supraprostatic structure.

Pitfalls

Artefacts, reactive lymphadenopathy (shortly after biopsy) cannot be distinguished from metastatic lymphadenopathy (→ overstaging), distinction between scar and tumor. Lymph node metastases may be < 5 mm (→ understaging).

2. Test Element: Ultrasound-Guided Biopsy

Purpose

Evaluation of extraluminal pathology ~2–8 cm proximal to anal verge.

Indication
Cancer surveillance: evaluation of possible recurrence.

Lymphadenopathy: confirmation of stage III disease.

Equipment and technique
Endosonic multiplane transducer with channel for needle insertion.

Automatic-release TruCut biopsy needles. Visualization of pathology with conventional ultrasound → biplanar verification with biopsy probe → positioning of pathologic lesion in target plane/beam.

Risks
Direct trauma during insertion of probe, pain/discomfort (size of the probe, needle through anoderm), bleeding, infection, rectourethral fistula.

Reference values
Obtained tissue adequate and reflective of the true nature of the problem.

Interpretation
Positive biopsy → proof of tumor spread.

Negative biopsy → possibility of false negative (sampling error).

Pitfalls
Sampling error. Limitation of probe insertion.

3. Test Element: Endoanal Ultrasound

Purpose
Evaluation of structural integrity and pathology in the anal canal.

Indication
Evaluation of fecal incontinence: sphincter defect, sphincter attenuation?

Fistula/abscess: location, course.

Equipment and technique
Ultrasound machine with rotating 10 (7) MHz hardcap probe.

Risks
Direct trauma during insertion of probe, discomfort.

Reference values
Anal canal (Figure 2–2B):
- IAS: hypoechogenic (ie, black) ring: does not extend as far distal as EAS.
- EAS: thicker hyperechogenic (ie, white) ring.
- Puborectalis muscle: hyperechogenic (ie, white) parabolic muscle.

Interpretation

- Sphincter morphology (IAS, EAS): segmental gap/defect of internal or external sphincter (need to be assessed separately); assessment of sphincter thickness and architecture (scarring? atrophy?).
- Fistula: hypoechogenic tract, positive identification if whitening (hyperechogenicity) of the tract results from peroxide injected into external fistula opening.
- Abscess: extrasphincteric localized hypoechogenicity.

Pitfalls

Artefacts, rectocele/short anal canal mistaken for anterior sphincter defect.

Further Steps

Correlation with other clinical, radiologic, intraoperative, and pathologic data.

Cross-reference

Topic	*Chapter*
Fecal incontinence	4 (p 189)
Rectal cancer	4 (p 265)
Recurrent rectal cancer	4 (p 271)
Follow-up for colorectal cancer	6 (p 660)
Tumor staging in TNM system	App II (p 740)

Evaluation Tools

CONVENTIONAL X-RAYS (PLAIN FILMS)

Overview

Despite the rapid evolution of sophisticated diagnostic imaging techniques, conventional x-rays (plain films) remain an important evaluation tool because of their universal availability, simplicity, and low cost. The radiation exposure of a single test is moderate (compared with, eg, natural background radiation exposure of 300 mrem [3 mSv]), but the cumulative dose of medical imaging is significant.

Expected Benefits

Baseline imaging studies in many instances are sufficient, or they give a clue to serve as guidance for targeted ordering of subsequent, more specific tests. Serial images for assessment of evolution/resolution of a particular pathologic process (eg, bowel distention).

Limitations

Generally unspecific; lack of anatomical detail; 2-dimensional image of 3 dimensions results in superimposed structures; magnification effects for structures farther away from the x-ray film; blurring of contact zones (silhouette signs).

1. Specific Tests: Chest X-Ray

Purpose

1. Cardiopulmonary and mediastinal assessment.
2. Search for pneumoperitoneum (upright chest x-ray), eg, hollow viscus perforation or anastomotic leak.
3. Evaluation of chest skeleton.

Equipment and technique

Posteroanterior (potentially lateral) upright chest x-ray; if patient mobility limited: perform anteroposterior supine chest x-ray.

Risks

Radiation exposure: 6 mrem (0.06 mSv)

Interpretation

• Free air (Figure 2–3A): after preceding abdominal exploration most commonly absorbed within 7–10 days; increase of free air after previously documented disappearance suggestive of perforation/leak.
• Pulmonary lesions: inflammatory vs neoplastic.

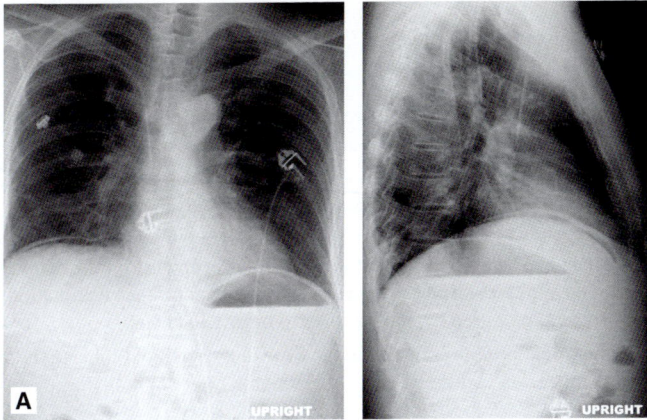

Figure 2–3A. Free air.

- Mediastinum: air, widening, lymphadenopathy.
- Atelectasis, pulmonary consolidations, pleural effusion, vascular congestion, pulmonary edema, pneumothorax, etc.

Pitfalls
Chilaiditi syndrome: suprahepatic colon loop mimicking free subdiaphragmatic air.

False negative for free air: small/early hollow viscus perforation may not show.

False positive (for perforation): benign causes of pneumoperitoneum.

2. Specific Tests: Abdominal Series

Purpose
Assessment of bowel gas pattern and diameter, extraintestinal air (eg, pneumobilia, hollow viscus perforation or anastomotic leak with local diffuse pneumoperitoneum), extraintestinal fluid (enlarged interloop space). Opacifications (gallstones, urolithiasis, pancreas calcifications, vascular, foreign bodies). At the same time, assessment of visible skeletal and soft tissue structures (eg, osteolysis, subcutaneous emphysema, etc).

Equipment and technique
Supine and upright abdominal views extending from diaphragm to pelvis. If patient mobility limited: perform supine and left lateral decubitus abdominal x-ray.

Evaluation Tools

Risks

Radiation exposure: 70 mrem (0.7 mSv); 20–30% false negative findings.

Interpretation

- Free peritoneal air: left lateral decubitus position (upright chest x-ray better if possible). Retroperitoneal air. Subcutaneous or subfascial gas.
- Fluid levels and bowel dilation (Figure 2–3B): consistent with obstruction; transition point suggestive of mechanical obstruction; air visible throughout to rectum suspicious for pseudoobstruction or enteritis.
- "Double bubble" sign (two air-filled structures in epigastrium, while little or no air is seen distally): duodenal obstruction, intestinal malrotation, obstruction produced by midgut volvulus or by Ladd bands.
- Colonic dilation with coffee-bean sign: volvulus of sigmoid colon (axis to LLQ) or cecum (axis to RLQ).

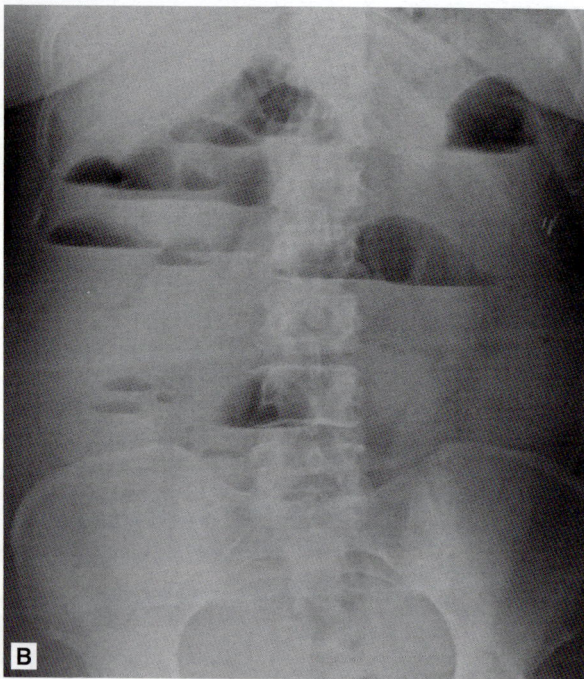

Figure 2–3B. Air-fluid levels in SBO.

- Diffuse colonic dilation: maximum 6 cm ($1\frac{1}{2}$ vertebrae) for transverse colon, 12 cm for cecum. Critical diameter depending on speed of evolving dilation.
- Pneumatosis: intestinal ischemia vs pneumatosis cystoides intestinalis.
- Air in the hepatic area:
  - Portal venous gas (liver periphery): ominous for intestinal necrosis or severe infection.
  - Pneumobilia (liver hilum): contact of intestinal lumen with biliary tree, eg, post-ERCP, gallstone ileus, hepaticojejunal anastomosis.
- Negative colonic contrast: limited intestinal air except for the colon occasionally allows clear visualization of colonic configuration.
- Displacement of intestinal gas: → mass effect?
- Calcifications: gallstones, kidney stones, arteriosclerosis, phleboliths, appendicolith, mesorectal calcifications → hemangioma.
- Foreign bodies.

Pitfalls
Normal abdominal x-ray does not exclude possibility of pathologic lesion or process, eg, bowel obstruction or viscus perforation.

Air-fluid levels: consistent with but not pathognomonic for bowel obstruction; can also be found in enterocolitis (diarrhea), postoperative ileus.

Rectal air after preceding rectal examination.

3. Specific Tests: Skeletal X-Rays

Purpose
Evaluation of skeletal anatomy and integrity. Not typically needed for colorectal questions but incidental findings when ordered for other indications.

Equipment and technique
Depending on target, x-ray in 2 separate projections.

Risks
Radiation exposure: skull, 3 mrem (0.03 mSv); limb, 6 mrem (0.06 mSv); pelvis, 70 mrem (0.7 mSv); spine, 30–70 mrem (0.3–0.7 mSv).

Interpretation
- Mandibular osteoma, dental abnormalities (number, form) → Gardner syndrome.
- Sacral destruction/malfusion (pelvic scimitar sign) → meningomyelocele, chordoma.
- Ankylosing spondylitis, sacroiliitis → IBD.

Pitfalls
None.

Further Steps

Depending on clinical circumstances and radiologic findings:

• Cross-sectional imaging studies: CT scan or MRI.

• Ultrasound: abdominal, chest.

• Specific contrast studies.

• PET not typically indicated as next step unless specific circumstances.

Immediate surgical exploration without further imaging: eg, free peritoneal air.

Cross-reference

Topic	*Chapter*
Contrast enema	2 (p 99)
Small bowel follow-through	2 (p 107)
CT	2 (p 117)

CONTRAST ENEMAS

Overview

Instillation of radiographic contrast material (with air = double contrast (Figure 2–4A), without air = single-column contrast) into hollow viscus or cavity to obtain anatomic road map and functional assessment. Evaluation of mucosal pathologies limited, contrast enema therefore only indicated if endoscopy is not possible, not successful, or because of patient preference.

Precontrast images (scout film) and postevacuation films mandatory. Particularly for evaluation of colon: bowel cleansing mandatory (screening), desirable (elective test for specific symptom), even though not always possible (emergency, eg, large bowel obstruction).

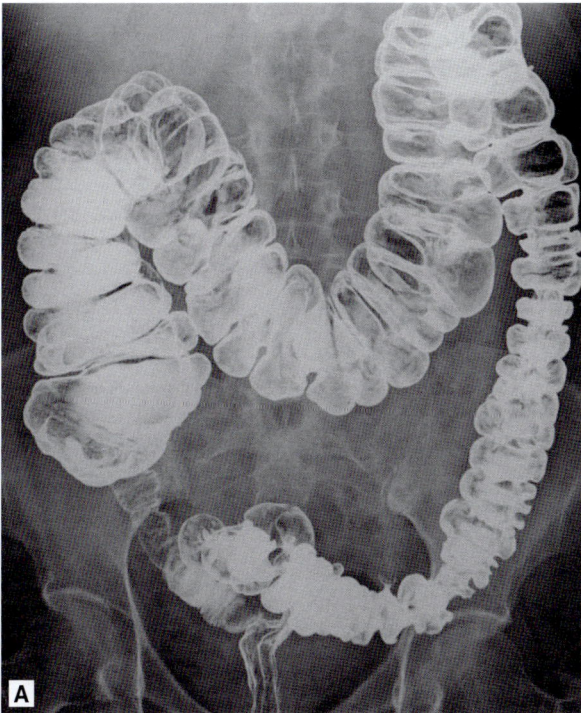

Figure 2–4A. Barium air double contrast enema.

Different types of contrast agents:

• Barium sulfate:

  – Pro: better image quality, better tolerability if aspirated.

  – Con: potentially fatal barium peritonitis ($\rightarrow$ contraindicated if perforation/leak suspected, confirmed, or imminent, or if surgery planned shortly after study), barium impaction in the colon (particularly if stasis (diverted/unused segments and contrast not washed out, prestenotic segments).

• Water-soluble contrast, eg, diatrizoate meglumine (Gastrografin), diatrizoate sodium (Hypaque):

  – Pro: no risk of contrast-induced peritonitis $\rightarrow$ contrast of choice for perforation/leak; cathartic effect.

  – Con: poorer image quality (less mucosal details, rapid dilution along the course of the intestines); aspiration $\rightarrow$ risk of chemical pneumonitis; hyperosmolar $\rightarrow$ dehydration and risk of rupture of closed segment with trapped contrast.

Caveat: Patients with "contrast allergy" are allergic to iodine-based contrast agents, but not to the above-mentioned barium!

Expected Benefits

1. Assessment of colonic anatomy, configuration (eg, haustration, tortuosity/redundancy, rigid pipe of burned out colitis), diameter, length of target pathology (eg, stricture), diverticula, malrotation, residual length after previous resections, etc.

2. Assessment of integrity (eg, leak, perforation), delineation of nonanatomic communication (fistula).

3. As guidance prior to or during intervention, eg, colonic stent placement.

Limitations

Limited ability to assess the mucosa.

Inability to perform therapeutic intervention for findings $\rightarrow$ subsequent colonoscopy (or surgery) may be necessary.

Lower sensitivity for small and even larger polyps.

False positive findings in inadequate colon cleansing.

1. Specific Test: Barium Enema

Purpose

Evaluation of colon polyps, cancer, diverticulosis $\rightarrow$ double-contrast study.

Evaluation of fistula or sinuses tracts, colonic obstruction $\rightarrow$ single-contrast enema.

Equipment and technique

Bowel cleansing. Rectal exam. Insertion of rectal tube and insufflation of balloon. Instillation of contrast by means of rectal tube. Single column study: images during in-flow and contrast distention; double contrast study: images after evacuation of contrast and insufflation of air until cecum dilated.

Risks

Radiation exposure: 700 mrem (7.0 mSv).

Barium peritonitis: contraindicated if concern about perforation/leak, and within 5–7 days after incomplete colonoscopy with biopsy.

Impaction of contrast precipitates in static or diverted colon may cause functional bowel obstruction.

Precipitation of toxic megacolon in active flare-up of IBD.

Interpretation

- Dolichocolon: axial elongation and tortuosity of the colon.
- Megacolon: radial distension of the colon; reference points: 6 cm ($1^1/_2$ vertebral heights) in transverse colon, 12 cm in cecum. Caveat: contrast study contraindicated in acute IBD or megacolon.
- Diverticula: distribution, size and number of limited clinical relevance; chronic diverticulotic stricture: smooth mucosal surface overall preserved (see Figure 4–18D) as opposed to ulceration/apple core in cancer.
- Cancer: characteristic "apple core" lesion (Figure 2–4B), mucosal integrity not preserved.

Evaluation Tools

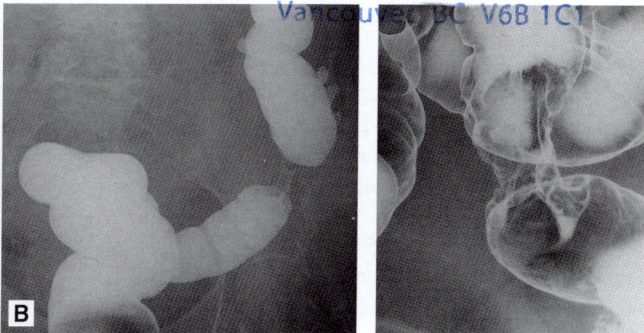

Figure 2–4B. Apple core lesions.

Pitfalls

Overlapping of contrast-filled colon segments (particularly sigmoid and cecum) → missing of relevant pathology.

False positive defects after inadequate cleansing.

Sensitivity of barium: colorectal cancer, 80–85%; large polyps (> 1 cm), 50%.

2. Test Element: Water-Soluble Contrast Enema

Purpose

Nonelective evaluation of colonic anatomy, configuration, search/rule out leak/perforation or point of obstruction (road map).

Elective evaluation of diverted segment (→ eliminates risk of contrast impaction).

Therapeutic (and diagnostic) intent: fecal impaction → taking advantage of hyperosmolar, ie, laxative properties to facilitate bowel movement.

Equipment and technique

Rectal exam. Insertion of rectal tube and insufflation of balloon. Instillation of contrast. Single column: images taken during inflow of contrast.

Risks

Radiation exposure: 700 mrem (7.0 mSv).

Colonic distention/rupture from hyperosmolar effect with suction of fluid into closed segment and trapped contrast (prestenotic).

Interpretation

As above for barium enema, in addition:

– Leak or perforation: extravasation of contrast.

– Intussusception → contrast enema potentially therapeutic.

– Volvulus: "bird's beak," "ace of spades."

Pitfalls

Lower detail and sharpness of contrast (compared with barium).

Overlapping of contrast-filled colon segments (particularly sigmoid and cecum) → risk of missing relevant pathology.

False positive defects from residual stool.

Further Steps

Depending on clinical circumstances and radiologic findings:

• Cross-sectional imaging studies: CT scan or MRI.

• Ultrasound: abdominal, chest.

• PET not typically indicated as next step unless specific circumstances. Obstruction/leak/perforation → surgical exploration/intervention?

Cross-reference

POUCHOGRAM

Overview

Instillation of radiographic contrast material into existing pouch (ileoanal pouch, continent ileostomy) for assessment of pouch configuration and functional evaluation. Conversely, endoscopy is preferable for assessment of mucosal pathologies (eg, pouchitis, ulcers, etc). Precontrast images (scout film) and post-evacuation films are mandatory to rule out unrelated findings and to assess adequate ability to evacuate.

Expected Benefits

• Assessment of pouch anatomy, configuration, size, obstruction, prolapse, in-/outlet, potentially valve segment (continent ileostomy).
• Assessment of integrity (eg, leak, perforation), delineation of nonanatomical communication (fistula).
• As guidance for intervention, eg, radiologic drain placement (continent ileostomy).

Limitations

Limited ability to assess the mucosa.

Interference with overlaying bowel loops.

1. Specific Test: Barium Pouchogram

Purpose

Fast, universally available, reasonably reliable examination.

Equipment and technique

Limited bowel cleansing/evacuation prior to exam.

– Ileoanal pouch: rectal exam, insertion of rectal tube and gentle insufflation of balloon, instillation of contrast → images in multiple projections, particularly lateral view.
– Continent ileostomy: insertion of Foley catheter into stoma/valve segment, instillation of contrast → images in multiple projections, particularly tangential to skin surface.

Risks

Radiation exposure: 300–700 mrem (0.3–7.0 mSv).

Barium peritonitis: contraindicated if concern about perforation/leak.

Interpretation

- Ileoanal pouch:
  - Intact pouch of normal size, no extravasation; lateral projection: pouch follows sacral curvature.
  - Pathology: leak, stricture, fistula; lateral projection: pouch does not follow sacral curvature → suspicion of presacral pathologic lesion or process (hematoma, abscess).
- Continent ileostomy:
  - Size, configuration of pouch reservoir, leak, etc.
  - Valve segment (negative imprint to pouch reservoir): assessment of length, course (kinking?), fistula? desintussusception, ie, valve outside reservoir (see Figure 4–15A).

Pitfalls

Radiologist often inexperienced with pouches → surgeon's presence helpful.

Overlapping of contrast-filled small bowel segments → risk of missing relevant pathology.

Suboptimal projections.

Covering of relevant pathology with catheter or balloon → false negative.

2. Test Element: CT-Pouchogram

Purpose

To assess 3-dimensional (3D) configuration and correlation to surrounding structures.

Equipment and technique

Enteral CT-contrast: instilled into pouch → high-resolution CT scan with 3D reconstruction.

Risks

Radiation exposure: 1000 mrem (10.0 mSv).

Interpretation

As above.

Pitfalls

Radiologist often inexperienced with pouches → surgeon's presence helpful.

Further Steps

Depending on clinical circumstances and radiologic findings:

• Pouchoscopy.

• Small bowel follow-through.

Obstruction/leak/perforation → surgical exploration/intervention?

Cross-reference

SMALL BOWEL FOLLOW-THROUGH *(SBFT)*

Overview

Instillation of radiographic contrast material to the upper GI tract (oral ingestion or via NGT), followed by sequential x-rays to observe the progression of the contrast through the small into the large bowel (Figure 2–5).

Expected Benefits

- Assessment of anatomy, configuration, diameter, length (eg, after previous resections), strictures, fistulae, mucosal abnormalities, etc.
- Assessment of functional integrity: passage time, delayed contrast progression.
- Identification of site of obstruction.

Evaluation Tools

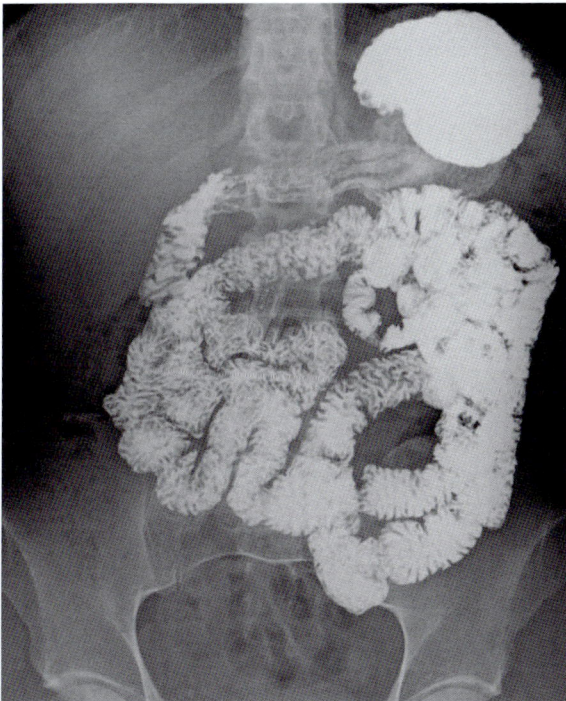

Figure 2–5. Small bowel follow-through.

Limitations

Limited ability to assess the mucosa due to overlay of loops.

1. Specific Test: Barium SBFT

Purpose

Evaluation of the small bowel with best contrast (elective setting).

Equipment and technique

Scout film. Administration of 2 bottles of liquid barium → serial images in appropriate time intervals (Figure 2–5). If colon is not reached within 4 hours → late films (eg, 24 hours later).

Risks

Radiation exposure: 300 mrem (3 mSv).

Barium peritonitis: → barium contraindicated if concern about perforation/leak.

Impaction of contrast precipitates in static bowel may result in functional bowel obstruction.

Interpretation

- Crohn disease: potentially visible mucosal alteration, presence and number of strictures, presence/characterization or absence of fistula.
- Enterocutaneous fistula: characterization of fistula-bearing bowel segment, identification of distal obstruction.
- Partial bowel obstruction: evidence and nature of transition point, additional distal obstructive sites.
- GI bleeding of unknown source: identification of altered bowel segment, tumor.

Pitfalls

Overlapping of contrast-filled colon segments → risk of missing relevant pathology.

False positive defects (air bubbles, enteric content).

2. Specific Test: Water-Soluble Contrast SBFT

Purpose

Evaluation of the small bowel while avoiding negative barium impact (subacute/nonelective setting).

Taking advantage of the cathartic (laxative) effect of the water-soluble contrast, the study may potentially result in opening up a partial bowel obstruction.

Equipment and technique

Scout film. Administration of 2 bottles of water-soluble contrast with serial images in appropriate time intervals. Late films not revealing due to dilution of the contrast.

Risks

Radiation exposure: 300 mrem (3 mSv).

Osmotic effect of hyperosmolar contrast → risk of perforation in closed loop (eg, colonic obstruction and competent ileocecal valve).

Interpretation

• Partial bowel obstruction: evidence and nature of transition point, additional distal obstructive sites.

• Enterocutaneous fistula: characterization of fistula-bearing bowel segment, identification of distal obstruction.

Pitfalls

Water-soluble contrast significantly diluted in the course of the small bowel → suboptimal resolution of structural details.

Overlapping of contrast-filled colon segments → risk of missing relevant pathology.

False positive defects (air bubbles, enteric content).

3. Specific Test: 50–50 SBFT

Purpose

Evaluation of the partially obstructed small bowel with a mixture of 50% water-soluble contrast and 50% barium. Goal: obtaining better contrast than with water-soluble contrast alone, but avoiding too much barium in partially obstructed bowel; taking advantage of the cathartic (laxative) effect of the water-soluble contrast that may potentially open up a partial bowel obstruction.

Equipment and technique

Scout film. Administration of 2 bottles of water-soluble contrast and barium mixed in a 1:1 ratio with serial images in appropriate time intervals. If colon is not reached within 4 hours → late films.

Risks

Radiation exposure: 300 mrem (3 mSv).

Osmotic effect of hyperosmolar contrast → risk of perforation if hyperosmolar contrast trapped in functionally closed loop.

Negative impact of barium.

Interpretation
• Partial bowel obstruction: evidence and nature of transition point, additional distal obstructive sites.

Pitfalls
This combination is of relatively limited value, not good enough to allow an accurate evaluation, but essentially carrying the same risks as a barium SBFT.

Further Steps

Depending on clinical circumstances and radiologic findings:
• Cross-sectional imaging studies: CT scan or MRI.
• Ultrasound: abdominal, chest.
Surgical exploration, depending on the circumstances.

Cross-reference

Topic	*Chapter*
SBO	1 (p 43)
CT enterography	2 (p 122)
IBD—Crohn disease	4 (p 327)
Enterocutaneous fistula	4 (p 395)

COLONIC TRANSIT STUDY (SITZMARK)

Overview

Qualitative and (semi-)quantitative assessment of unassisted colonic transit time. Useful tool for evaluation of patients with constipation and abdominal bloating to distinguish between etiopathogenetic subtypes and serve as guidance for further diagnostic and treatment options.

Classical method: ingestion of radiopaque markers (commercial: Sitzmarks, or hand-made: cut radiopaque tubes) with scheduled x-rays: inexpensive, safe, and simple, does not require infrastructure.

Alternative method: scintigraphy with oral radioisotope markers.

Expected benefits

Assessment of colonic transit function in patients with chronic constipation for distinction between:

- Slow transit constipation (colonic inertia).
- Pelvic floor dysfunction/fecal outlet obstruction.
- Normal transit constipation, eg, IBS.

Limitations

Noncooperative patients: continuation of laxatives, lack of fiber supplementation.

1. Specific Test: Sequential Sitzmark Study (3-Day Variant)

Purpose

Qualitative and semi-quantitative assessment of colonic transit time.

Equipment and technique

General patient instructions:

- Temporary discontinuation of any laxatives or enemas for the duration of the study.
- Daily fiber supplement 4 times per day.
- At least six 8-ounce glasses of water every day.
- Otherwise regular diet (no special adjustments).

Sitzmark capsules: 1 capsule in the morning on days 1, 2, and 3.

Abdominal x-rays: on days 4 and 7.

Risks

Radiation exposure: 140 mrem (1.4 mSv).

Fecal impaction.

Interpretation

Three distribution patterns:

1. All markers accumulating in the pelvis: pelvic outlet obstruction → defecating proctogram.

2. Markers diffusely distributed throughout colon: slow transit constipation (see Figure 4–24).

3. All markers disappeared: normal-transit, constipation-predominant IBS.

Semi-quantitative calculation of total and segmental transit times.

Pitfalls

False negative test: noncompliant patient cheating (eg, not taking pills, taking laxatives) → normal-appearing study with all markers eliminated.

False positive: too-short interval between tablet ingestion and abdominal x-ray.

2. Test Element: Simplified Sitzmark Study (1-Day Variant)

Purpose

Qualitative assessment of colonic transit time.

Equipment and technique

General patient instructions:

• Temporary discontinuation of any laxatives or enemas for the duration of the study.

• Daily fiber supplement 4 times per day.

• At least six 8-ounce glasses of water every day.

• Otherwise regular diet (no special adjustments).

Sitzmark capsules: 1 capsule in the morning on day 1.

Abdominal x-rays: on day 5.

Risks

Radiation exposure: 70 mrem (0.7 mSv).

Fecal impaction.

Interpretation

Three distribution patterns: as above.

Pitfalls
As above.

Further Steps

Defecating proctogram.

Anophysiology studies.

Decision-making about treatment options, eg, subtotal colectomy?

Cross-reference

Topic	*Chapter*
Defecating proctogram	2 (p 114)
Pelvic floor dysfunction	4 (p 420)
Constipation	4 (p 427)
IBS	4 (p 434)
Selected colorectal reference values	App II (p 732)

Evaluation Tools

DEFECATING PROCTOGRAM (DEFECOGRAPHY)
Overview

Evaluation of patients with defecation disorders: ie, outlet obstruction, pelvic floor dysfunction, rectal or pelvic organ prolapse, distal marker distribution on Sitzmark study. Instillation of radiographic contrast paste with viscosity that more closely resembles stool than regular contrast. Imaging with static images or video defecography while the patient sits on a special toilet chair and attempts to evacuate the contrast. Assessment includes dynamic observation of structural and functional alterations in the process as well as rate and completeness of the defecation.

Normal sequence (Figure 2–6): correct anorectal position above pubococcygeal line; puborectalis muscle tone with anterior traction causes anorectal angle (normal: 90–110 degrees at rest); squeezing results in elevation of pelvic floor and the anorectal angle becomes more acute; conversely, straining results in widening of anorectal angle (relaxation of puborectalis muscle), evacuatory force, opening of anal canal, and complete evacuation.

Expected Benefits

Continuous assessment of dynamic interaction between rectum and rectal content during evacuation effort proves useful to identify rectal intussusception, rectocele with retention of stool, pelvic floor dyssynergia, and extent of rectal emptying.

Limitations

Generally unspecific information, indirect evidence. Interobserver variability of different parameters, particularly measurement of anorectal angles or agreement for intussusception and anismus.

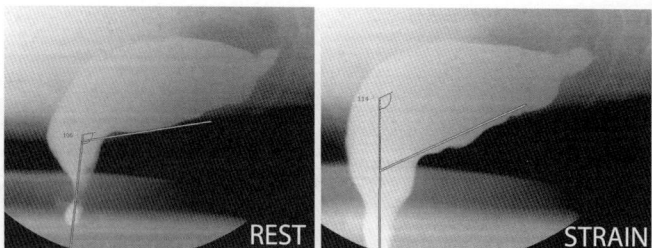

Figure 2–6. Defecating proctogram with anorectal angle at rest and during straining.

Lack of information about extraluminal pathology → MRI defecography or dynamic pelvic MRI.

Incontinence: loss of contrast before adequate completion of test.

Negative diagnostic impact of noncooperative patient.

1. Specific Test: Conventional Defecating Proctogram (Defecography)

Purpose
As stated above: technique relatively simple, cheap, unlimited length of sequence.

Equipment and technique
Instillation of radiographic contrast paste; patient then positioned on radio-transparent Brunswick chair → sequence of resting, squeezing, straining, evacuation.

Imaging: fluoroscopy with static images or preferably video defecography.

Risks
Radiation exposure: 450–700 mrem (4.5–7.0 mSv).

Interpretation
Pathology of primary relevance: quality of dynamic changes, transition, effective evacuation, pelvic floor descent (below pubococcygeal line), puborectalis relaxation vs paradoxical contraction, rectocele, intussusception, prolapse, enterocele, incomplete evacuation.

Pathology of minor relevance: absolute values for anorectal angle (high inter-observer variability!).

Pitfalls
False negative: presence of significant fecal incontinence results in loss of contrast without adequate expansion of rectal reservoir.

Prevalence of "pathologic" findings in asymptomatic patients: eg, rectocele ~25–50%.

Overinterpretation of findings: rectocele, angle, mucosal folds → always clinical correlation needed to determine whether the documented findings are truly relevant for the patient's complaints.

2. Specific Test: MRI Defecography

Purpose
If available, MRI is the preferred technique as both endoluminal and extraluminal events are visible during whole course of evacuation. In contrast to "dynamic MRI" (in supine patient), open interventional MRI defecography

examines patient in the more relevant sitting position and during the actual evacuation process.

Equipment and technique

Requires very expensive infrastructure and equipment: superconducting open-configuration MRI system: allows patient to sit within. Instillation of MRI-opaque contrast paste (gadolinium 2.5 mmol/L): 300 mL of synthetic stool (mashed potato starch) mixed with 1.5 mL of gadopentetate dimeglumine (377 mg/mL). Patient positioned on MRI-transparent chair in center of open-configuration MRI. MRI image sequence of resting, squeezing, straining, evacuation (with static images or preferably video defecography).

Risks

MRI related (contraindications: magnetic implants, etc), gadolinium side effects.

Interpretation

Pathology of primary relevance: quality of dynamic changes including assessment of other pelvic and abdominal organs: transition, effective evacuation, pelvic floor descent (below pubococcygeal line), pelvic organ and rectal prolapse, enterocele, puborectalis relaxation vs paradoxical contraction, rectocele, intussusception, incomplete evacuation.

Pathology of minor relevance: absolute values for anorectal angle (high inter-observer variability!).

Pitfalls

Limited availability of infrastructure.

Other pitfalls: as above.

Further Steps

Depending on clinical circumstances and radiologic findings:
• Anophysiology studies.
• Contrast enema.
• Dynamic MRI.

Cross-reference

COMPUTED TOMOGRAPHY (CT SCAN)

Overview

Cross-sectional imaging studies (CT, MRI, ultrasound) have become a cornerstone of modern medicine. All specialties (including surgery, oncology) rely on a noninvasive and reproducible evaluation. Computed tomography (CT scan) is by far the most universal and fastest tool to evaluate and quantitate tumor burden and infections, to plan surgical resection, to perform precise interventions, to detect comorbidities.

Increased resolution and slice thickness allows complete reconstruction and evaluation in different planes and to filter areas of interest. Ability to read CT scans is mandatory for colorectal surgery.

Alternatives

MRI.

Abdominal ultrasound.

Surgical exploration.

Indications

- Cancer staging: local extent (particularly for rectal cancer), secondary pathology (evidence of perforation/obstruction, liver metastases, hydronephrosis, paraaortic lymph node involvement, etc).
- Assessment of cancer response or progression (during neo-/adjuvant treatment)
- Evaluation of infections, sepsis, peritonitis, respiratory dysfunction, postoperative complications, etc.
- Detection of coexistent pathology: liver cirrhosis, ascites, anatomic variants, inflammatory changes, gallstones, kidney stones.
- Evaluation of unexplained abdominopelvic symptoms: pain, distention, abdominal wall hernia (Figure 2–7), etc.
- CT colonography and CT enterography (see respective sections later in this chapter).
- Helical CT scan: workup of active GI bleeding; vascular extravasation of contrast?

Advantages

Universal availability.

High sensitivity and specificity for detecting liver lesions > 1 cm (90% and 95%).

Not examiner-dependent, more reproducible than ultrasound.

Evaluation Tools

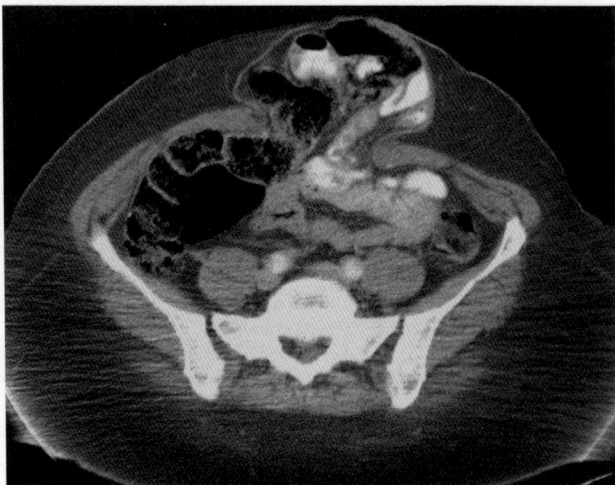

Figure 2–7. CT scan showing large incisional hernia.

Risks and Limitations

• Risks: radiation exposure (2000 mrem [20.0 mSv]), contrast allergy.
• Adequate imaging requires administration of oral and IV contrast: not possible in renal insufficiency and contrast allergies.
• Correlation with other evidence needed.
• Distinction between benign and malignant lesions frequently is not possible.

Characteristic Features

• Cancer: visible mass (primary colon tumor not necessarily visible on CT), evidence for metastatic spread, invasion of other structures, critical proximities, etc.
• Peritonitis/abdominal crisis: abscess formation (pelvic, pericolonic, subhepatic, subphrenic, interloop, etc), evidence of contrast extravasation (leak, perforation), extraluminal air?
• Diverticulitis: important for staging/possible intervention: phlegmon, wall thickening, fat stranding, abscess formation (pericolonic, pelvic), confined extracolonic air, free air, ascites.

- Appendicitis: increased diameter (> 6 mm), fecalith? Perifocal inflammatory changes (fluid, stranding, limited wall thickening, free fluid.
- IBD:
  - Crohn disease: bowel wall thickening, skip areas, fat stranding, abscess formation, fistulas (short-cut of oral contrast, air in bladder), lymphadenopathy.
  - Ulcerative colitis: typically no specific pathology on CT, occasionally marked enhancement of mucosa.
- Colitis: marked enhancement of mucosa, possible colonic wall thickening (eg, *C difficile* colitis), thumbprinting (mucosal edema).
- Ischemic colitis: altered enhancement of bowel wall (increased/decreased), pericolonic stranding, incomplete course of visceral blood supply, pneumatosis (air in bowel wall: suggestive of necrosis), portal vein gas (from gangrenous process), free air.
- Bowel obstruction: air/stool distribution, transition point, colonic wall thickening, evidence of causative pathology (tumor, adhesion), signs of perforation, cecal diameter (> 12 cm?), transverse colon diameter (> 6 cm?), pneumatosis?
- Active GI bleeding: vascular extravasation of contrast, contrast enhancement of bowel wall, thickened bowel wall, vascular dilations.

Cross-reference

Evaluation Tools

CT COLONOGRAPHY ("VIRTUAL COLONOSCOPY")

Overview

Noninvasive imaging of entire colon by means of high-resolution CT scan with digital 3D-reconstruction of colon, allowing for a virtual fly-through (Figure 2–8). In addition visualization of extracolonic structures. Test still requires full bowel cleansing, which is biggest hurdle to wide screening. During procedure: rectum is pumped with air, which causes significant discomfort and rarely perforation.

Data somewhat divergent: some studies showing similar sensitivity as standard colonoscopy (> 90% for polyps > 8 mm), others showing only moderate sensitivity/specificity and high inter-observer variability. Therefore CT colonography promising, but not yet "prime time" test.

Future: rapid technologic progress is expected, leading to better resolution, better distinction between stool and pathology, and no need for bowel prep.

Alternatives

Colonoscopy.

Barium-air contrast enema.

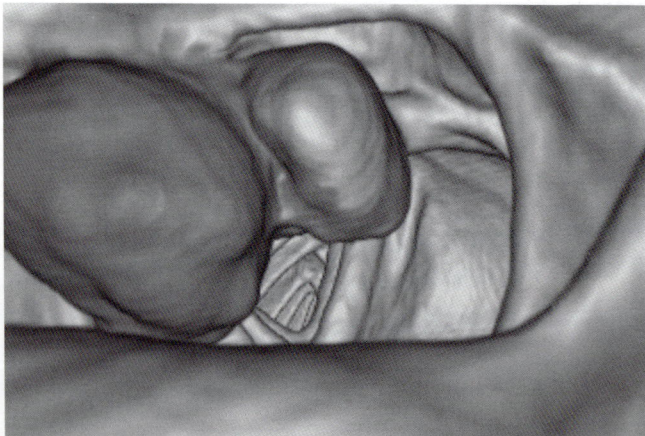

Figure 2–8. CT colonography showing colonic mass.

Indications

Failed colonoscopy.

Primary screening (not yet recommended).

Advantages

Fast (10–15 minutes), avoidance of instrumentation, overall safe.

Sedation not required → patients are not dependent on other people (eg, driving).

Better patient acceptance.

Detection of significant extracolonic pathology: aortic aneurysms, renal cell carcinomas, etc.

Risks and Limitations

Risks: risk of perforation low but not zero, radiation exposure (> 2000 mrem [20.0 mSv]).

Abnormal findings → further testing with colonoscopy needed.

Frequent unnecessary evaluations/surgeries for incidental findings.

Need for bowel prep (like colonoscopy).

Insufflation of air through rectal tube associated with cramping: more uncomfortable than standard colonoscopy (as no sedation given).

May not be covered by insurance for screening (unless colonoscopy failed).

Characteristic Features

Colonic: polyps, mass, stricture, diverticulosis, colonic road map.

Extracolonic: mass (kidney, adrenals, pancreas, etc), gallstones, vascular abnormalities, etc.

Cross-reference

Topic	*Chapter*
Colorectal cancer screening	2 (p 64)
Colonoscopy	2 (p 71)
Contrast enema	2 (p 99)
Polyps	4 (p 236)
Polyposis syndromes	4 (p 240)
Colorectal cancer	4 (p 252)
Bowel preparation/cleansing	7 (p 700)

Evaluation Tools

CT ENTEROGRAPHY ("VIRTUAL SMALL BOWEL FOLLOW-THROUGH")

Overview

Noninvasive imaging of the small bowel by means of high-resolution CT scan with improved spatial and temporal resolution to allow digital 3D-reconstruction of small intestine. The technique involves administration of large volume oral contrast (to achieve bowel distention) in conjunction with IV contrast to enhance the mucosa.

Future: rapid technologic progress is expected with better resolution, fly-through.

Alternatives

Small bowel follow-through.

Capsule endoscopy.

Indications

Crohn disease.

Enterocutaneous fistula.

Partial/intermittent small bowel obstruction.

GI bleeding of unknown source.

Advantages

Fast (10–15 minutes), noninvasive, safe.

Accurate visualization of extent/distribution of disease, separation of intestinal overlay projections, demonstration of extraluminal pathology.

Risks and Limitations

• Risks: radiation exposure (2000 mrem [20.0 mSv]).

• Relatively new modality: not universally available, still in learning curve.

• Contraindicated in: contrast allergy, renal insufficiency.

Characteristic Features

• Crohn disease: small bowel inflammation with increased wall enhancement, thickening, inflammatory mass, presence and number of strictures, enlarged vessels, perienteric inflammatory changes and abscess, presence/characterization or absence of fistula.

• Enterocutaneous fistula: characterization of fistula-bearing bowel segment, identification of distal obstruction, assessment of extraluminal scar tissue.

- Bowel obstruction: evidence and nature of transition point, additional distal obstructive sites.
- GI bleeding of unknown source: identification of altered bowel segment, inflammatory signs, tumor.

Cross-reference

Evaluation Tools

MAGNETIC RESONANCE IMAGING *(MRI)*

Overview

MRI—like other cross-sectional imaging studies (CT, ultrasound)—provides reproducible high-resolution imaging, but with the advantage of being examiner-independent and avoiding radiation exposure. MRI is based on detection and mapping of radio signals emitted by alignment of spins of hydrogen atoms that are exposed to strong magnet fields and stimulated by radio waves. The different hydrogen (ie, water) content of tissues allows creation of anatomic images.

- T1: realignment of nuclear spins with magnetic field → T1-weighted images show fluid black, fat white; contrast improvement with gadolinium-enhancement (ie, vascularity) and fat suppression: abdominal MRI.
- T2: dephasing of nuclear spins with transverse field → T2-weighted images show fluid white, fat dark; pelvic MRI.

MRI and CT scan are exchangeable to some degree but complementary for specific areas. MRI typically has an advantage in distinguishing soft tissue structures and processes with different water content, eg, inflammatory or neoplastic processes, muscular and fascial anatomy, etc.

Increased contrast and resolution in dynamic protocols allow noninvasive reconstruction and visualization of vascularization (MRI angiogram), duct structures (eg, MRCP), pelvic floor dynamic during straining-squeezing sequences and defecation (MRI defecography).

Alternatives

CT scan.

Abdominal ultrasound.

Surgical exploration.

Indications

- Cancer staging: local extent, radial margin of rectal cancer.
- Discrimination between liver cysts, metastases, hemangiomas.
- Evaluation of abdominal wall pathology.
- MRCP: noninvasive ERCP for evaluation of biliary disease, cholestasis.
- MRI angiography: noninvasive angiogram.
- Pelvic MRI with dynamic sequences: pelvic organ prolapse syndrome, MRI defecography.
- Anorectal pathology, MRI fistulography.

Advantages

No radiation exposure.

Better resolution for soft-tissue pathology.

Not examiner-dependent, more reproducible than ultrasound.

Risks and Limitations

- Contraindications: pacemaker, metallic implants, patient claustrophobia.
- Adequate imaging may require administration IV gadolinium.
- Correlation with other evidence is needed.
- Distinction between benign and malignant lesions is not always possible.
- Nonradiologists are still less familiar with MRI than with CT images.

Characteristic Features

- Tumor: T2-weighted $\rightarrow$ intense (white); T1-weighted $\rightarrow$ dark, early enhancement with gadolinium.
- Scar tissue: T1- and T2-weighted $\rightarrow$ low signal intensity, no gadolinium enhancement.
- Inflammation: T2-weighted $\rightarrow$ intense (white), T1-weighted $\rightarrow$ dark, delayed enhancement with gadolinium.
- Dynamic pelvic MRI: lubricant gel used as rectal and vaginal contrast; dynamic evaluation during rest, squeeze, strain, evacuation: assessment for perineal descent, rectocele, cystocele, vaginal prolapse, enterocele (comparison to pubococcygeal line).

Cross-reference

Evaluation Tools

POSITRON EMISSION TOMOGRAPHY
(PET / PET-CT)

Overview

Positron emission tomography—either alone or in conjunction with CT—provides imaging based on metabolic tissue activity. PET substrate is an 18F-glucose analogue that is taken up into the cell but cannot be further metabolized and therefore accumulates intracellularly. Imaging with a whole body scanner allows for identification of foci with increased metabolism. Of particular interest are tumors, which are generally metabolically more active than normal tissue as they take up and burn large amount of glucose.

Expected Benefits

Detection of previously unidentified tumor foci.

Qualitative differentiation between scar tissue and tumor recurrence or metastases.

Limitations

Generally unspecific, potentially altered/suppressed by chemotherapy. False positive activity possible in GI mucosa ($\rightarrow$ repeat study).

1. Test Element: Whole Body PET

Purpose

1. Differentiation of local recurrence from unspecific scar tissue.

2. Detection of distant metastasis, eg, before deciding on surgical management of proven local recurrence.

Equipment and technique

PET scanner. 18F-fluoro-deoxyglucose (FDG).

Risks

Minimal radiation exposure: 14–20 mrem (0.14–0.2 mSv).

Pitfalls

Distinction between neoplastic and inflammatory changes not sufficiently reliable.

False negative: tumor suppression during concomitant chemotherapy, tumors without significant FDG uptake; false positive: GI mucosa.

Interpretation

Areas of normally increased activity: bladder, brain, occasionally GI mucosa.

Tumor generally more active than scar tissue.

2. Test Element: PET/CT

Purpose

Improved diagnostic accuracy through combination of the activity assessment (PET) with imaging (CT) to directly correlate hypermetabolic areas with the respective morphology.

Equipment and technique

PET and CT scanner. 18F-FDG.

Risks

Significantly higher radiation exposure than PET alone: 2000–2500 mrem (20–25 mSv).

Pitfalls

As above.

Interpretation

Independent analysis of PET and CT and overlap correlation of areas with increased metabolic activity to morphologic changes on CT.

Further Steps

Other imaging modalities.

CT-guided or open biopsy of suspicious areas vs surgical exploration.

Watchful waiting with repeat exams to assess temporal change.

Cross-reference

Evaluation Tools

ANGIOGRAPHY WITH POSSIBLE EMBOLIZATION

Overview

Selective mesenteric (visceral) angiography remains an important tool in the management of acute severe GI bleeding. Diagnostic value: extravasation of contrast material to identify bleeding site. Potentially therapeutic value through direct intervention (eg, embolization).

Mesenteric angiography (Figure 2–9): sequential injection of contrast into IMA, SMA, celiac trunk.

False negative examinations due to intermittent nature of hemorrhage, transient vasospasms, intermittent clotting. Pharmacologic agents that actively trigger bleeding (eg, heparin, urokinase/streptokinase, etc) may improve sensitivity, but also lead to increased bleeding complications.

Expected Benefits

Direct visualization of arterial perfusion, identification of pathologic lesion and bleeding site (30–50%), possible intervention with superselective embolization.

Limitations

Intermittent bleeding: most bleeding will have stopped before initiation of diagnostic imaging or intervention.

Active bleeding > 1.0 mL/min.

Venous bleeding source may escape detection.

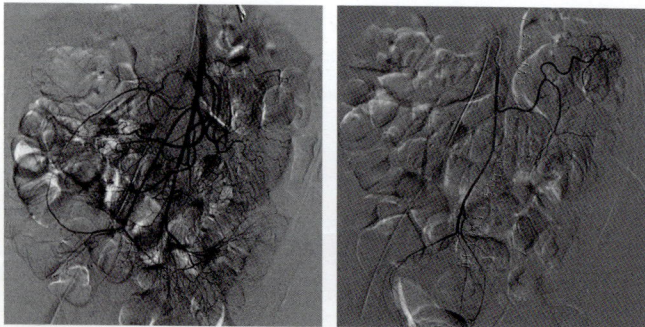

Figure 2–9. Angiogram SMA (left) and IMA (right).

1. Specific Test: Angiography with Pharmacologic Intervention

Purpose
After identification of bleeding site induction of vasoconstriction with selective vasopressin drip → ability for hemodynamic stabilization, bridge to surgery rather than final treatment.

Equipment and technique
Intravascular injection of contrast via transfemoral access catheter, phased fluoroscopic visualization.

Risks
Radiation exposure: 750–5000 mrem (7.5–50.0 mSv).

Procedure-related complication: 2%.

30–50% false negative findings; risk of rebleeding; risk of myocardial or peripheral vascular ischemia → contraindicated in coronary artery or peripheral vascular disease.

Interpretation
Cessation of extravasation at identified bleeding site, decreased hemodynamic instability.

Pitfalls
Vasopressin infusion successful in 70–90%, but high risk of rebleeding after cessation of drip.

2. Test Element: Angiography with Superselective Embolization

Purpose
After identification of bleeding site superselective embolization with gel foam, microcoils, or polyvinyl alcohol particles → decreased perfusion pressure to stop hemorrhage without causing segmental devascularization.

More durable than pharmacologic intervention, avoidance of systemic side effects.

Equipment and technique
Intravascular injection of contrast via transfemoral access catheter, phased fluoroscopic visualization → insertion of 3-F microcatheter.

Risks
Radiation exposure: 750–5000 mrem (7.5–50.0 mSv).

Procedure-related complication: 2%.

Evaluation Tools

Thirty to fifty percent false negative findings; recurrent bleeding; with modern technique only 5–10% risk of intestinal ischemia/infarction.

Interpretation
Superselective embolization of identified bleeding site: 75–85% successful.

Pitfalls
Intestinal ischemia/infarction → need for repeated clinical monitoring and surgery if evidence of deterioration.

Further Steps

- Identified bleeding site and successful intervention → monitoring for possible complication → surgery.
- Identified bleeding site and intervention not successful → surgery, eg, segmental resection.
- Bleeding site not identified, but bleeding stopped and patient stable → watchful waiting, colonoscopy, repeat tests if bleeding recurs, etc.
- Bleeding site not identified and ongoing bleeding with patient instability → surgery, ie, subtotal colectomy.

Cross-reference

NUCLEAR SCINTIGRAPHY

Overview

Nuclear scintigraphic provides noninvasive functional imaging based on dynamic changes within a target tissue or organ compared with the surrounding environment. Examples increased metabolic tissue activity, changes in passage, extravasation. Substrates are generally gamma-emitting radioisotopes linked to a carrier. The change in activity is captured by serial images with a whole body gamma camera. Radioactivity half-life is dependent on the physical half-life of the radioisotope and the biologic half-life of the whole substrate (excretion, metabolism, etc).

Expected Benefits

Noninvasive detection of pathology.

Limitations

Generally unspecific information, anatomic uncertainty (2-dimensional image), indirect evidence → need for careful interpretation and potentially for follow-up tests.

1. Specific Test: Tagged Red Blood Cell Scan ("Bleeding Scan")

Purpose
Sensitive diagnostic tool (50–90%) to detect bleeding > 0.1–0.5 mL/min: it is therefore the test of choice for first evaluation of significant lower GI bleeding.

Indication
Lower GI bleeding.

Equipment and technique
- Technetium-99m scanning: sensitivity 50–90%.
- Technetium-99m–labeled red blood cells: allows late scanning after 24 hours.
- Indium-111–labeled red cells: more expensive and labor-intensive technology, long half-life causing blurring of images; advantage: detection of intermittent bleeding.
- Sulfur-99m colloid: immediately available.
- Cinematic technetium-99m red blood cell scintigraphy for real-time scanning.

Risks
Radiation exposure: > 570 mrem (5.7 mSv).

Interpretation
Immediate blush (within 10 min): highly predictive for accurate identification of bleeding segment (Figure 2–10). Late images less reliable (cumulative effect, diffusion).

Pitfalls
Low specificity (50%), limited anatomic resolution → false localization of bleeding site in 10–60%. Pathology in hepatic and splenic flexure potentially obscured if substrate (eg, sulfur-99m colloid) phagocytosed in reticuloendothelial system (liver, spleen).

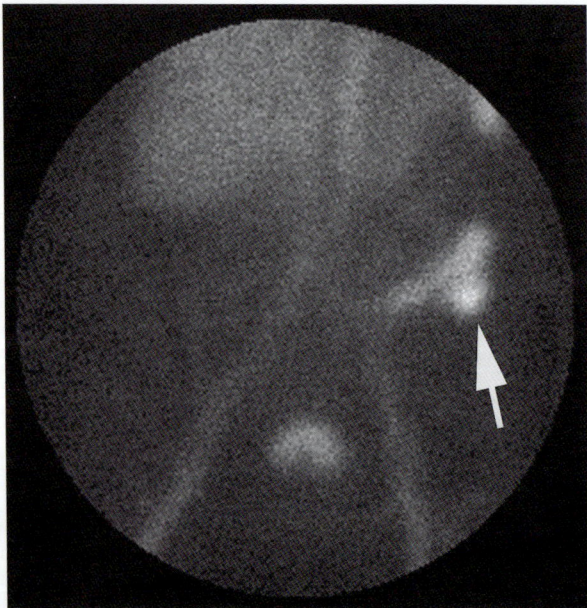

Figure 2–10. Bleeding scan.

2. Specific Test: Meckel Scan

Purpose
Detection of ectopic gastric mucosa in a Meckel diverticulum: IV technetium-99m (^{99m}Tc) pertechnetate is secreted by gastric mucosa tissue, both in the stomach and in ectopic locations.

Indication
Lower GI bleeding: suspicion for Meckel diverticulum, lack of other bleeding source.

Equipment and technique
IV ^{99m}Tc pertechnetate. Gamma camera.

Risks
Radiation exposure: 635 mrem (6.35 mSv).

Interpretation
Early abdominal images with localized activity in RLQ in addition to the gastric activity (which serves as positive control).

Pitfalls
False negative, if no functioning gastric mucosa in Meckel diverticulum: however, this is clinically not relevant because of low risk of bleeding in absence of gastric mucosa.

3. Test Element: Octreotide Scan

Purpose
Detection of neuroendocrine tumor activity with specific uptake of indium-111–labeled somatostatin-analogue octreotide: 80–90% sensitivity.

Equipment and technique
Indium-111–labeled somatostatin-analogue octreotide. Gamma camera.

Risks
Radiation exposure: 1810 mrem (18.1 mSv).

Interpretation
Detection of foci of increased activity: suspicious for metastatic carcinoid.

Pitfalls
Lack of anatomic resolution $\rightarrow$ cross-sectional imaging needed.

4. Test Element: Scintigraphic Emptying and Transit Studies

Purpose
Ingestion/delivery of carrier-linked isotope and observation of material progression through stomach, small intestine, colon and eventually anorectal evacuation: quantitative measurement of gastric, small bowel, and colonic transit time.

Equipment and technique
Indium-111, technetium-99m, iodine-131 linked to carrier (eg, diethylenetriamine pentaacetic acid [DTPA]).

Risks
Radiation exposure: 100–500 mrem (1.0–5.0 mSv).

Interpretation
Measurement of active transit time.

Further Steps
Depending on the results (positive/negative) and the clinical circumstances:
- Further radiologic studies: PET, CT/MRI, etc.
- Surgical planning or exploration without further imaging.
- No immediate action necessary, watchful waiting.

Cross-reference

Topic	Chapter
Colonic transit study	2 (p 111)
CT	2 (p 117)
MRI	2 (p 124)
PET	2 (p 126)
Carcinoid tumor	4 (p 287)
Acute lower GI bleeding	4 (p 391)
"Incidentalology"	4 (p 445)

Chapter 3

Anatomy and Physiology

EMBRYOLOGIC COLORECTAL DEVELOPMENT

Overview

Knowledge of embryologic development facilitates the understanding of congenital malformations and many other disease processes.

Embryonic period: first 8 weeks; fetal period: from 9th week to birth.

Landmarks

- Ectoderm → epidermis, nervous system.
- Mesoderm → mesenchymal tissues: muscular and connective tissue component of intestinal tract.
- Endoderm → GI tube to form epithelia and parenchymatous tissues of visceral/thoracic organs.
- Fusion zones:
  - Cephalad endo-/ectoderm: stomatodeum.
  - Caudad endo-/ectoderm: proctodeum.

Developmental Details

Weeks 2–4 (embryonic disc → early organ layout)

- Three germ layers: ectoderm, mesoderm, endoderm.
- Notochord: primordial axis of the embryo → axial skeleton and inductor of neural plate (→ neuroectoderm).
- Day 21: heart begins to beat → circulation.
- Craniocaudal and lateral folding of 3 layers → formation of cranial and caudal ends → head fold (stomatodeum), tail fold (proctodeum).

Weeks 4–8 (morphogenesis/organogenesis)

- Week 4: formation of primordial gut: foregut, midgut, hindgut → cloacal membrane.
- Formation of cloaca → urinary, genital, and rectal tracts empty through the same opening.
- Week 5: migration of neural crest cells along spinal cord → sympathetic ganglia; proximal to distal migration of neural crest cells to internal organs.
- Week 6: formation of levator ani.
- Week 7: fusion of urorectal septum with cloacal membrane (perineal body) → partitioning of cloaca into dorsal and ventral part; division of cloacal sphincter into posterior (external anal sphincter) and anterior (bulbocavernosus, transverse perinei muscles) parts.

- Week 8: rupture of anal membrane → communication of hindgut with amniotic cavity; formation of internal anal sphincter (hindgut).

Weeks 9–12 (tissue and organ differentiation)

- Midgut → small intestine including most of duodenum, colon from cecum to splenic flexure: arterial supply by SMA.
  - Week 9: physiologic umbilical herniation → 90-degree counterclockwise rotation.
  - Week 10: return of intestines to the abdomen → 180-degree counterclockwise rotation, 90-degree horizontal rotation of duodenum/pancreas to the right.
- Hindgut → colorectum from splenic flexure to anus, bladder, most of the urethra: arterial supply by IMA.
  - Formation of anal canal: proctodeum = fusion zone between hindgut (proximal) and ectoderm (distal) → dentate line, separate blood supply above/below.

Clinical Focus and Pathology

- Remnant of primitive streak → sacrococcygeal teratoma.
- Remnants of notochord → chordoma.
- Intestinal malrotations → incomplete rotation, incomplete fixation (eg, mobile cecum), volvulus.
- Incomplete return of intestines → omphalocele, umbilical hernia.
- Persistent yolk stalk → Meckel diverticulum, omphaloenteric fistula.
- Failure of recanalization → intestinal duplication.
- Failure of neural crest cells to migrate to distal bowel → Hirschsprung disease.
- Abnormal partitioning of urorectal septum → anorectal malformations.

Cross-reference

Aantomy and Physiology

VASCULAR ANATOMY

Overview

Knowledge of the vascular anatomy is prerequisite for the performance of safe and oncologically correct surgery. Vascular anatomy to the colorectal organs is characterized by 3 circulatory systems: systemic arterial network, systemic venous network, and portal venous network.

Landmarks

- SMA/SMV: at duodenum part III.
- IMA: at the aorta.
- IMV: at the inferior edge of the pancreas.
- Splenic flexure: transition from superior to inferior mesenteric vessels.
- Dentate line: border between visceral and systemic circulation.

Anatomic Details

Small intestine

Arterial:

- Supply mostly from SMA, partly from celiac trunk, some proximal collateralization, but end arteries at the level of the bowel.
- SMA: 1st branch: pancreaticoduodenal artery, 2nd: mid-colic artery, 3rd: vascular arcades to small bowel.

Venous:

- Paralleling the arterial supply → SMV → portal vein.

Colon (Figure 3–1)

Arterial:

- Supply from SMA and IMA → 3–4 major (named) vessels with significant anatomic variation.
- Ileocolic artery/right colic artery: last branch of SMA → terminal ileum, right colon, hepatic flexure.
- Mid-colic artery: 2nd branch of SMA → transverse colon (1st branch = pancreaticoduodenal artery). Anatomically special situation: transverse colon more distal to small bowel, but its arterial run-off more proximal than blood supply to small bowel.
- Left colic artery: 1st branch of IMA → splenic flexure to descending colon.
- Superior hemorrhoidal (superior rectal) artery: 2nd branch of IMA → sigmoid colon/upper rectum.

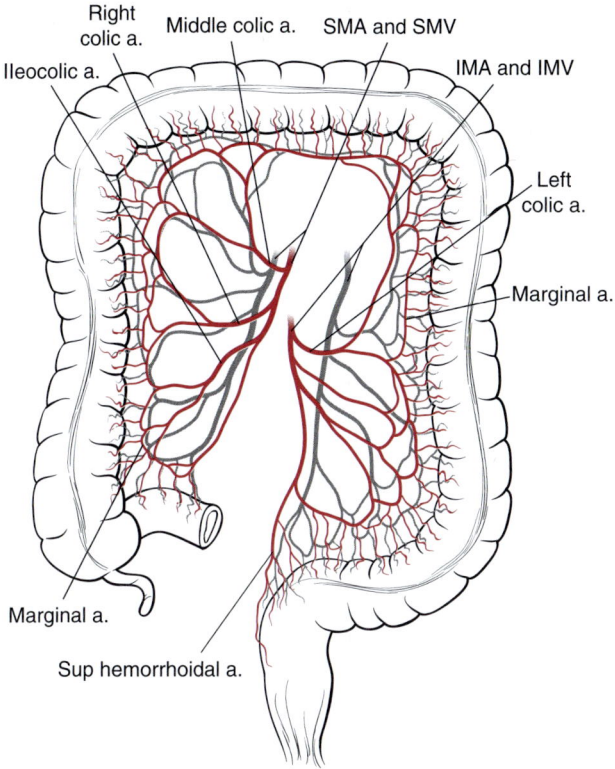

Figure 3–1. Vascular anatomy of the colon.

- Critical watershed areas: marginal artery of Drummond (variability on both the left and right colon). Griffith point (at splenic flexure): diminutive or absent (5%) marginal artery junction between SMA and IMA; extra connection between SMA and IMA: arch of Riolan (60%). Sudeck point: watershed between sigmoid colon and rectum.

Venous:

- Drainage through SMV or IMV to portal vein system. Limited collaterals to systemic circulation.
- Right colon to transverse colon: drainage collecting into SMV → parallel course to SMA → fusing with splenic vein at portal vein confluens.

- Splenic flexure to rectosigmoid colon: drainage collecting into IMV → course separating from IMA but targeting to pancreas tail → fusion with splenic vein.

Rectum

Arterial:

- Blood supply to rectum from two sources: IMA and internal iliac arteries.
- IMA: → superior rectal artery (synonym: superior hemorrhoidal artery) → rich reticular anastomotic network in the rectal submucosa with extensive collaterals.
- Internal iliac (hypogastric) arteries:
  - Middle rectal arteries (synonym: middle hemorrhoidal artery): abundant interconnecting network of dual blood supply → distinct reticular vascular pattern on endoscopy.
  - Inferior hemorrhoidal arteries.
- Variably present: median sacral artery (arises from posterior surface of the aorta and descends behind rectum to tip of the coccyx).

Venous:

- Blood from anorectum collects in arteriovenous plexuses → drainage through:
  - Single superior hemorrhoidal vein → splenic vein → portal vein.
  - Bilateral middle hemorrhoidal veins → internal iliac veins → IVC.
  - Bilateral inferior veins: external and internal hemorrhoidal plexus communicate → partial blood flow from internal hemorrhoidal plexus → pudendal veins → IVC.
  - Caveat: close proximity to rectum, but not associated with it: presacral veins!

Anal canal and pelvic floor

Arterial:

- Blood supply mostly from internal iliac artery.
- Middle hemorrhoidal artery → wide intramural network of collaterals.
- Extrapelvic pudendal artery → inferior hemorrhoidal artery.

Venous:

- Via wide venous network of middle and inferior hemorrhoidal veins: not exposed to effects of portal hypertension.

Clinical Focus

- Oncologic resection: to follow arterial supply and lymphatic and venous drainage.

- Hematogenous tumor spread: colon: portal vein system ($\rightarrow$ liver); rectum: portal vein system ($\rightarrow$ liver) and systemic circulation ($\rightarrow$ lungs).
- Intestinal ischemia: colon: watershed areas at splenic flexure, rectosigmoid junction, right colon; rectum: because of extensive collaterals virtually no risk for ischemia (unless previous surgical interruption of routes or complete aortic occlusion).

Pathology

- Ischemic colitis.
- Anatomic variability.
- Rectal varices.
- Hemorrhoids.

Cross-reference

Topic	*Chapter*
Angiography with possible embolization	2 (p 128)
Ischemic colitis	4 (p 303)
Colon resections	5 (pp 544–557)
Low anterior resection	5 (p 610)

ANORECTAL LANDMARKS

Overview

Anatomy of the pelvis and anorectum is complex. Thorough knowledge and use of precise terminology are a key distinction of the colorectal specialty.

Landmarks

• Anus: anal verge, intersphincteric groove, dentate line, anorectal ring.
• Rectum: valves of Houston, confluens of teniae.

Anatomic Details

Anorectum (terminal portion of GI tract)

• Embedded in osseous pelvis, surrounded by urogenital organs, muscular, ligamentous, and connective tissue structures.
• Maintenance of fecal continence: stopper-equipped reservoir, controlled expulsion mechanism for feces.

Rectum (pelvic segment of large intestine)

• Partially extraperitoneal.
• Proximal start: rectosigmoid junction, defined as:
  – Confluence of teniae.
  – Endoscopic (rigid sigmoidoscope) 12–15 cm proximal to anal verge.
  – Inadequate definitions: position of peritoneal reflection, level of sacral promontory
• Distal end: pelvic floor, upper end of anal canal.
• Nonmobilized rectum: 3 distinct endoluminal curves that form folds: valves of Houston.
• Lymph drainage: upper two-thirds of the rectum → primarily draining to inferior mesenteric and paraaortic nodes; lower one-third of the rectum → multidirectional drainage: along superior hemorrhoidal artery and IMA, along middle hemorrhoidal vessels to lateral pelvic side wall to internal iliac lymph nodes.

Anal canal

• Definitions:
  – Surgical: approximately 2–4 cm long: between anal verge and anorectal ring (proximal level of levator-external anal sphincter complex) → correlates with digital or sonographic exam.
  – Anatomic: based on histologic architecture along the canal.
  – Functional: high-pressure zone (manometry).

- Intersphincteric groove between internal and external anal sphincter around level of anal verge.
- Narrowing of rectum into anal canal → change of smooth mucosal lining to plicated appearance: columns of Morgagni, crypts.
- Dentate line: ~ 1–2 cm proximal to anal verge = embryologic fusion point between endoderm and ectoderm:
  – Separation between innervation, arterial/venous blood supply.
  – Separation of lymphatic drainage: above dentate line → drainage to inferior mesenteric and internal iliac nodes; below dentate line → drainage to superficial inguinal lymph nodes.
- Crypts: cryptoglandular complex with 4–8 apocrine anal glands from intersphincteric space that empty via anal ducts through IAS into anal canal.
- Epithelia:
  – Anal transition zone (ATZ, cloacogenic zone) above dentate line: combination of columnar, transitional-cuboidal, and squamous epithelium.
  – Anal canal between dentate line and anal verge: anoderm, ie, modified squamous epithelium without appendages.
  – Anal margin (outside anal verge): radial skin folds, thicker skin, pigmentation, skin with adnexal tissues.

Anus
- Virtual orifice, ie, anal canal not visible from outside; even with lateral traction, the sphincter reflex results in an immediate contraction that keeps it closed.
- Normal position: midline, ~ 60% of distance from coccyx to posterior vulva/scrotal base.

Clinical Focus
- Neoadjuvant chemoradiation for rectal cancer requires nonsurgical definition of rectum → endoscopic length definition for the purpose of uniformity in clinical trials.
- Rectal cancer: sphincter preservation (complete/partial) vs need for abdominoperineal resection, no oncologic benefit of removing sphincter muscle unless it is involved.
- Anal cancer → inguinal lymph node spreading pathway.

Pathology
- Cancer: adenocarcinoma above dentate line or anal glands; squamous cell cancer at ATZ and below.

Aantomy and Physiology

- Anal ducts serve as conduit for contamination of the perianal and perirectal tissues → cryptoglandular abscess and fistula.
- Patulous anus: lax anus with open view into anal canal; gaping to lateral traction: diminished reflex contraction.

Cross-reference

PELVIC MUSCLES

Overview

Management and understanding of fecal incontinence, pelvic floor dysfunction, and planning of surgical intervention is based on a fundamental knowledge about muscular pelvic structures.

Landmarks

- Intersphincteric groove: between EAS and IAS: palpated ~1 cm below to the dentate line.
- Anal sphincter complex: internal, external sphincter muscle, puborectalis muscle.
- Puborectalis muscle: upper end of surgical anal canal, anorectal angle (defecography).
- Pelvic floor muscles: ischiococcygeus, iliococcygeus, pubococcygeus, puborectalis.

Anatomic Details

Three categories of muscular structures:

1. Muscles lining sidewalls of the osseous pelvis:
   a. Obturator internus muscle.
   b. Piriformis muscle.
2. Pelvic floor muscles (pelvic diaphragm):
   a. Funnel-shaped musculotendinous termination of pelvic outlet.
   b. Innervation: branches of ventral primary rami of spinal nerves S3–S4.
   c. Function: mechanical support to abdominal/pelvic organs, passage for anorectal and urogenital viscera (two hiatal openings).
   d. Layout: symmetric array of paired striated muscles: originate at arcus tendineus (obturator fascia with extension anteroposteriorly from pubic bone to ischial spine at S3–S4).
   e. Subunits: ischiococcygeus muscle, iliococcygeus muscle, pubococcygeus muscle, puborectalis muscle; anococcygeal raphe: fibrous condensation of iliococcygeus muscle in posterior midline with fibers crossing over from one side to the other.
   f. Perineal body anterior to anus: superficial and deep transverse perinei muscles, some fibers of external sphincter muscle fusing with bulbocavernosus muscle → tendinous intersection.
3. Anal sphincter complex:
   a. Puborectalis muscle:

Aantomy and Physiology

- **(1)** Most medial portion of levator ani complex, cephalad to deep component of external anal sphincter muscle.
- **(2)** Endorectal ultrasound: anteriorly open, hyperechogenic U-shape 5–10 mm in thickness.
- **(3)** Innervation: inferior rectal nerve (branch of pudendal nerve).
- **(4)** Function: U-shaped, striated muscle part of sphincter mechanism and levator floor that pulls/angulates distal rectum towards pubic bone.

b. EAS: external anal sphincter muscle (→ forms functional unit with IAS):

- **(1)** Slow-twitch striated skeletal muscle cylinder surrounding anal canal and IAS; superficial EAS portion fixed to the coccyx via dense connective tissue and anococcygeal ligament, deep EAS portion without posterior attachments, inserts anteriorly into perineal body.
- **(2)** Endorectal ultrasound: circumferential hyperechogenic ring 5–10 mm in thickness.
- **(3)** Innervation: inferior rectal branch of pudendal nerve.
- **(4)** Function: state of continuous contraction → contributes 20–30% of resting anal sphincter tone, reflexive or voluntary contraction of EAS/puborectalis active fecal control; voluntary contraction limited to 30–60 seconds.

c. IAS: internal anal sphincter (→ forms functional unit with EAS):

- **(1)** Specialized smooth muscle condensation in continuation of circular muscularis propria of the rectum, does not extend as distally as EAS (→ forms intersphincteric groove).
- **(2)** Endorectal ultrasound: circumferential hypoechogenic ring 2–3 mm in thickness.
- **(3)** Innervation: autonomic sympathetic and parasympathetic nerves.
- **(4)** Function: state of continuous contraction → contributes 55% of resting anal tone.

d. Conjoined longitudinal muscle and corrugator cutis ani:

- **(1)** Longitudinal rectal muscles fuse with striated levator ani and puborectalis fibers at anorectal ring to form conjoined longitudinal muscle.
- **(2)** Fibers descend between internal and external anal sphincters → continuation through lower portion of EAS → form corrugator cutis ani, which inserts in perianal skin.

Clinical Focus

- Puborectalis muscle as distal reference for sphincter-preserving low anterior resection for rectal cancer.
- Function: puborectalis "sling" relaxation during defecation → widening of anorectal angle; contraction of levator ani complex → elevation of the pelvic floor and widening of levator hiatus.
- Intersphincteric dissection for ultralow anterior dissection.

Pathology

- Obturator internus muscle: open communication to extrapelvic tissue allows for tracking of pelvic infections: eg, cryptoglandular complex in posterior midline → deep postanal space → along obturator internus fascia to ischioanal fossae.
- External sphincter defect → fecal incontinence.
- Pelvic floor descent.
- Paradoxic/nonrelaxing puborectalis contraction.

Cross-reference

Topic	Chapter
Endorectal ultrasound	2 (p 89)
Fecal control	3 (p 153)
Fecal incontinence	4 (p 189)
Rectal cancer	4 (p 265)
Pelvic floor dysfunction	4 (p 420)
Constipation	4 (p 427)

Aantomy and Physiology

PELVIC FASCIAL STRUCTURES AND SPACES

Overview

Defined planes of muscles and tense fibrous tissue delineate several real or virtual compartments and space entities in the pelvis. These spaces are filled with adipose or a fine areolar connective tissue; some contain blood vessels, nerves, and lymphatics.

The spaces define routes for the propagation of disease processes (eg, abscesses); the fascial planes represent important barriers of the compartment in which rectal neoplasms primarily extend. From a surgical standpoint, these are anatomic landmarks that define the course of an anatomic dissection for an oncologic total mesorectal excision.

Landmarks

- Waldeyer fascia.
- Denonvillier' fascia.
- Postanal space of Courtney.
- Supra- vs infralevator spaces.

Anatomic Details

1. Posterior: endopelvic fascia with two components:
   a. Visceral layer (fascia propria of the rectum): thin transparent layer maintaining integrity of the mesorectum.
   b. Parietal layer (presacral fascia): covering sacrum and presacral veins.
   c. Fine areolar tissue in between anterior surface of parietal layer and posterior surface of visceral layer; fusion of the two layers a few centimeters above the coccyx forms the Waldeyer fascia.
2. Lateral: fascial interruption by hypogastric and pelvic nerves and plexuses, hypogastric blood vessels medial to the pelvic sidewalls.
3. Anterior to rectum: Denonvillier' fascia interposed between bladder and rectum: virtual space rather than distinct fascial structure → separation of anterior rectum below peritoneal reflection from bladder, prostate, and seminal vesicles or vagina; contains neurovascular bundles originating from pelvic plexus and hypogastric circulation.
4. Levator ani: muscular division of pelvis into:
   a. Supralevator space: between peritoneum and pelvic diaphragm.
   b. Infralevator (extrapelvic) spaces: ischioanal fossae, perianal, intersphincteric, submucosal, superficial and deep postanal spaces. Caveat: not "ischiorectal" because rectum is not part of its boundaries.

   c. The two compartments are almost completely separated from each other, except: communication of supralevator space with ischioanal space via fascia of the obturator internus (medial to ischial spine) → conduit for supralevator infections to extrapelvic sites.

5. Ischioanal fossae: superiorly defined by levator ani muscle fascia, medially by external anal sphincter complex at level of anal canal, laterally by obturator fascia, inferiorly by thin transverse fascia separating it from perianal space; contains neurovascular structures including pudendal nerve and internal pudendal vessels, which enter through pudendal (Alcock) canal.

6. Deep postanal spaces of Courtney: located behind anal canal with bilateral communication to ischioanal fossa → route for formation of a horseshoe abscess. Superficial postanal space: located between the anococcygeal ligament and skin; deep postanal space: located between anococcygeal ligament and anococcygeal raphe.

7. Intersphincteric space: located between internal and external sphincter muscles: location of anal glands; distal communication with perianal space.

8. Perianal space: surrounds lower part of anal canal and extends laterally to subcutaneous buttock fat; contains communicating hemorrhoidal plexus: external ↔ mixed ↔ internal hemorrhoid plexus; also contains the most distal part of EAS, IAS, and fibers of corrugator ani muscle → septa-like division of perianal space into compact and inelastic subcompartments.

9. Submucosal space: between IAS and rectal mucosal at the dentate and continuing into submucosal layer of distal rectum: contains internal hemorrhoidal plexus and the muscularis mucosa.

Clinical Focus

- Total mesorectal excision for rectal cancer: complete rectal mobilization to the pelvic floor requires division of Waldeyer fascia behind the rectum at S3 level; anterior dissection with/without inclusion of Denonvillier' fascia.

- Damage to compartmental integrity (eg, tumor, poor surgical technique) → cancer contamination of operative field with increased risk for local recurrence.

- Violation of presacral fascia → injury to presacral veins with massive bleeding during rectal dissection.

- Pelvic CT/MRI: identification of triangular pyramid-shape of ischioanal fossa.

• Inelastic perianal spaces → little room for expansion such that hematoma/abscess result in rapid pressure increase with dramatic pain.

Pathology

• Perirectal abscesses: location defined by spaces.
• Rectal cancer: lymph node compartment.
• Postsurgical autonomic nerve dysfunction: prevention by following fascial planes.

Cross-reference

Topic	*Chapter*
Perianal/-rectal abscess	4 (p 174)
Modified Hanley procedure	5 (p 479)
Proctocolectomy	5 (p 560)
LAR/TME	5 (p 610)

PELVIC AND ANORECTAL INNERVATION

Overview

Somatic and autonomic innervation to viscera and pelvic/anorectal region.

Landmarks

- Inferior mesenteric nerve → 2 hypogastric nerves.
- Pudendal nerves: S2–S4 → Alcock canal.
- Sympathetic: thoracolumbar ganglia.
- Parasympathetic: S2–S4.

Anatomic Details

- Colon and rectum: autonomic nerves (sympathetic, parasympathetic).
- IAS: autonomic nerves (sympathetic, parasympathetic).
- EAS: somatic nerves.
- Anal canal: somatic nerves.

Anatomic nerve structures

- Pelvirectal autonomic nerves (hypogastric plexus, pelvic neural plexus):
  - Sympathetic: postganglionic fibers from thoracolumbar ganglia (retroperitoneal course anterior to abdominal aorta) → inferior mesenteric nerve (at level of distal aorta) → bifurcation into two hypogastric nerves at level of aortic bifurcation → travel behind the rectum toward lateral pelvic sidewalls → pelvic nerve plexuses.
  - Parasympathetic: preganglionic visceral fibers exit bilaterally from sacral foramina S2, S3, S4 → pelvic nerve plexus (nervi erigentes) near root of middle rectal artery on medial side of hypogastric blood vessels.
  - Conjoining of parasympathetic pelvic nerves and sympathetic hypogastric nerves → pelvic plexuses → continue anterolaterally to prostate, seminal vesicles, vagina, urethra.
- Pudendal nerves: bilaterally originate from sacral roots S2–S4 → passing through pudendal canal (Alcock canal) formed by fascia on medial surface of obturator internus muscle → infralevator space (ischioanal fossa) → branching into:
  - Inferior rectal nerve (S2, S3).
  - Perineal nerve (S4) → dorsal nerve (penis, clitoris).

Motor innervation

- Pelvic floor muscles:
  - Pelvic surface: S2–S4 fibers.
  - Inferior surface: perineal branch of pudendal nerves.

- Puborectalis muscle: inferior rectal branch of pudendal nerves.
- EAS: inferior rectal branch and perineal branch of pudendal nerves.
- IAS: sympathetic (L5) , parasympathetic (S2–S4).

Sensory innervation
- Anal canal: demarcation line 0.3–1.5 cm above dentate line:
  - Rectum proximal only sensitive to distention (afferent fibers along parasympathetic nerves and pelvic plexus to S2–S4).
  - Anal canal: inferior rectal branch of the pudendal nerve → sensation relevant for continence mechanism: touch, pinprick, heat, and cold.

Clinical Focus
- Identification of inferior mesenteric and hypogastric nerves in presacral space upon opening the peritoneal reflection or just dorsal to origin of IMA → care must be taken to avoid injury to neural structures when dividing superior rectal or inferior mesenteric arteries.
- Nerve function: ejaculation = sympathetic; erection and bladder emptying = parasympathetic.
- Evaluation of PNTML for workup of fecal incontinence.
- Hemorrhoid banding and stapled hemorrhoidectomy: less pain because done above dentate line.

Pathology
- Autonomic nerve injury: postradiation, surgical dissection (electrocautery) of anterior/anterolateral plane along Denonvillier' fascia → urinary retention, retrograde ejaculation, erectile dysfunction.
- Pudendal nerve damage: stretching injury during pregnancy, direct injury during perianal dissection, but cannot occur during LAR (as pudendal nerve located below levators).

Cross-reference

Topic	*Chapter*
Anophysiology studies	2 (p 78)
Fecal control	3 (p 153)
Fecal incontinence	4 (p 189)
Recurrent rectal cancer	4 (p 271)
LAR/TME	5 (p 610)

FECAL CONTROL (CONTINENCE)

Overview

An adequate control mechanism for stool and urine provides a fundamental quality of life allowing for a conscious selection of the appropriate timing, location, and privacy for voiding and moving the bowels. Continence is the result of a balanced interaction between the anal sphincter complex ("plug"), stool consistency, the rectal reservoir function, and neurological function. Disease processes or structural defects that alter any of these aspects can lead to fecal incontinence. While fecal control is often thought to be synonymous with normal sphincter muscles, other factors are equally important.

Elements

1. Plug function: structures and function in place to create sufficient outlet resistance against the intrarectal pressure of the feces at rest, against increased intra-abdominal pressure, during a peristaltic wave, or during physical stress/activity:

   a. Puborectalis sling and external anal sphincter: striated muscles, slow-twitch, fatigue-resistant muscle fibers, innervated by inferior branch of the pudendal nerve (S3–S4) → voluntary sphincter contraction with doubling of resting pressure (20–30% of anal resting tone).

   b. IAS: smooth muscle, autonomic innervation → 55% of resting tone of the anal canal.

   c. Hemorrhoidal cushions: expansion → 15–25% of overall control.

   d. Configuration of anal canal: length of high-pressure zone, concentric appearance without focal defects (eg, keyhole deformity).

2. Stool quality:

   a. Formed stool easier to control than liquid.

   b. Extent of gas production.

3. Rectal capacity: ability to provide a low-pressure storage area for feces to accumulate until an evacuation is desired:

   a. Overall size of reservoir.

   b. Distensibility, as measured by rectal compliance.

4. Neurologic sensory or motor function:

   a. Central nervous system: conscious (awareness) and subconscious networking of information from and to the anorectum.

Aantomy and Physiology

b. Intact peripheral nerve function: transmission of nerve input to muscle complex, transmission of sensory receptor information (rectal pressure, sphincter pressure.

c. Functional dysfunction: visceral hypersensitivity (IBS).

Physiologic Sequence

Interaction of the various mechanical factors contributing to fecal control expressed in a mathematical formula:

$$\frac{C \cdot \mu \cdot L \cdot P_{max}}{r} > V_{rectum}$$

where C = compliance, μ = stool viscosity, L = length of anal canal, P_{max} = maximal pressure, r = radius of anal canal, and V_{rectum} = volume in rectum. Continence is achieved if the formula returns a true solution when the patient's data are entered. Hence, continence is directly correlated with compliance, viscosity (or firmness), length of anal canal, and maximal pressure but inversely correlated with anorectal diameter.

Control and Coordination

Fecal and urinary control is acquired in the first 2–4 years of life: the term *incontinence* is therefore only applicable to the time after unless morphologic defects are obviously preventing development of control (eg, meningomyelocele, etc).

Control occurs subconsciously even at sleep, reinforced through conscious contraction on demand.

Examples and Symptoms of Dysfunction

• Plug: sphincter defect, sphincter dysfunction, anal disconfiguration:
  - Absent puborectalis function   →   complete incontinence
  - Deficient EAS   →   impaired voluntary control
  - Deficient IAS   →   impaired fine tuning
  - Keyhole deformity   →   seepage
• Reservoir: decreased volume after LAR, pelvic radiation, tumors, stricture, ongoing inflammation.
• Stool quality: diarrhea, IBS, IBD, radiation proctitis.

Associated Pathology
• Pelvic floor dysfunction.
• Pelvic organ prolapse syndrome.
• Obstetric/surgical trauma.

Associated Problems
Functional incontinence → absence of any measurable or visible deficiency.

Cross-reference

Topic	*Chapter*
Anophysiology studies	2 (p 78)
Fecal incontinence	4 (p 189)

Aantomy and Physiology

CARCINOGENESIS

Overview

Tumor: abnormal growth or mass of cells no longer linked to physiologic function or demand.

Cancer: characteristic growth patterns:

- Invasiveness: disrespect of tissue boundaries → invasion of other structures.
- Size-dependent potential to metastasize: access to blood/lymph vessels or other structures → tumor spread to distant locations.

Cancer is a genetic disease: series of mutations that result in a growth advantage: (a) germline mutation → transmission to the next generation (inherited defect); (b) somatic mutation (more common) → spontaneous mutation during tissue/organ growth, development, and maintenance.

Elements

Gatekeeper genes (oncogenes/tumor-suppressor genes)

- *APC* gene (adenoma-polyposis coli, 5q): tumor-suppressor gene → control of cell-to-cell adhesions and intercellular communication; found in 60% of even small adenomatous polyps and carcinomas → early event in carcinogenesis.
- *MCC* gene (mutated in colon cancer): tumor supressor gene
- *K-ras* (12p): normal function in intracellular signal transduction and stimulated cell division; found in larger adenomas and carcinomas → stimulates cell growth.
- *DCC* (deleted in colon cancer, 18q): tumor-suppressor gene → progression from benign polyp toward malignant growth.
- *p53* (17p): tumor-suppressor gene → among most frequent gene mutations in human cancers → late event in the development of the invasive phenotype.

Caretaker genes

- Mismatch repair genes: *hMLH1, hMSH2, hMSH6, PMS1, PMS2* → encode proteins for repair of nucleotide mismatches.
- Microsatellites: stretches in the DNA with several-fold repetition of a short sequence of 1–5 nucleotides → microsatellite instability: loss or gain of repeat units in germline microsatellite allele: found in 15% of sporadic colorectal cancer, in > 90–95% of HNPCC.

Physiologic Sequence

- Normal cell division: multiplication of cells as defined by tissue demand: once demand is satisfied → increased production is redirected to maintenance production to uphold steady state.
- Normal cell cycle: high number of spontaneous gene mutations without biologic or growth advantage → repair mechanism or inherent suicide program (apoptosis, if cell damage too severe).

Pathophysiology

- Adenoma-Carcinoma Model (Vogelstein, 1988): colorectal tumorigenesis as multistep process related to accumulation of genetic events → uninhibited cell growth → proliferation and clonal expansion.
- Carcinogenesis: → several independent accidents → failure to recognize and correct DNA damage → continued replication → accumulation of faulty gene products within cell → survival advantage → proliferative response:

$$GR_{tumor} - DR_{tumor} > GR_{normal} - DR_{normal}$$
$$[GR = growth\ rate,\ DR = death\ rate]$$

- DNA mismatch repair (MMR) systems:
  - Cell division: DNA duplication with original DNA serving as template for replicated copy, DNA polymerase serves as proofreader → recognition of mismatch genes → halt to DNA synthesis and removal of defective sequence.
  - Failure of DNA mismatch repair system → development of mutations.
  - Increased proliferation → increased genetic instability → malignant cells without feedback-controlled growth regulation.
- Two types of genetic instability:
  - Chromosome level: loss of chromosomal material, ie, chromosomal instability (CIN), asymmetric chromosome distribution (mitosis) → gel electrophoresis with loss of one or more bands = loss of heterozygosity (LOH).
  - DNA level: replication errors in repetitive short polymorphisms → additional band or bands = microsatellite instability (MSI).

Examples and Symptoms of Dysfunction

- FAP: APC gene mutation 5q21
- Attenuated FAP (AFAP): APC gene mutation in proximal 5′-end, exon 9, or distal 3′-end → fewer polyps, later age for cancer, more proximal polyp distribution.
- HNPCC: defective mismatch repair genes.

Associated Pathology

Extracolonic pathology (eg, desmoid tumors): more frequent with distal APC gene mutations.

Associated Problems

• Accelerated carcinogenesis in HNPCC: adenoma-carcinoma sequence shortened to 2–3 years (vs 8–10 years in sporadic colorectal cancer) → earlier screening, shorter interval.

• Genetic testing.

Cross-reference

Topic	*Chapter*
Polyps	4 (p 236)
Polyposis syndromes	4 (p 240)
FAP	4 (p 244)
HNPCC	4 (p 248)
Colorectal cancer	4 (p 252)
Amsterdam criteria	App II (p 738)
Bethesda criteria	App II (p 739)

Chapter 4

Diseases and Problems

ANAL FISSURE *(565.0)*

Overview

Anal fissures are frequent, simple to diagnose, and often overlooked. A fissure is a longitudinal tear/wound/ulceration between the dentate line and the anal verge, typically located in the midline, associated with high anal sphincter tone. Risk factors: constipation, chronic diarrhea (idiopathic, IBD, post–gastric bypass), but fissure may also occur with normal bowel movements.

- Acute fissure is defined as new onset, no signs of chronicity, typically related to identifiable acute episode of constipation or diarrhea.
- Chronic fissure is defined as either > 3 months of symptoms or morphologic signs of chronicity (elevated/indurated wound edges, exposed sphincter muscle, sentinel skin tag, hypertrophic anal papilla).

Complications are rare: development of a perirectal fistula/abscess, chronic pain (even if fissure healed), ie, anismus.

Pathophysiology: acute or chronic stress/trauma to the anal canal (constipation, diarrhea) results in superficial tear; acute fissure will heal in 40–60% with appropriate improved stool management, or may turn into chronic anal fissure and result in a vicious circle: increasing sphincter tone, hypertonicity of internal anal sphincter muscle (resting tone) → fissure hiding between anal canal folding such that it cannot clean out → pain → increased sphincter spasm → etc.

Treatment of fissure aims at normalizing stool regularity and decreasing sphincter tone.

Epidemiology

Exact prevalence and incidence are unknown (referral bias); in a specialist clinic, 3–5% of patients have a fissure as presenting symptom. More common in young and middle-aged adult patients; most frequent cause of rectal bleeding in children.

Symptoms

Patients often present with "painful hemorrhoids" as they feel the sentinel skin tag and notice the pain during and after bowel movements.

Pain: typically post defecation, varying degrees, ranging from mild itching to discomfort to massive excruciating pain periods. But an estimated 10% of patients do not complain of pain, or they just have pruritus or mild discomfort.

Duration of pain: typically during and post bowel movements, occasionally several hours thereafter, or permanent/constant pain.

Bleeding: acute fissure—sometimes significant bright red bleeding; chronic fissure—more often just traces of blood on toilet paper. Severe hemorrhage or anemia unlikely related to fissure.

Lump: "irritated" external hemorrhoids (sentinel skin tag), but absence of dynamic protrusion during bowel movement.

Differential Diagnosis

Pain: thrombosed external hemorrhoid, abscess, levator ani spasm, anismus.

HIV-associated ulcer: HIV infection+; ulceration: often in the same location and/or eccentric; sphincter tone typically not increased, or even decreased.

Crohn disease: anal symptoms may be the only manifestation or be associated with other signs/locations of active Crohn disease.

STDs: syphilis, herpes.

Perirectal fistula/abscess: particularly horseshoe fistula characteristically originates from posterior midline.

Tuberculosis: clinical suspicion, atypical presentation, associated pulmonary symptoms, positive PPD test.

Malignancy-associated lesion: cancer, melanoma, leukemia, lymphoma, plasmocytoma.

Pathology

Epithelial ulceration, unspecific acute and chronic infiltrates.

Evaluation

Required minimal standard

History: onset/pattern of symptoms, reversible prolapse or persistent "lump," bowel habits, preexisting incontinence?

Clinical examination:

- External inspection (skin tags, thrombosed external hemorrhoid, erythema/induration)? Lateral traction to the buttocks → exposure of posterior and anterior midline: often sufficient to diagnose the fissure (Figure 4–1). If fissure confirmed and significant pain reported, digital exam or instrumentation at the first presentation is not indicated!

- External palpation: tight sphincter tone, hypertonic internal sphincter muscle with well-palpable intersphincteric groove.

Full/partial colonic evaluation as per general screening guidelines (if history and findings consistent: may be deferred for 3–4 weeks until acute symptoms controlled).

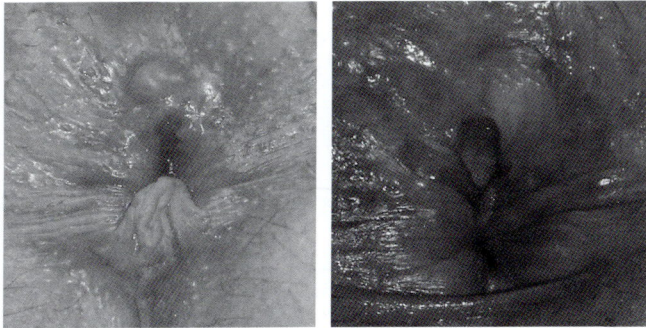

Figure 4–1. Chronic anal fissure with and without sentinel skin tag.

Additional tests (optional)

Anoscopy/proctoscopy: rule out tumor, hemorrhoids, proctitis, etc; if fissure is confirmed, these exams are only indicated if there are inconsistencies of complaints and findings!

Atypical (eccentric) fissures: cultures, biopsy.

Classification

Acute vs chronic anal fissure.

Nonoperative treatment

Improving stool regularity (increased supplemental fibers, increased fluid intake, stool softener, temporary mild laxative).

Sitz baths: to help patient relax, to wash off area.

Chemical sphincterotomy:

- Topical 0.2% nitroglycerin ointment (fingertip amount applied to anal verge twice daily): 40–60% chance of healing fissure within 4–8 weeks; side effects: headaches (particularly in the beginning, may respond to acetaminophen), tachycardia. Contraindicated with concomitant sildenafil (Viagra): risk of malignant arrhythmias. If no improvement/healing in 4–8 weeks, or significant side effects → Botox.

- Topical 2% diltiazem or 0.2% nifedipine ointment: applied twice or three times per day to anal verge; same cure rate as NTG, less headache, but local irritation may occur.

- Injection of Botox into internal anal sphincter muscle: local disinfection and injection of 10–20 units of botulinum toxin A (suspended in 1 mL 0.9% NaCl) directly into internal anal sphincter muscle on each side (total amount: 20–40 units): estimated 80–85% chance of curing the fissure within 6–12 weeks; may repeat one time.

Operative Treatment

Indication
• Severe acute symptoms: surgery by far providing the fastest relief.
• Failure of nonoperative management (including pharmacologic sphincterotomy).

Operative approach
• Lateral internal sphincterotomy (gold standard): 95% cure, 5(–15)% incontinence to stool or gas (often recovering within 1 year).
• Lateral internal sphincterotomy with excision of fissure and sentinel skin tag: indicated if fissure is very deep and/or hiding underneath a large redundant sentinel skin tag.
• Fissurectomy alone in combination with injection of Botox, potentially with external skin flap: in patients in whom weakening of the sphincter should be avoided (preexisting incontinence, chronic diarrhea, status post gastric bypass, IBD with potential need for future IPAA).
• Obsolete procedure: manual anal dilation; uncontrolled dilation results not only in stretching of the internal sphincter muscle but also of the external sphincter muscle → high risk of fecal incontinence. Possible renaissance of concept with use of controlled dilatation?

Comment: fissurectomy and sphincterotomy in the area of the ulcer/fissure → risk of keyhole deformity, generally better to perform sphincterotomy through separate lateral incision.

Outcome

Combined efforts should result in 95–100% of healing. Benchmark: < 10% problems with fecal control, rapid ability to return to workforce.

Follow-up

Recheck patient after 4–6 weeks of initiated treatment. Order appropriate tests (eg, cultures/biopsies) if no response or atypical presentation. Once resolved, no specific follow-up needed.

Cross-reference

ANAL SKIN TAGS *(455.9)*

Overview

Skin tags represent focal redundancy of the perianal skin. They may be solitary or form excessive changes of the anal landscape with deep troughs, hence causing a potential problem for local hygiene. Uncomplicated skin tags may develop spontaneously or result from known episodes of thrombosed external hemorrhoids. Sentinel skin tags result from a persistent chronic problem (eg, chronic anal fissure). Most commonly, anal skin tags have no disease character and, if a problem, are more a cosmetic/emotional one.

Epidemiology

Prevalence: very frequent, statistics unavailable/unreliable.

Symptoms

Most commonly asymptomatic. Occasionally negative interference with local hygiene.

Occasionally itching/irritation or "painful hemorrhoid" → high index of suspicion that chronic fissure is hiding underneath.

Differential Diagnosis

Sentinel skin tags (with underlying chronic anal fissure).

External hemorrhoid (visible vascular component with continuum to internal hemorrhoids).

Condylomata.

Tumor (malignant, benign).

Pathology

Squamous cell epithelium covering paucicellular stroma (eg, minimal inflammatory elements).

Evaluation

Required minimal standard

History: patient to define the actual problem: constant vs dynamic presence, need for reduction, associated symptoms (bleeding, pain, itching etc), daily bowel habits, constipation? Previous colonic screening?

Clinical examination: anal configuration (location and number of skin tags)? Underlying pathology (fissure, fistula, hemorrhoids, rectal prolapse)? Sphincter tone?

Anoscopy/proctoscopy: tumor, hemorrhoids, proctitis, etc.

Full/partial colonic evaluation: not because of the tag as such but as indicated per general screening guidelines.

Classification

- Uncomplicated skin tag.
- Symptomatic skin tag: sentinel skin tag, irritated skin tag.

Nonoperative treatment

No treatment needed for uncomplicated skin tag.

Treatment of underlying fissure in sentinel skin tag.

Operative Treatment

Indication

- Patient desire to have skin tag removed (no medical necessity).
- Patient desire to improve local hygiene (medically justifiable for extensive tags).
- Sentinel skin tag in treatment-refractory anal fissure.

Operative approach

- Simple excision (office vs OR setting).
- Fissure: sphincterotomy alone vs sphincterotomy with fissurectomy and excision of skin tag.

Outcome

In patients bothered aesthetically by the presence of a skin tag: low success rate of talking them out of a medically unnecessary surgical excision.

Follow-up

None for uncomplicated skin tag.

Cross-reference

Topic	*Chapter*
Lump or mass	1 (p 30)
Anal fissure	4 (p 161)
Hemorrhoids	4 (p 167)
Pruritus ani	4 (p 195)
Anal condylomata	4 (p 215)

HEMORRHOIDS *(455.X)*

Overview

"Hemorrhoids" remain the most common colorectal complaint; however, a majority of patients associate any type of anorectal symptoms with "hemorrhoids" even though they do not necessarily have a hemorrhoid problem. "Hemorrhoidal cushions" are a component of normal anal anatomy and contribute to physiologic continence mechanism. Anatomic primary locations: right anterior, right posterior, left lateral.

Hemorrhoidal disease: pathologic engorgement of submucosal vascular plexus, often asymptomatic, increasingly resulting in bleeding (superficial erosions), progressive prolapse, less commonly, pain. Contributing factors: constipation with straining, diarrhea, pregnancy, familial clustering, age.

Important distinction between internal/mixed hemorrhoids and external hemorrhoids (Figure 4–2A).

Appropriate hemorrhoid treatment depends on (1) a correct clinical diagnosis that rules out alternative differential diagnoses, (2) the patient's type and severity of symptoms, and (3) the grade, extent, and location of the hemorrhoid at the time of presentation.

Special circumstances: pregnancy, HIV infection, IBD, liver disease.

(Note: liver cirrhosis is not associated with increased incidence of hemorrhoids but may result in rectal varices!)

Epidemiology

Prevalence: 3–6%; peak age: between 45 and 65 years, unusual before adolescence; approximately one-third of patients will seek medical treatment.

Symptoms

Internal hemorrhoids: bleeding and dynamic prolapse associated with bowel movement. Other symptoms generally unspecific: pain/discomfort (only when partially thrombosed or incarcerated (grade IV, Figure 4–2B), itching (from moisture).

External hemorrhoids: most commonly no symptoms; pain (only if thrombosed); difficulty with hygiene (if very redundant); psychological aversion; bleeding only if spontaneous rupture of acute thrombosis.

Differential Diagnosis

Rectal prolapse (concentric pattern).

Skin tags.

Anal fissure with sentinel skin tag ("painful hemorrhoid").

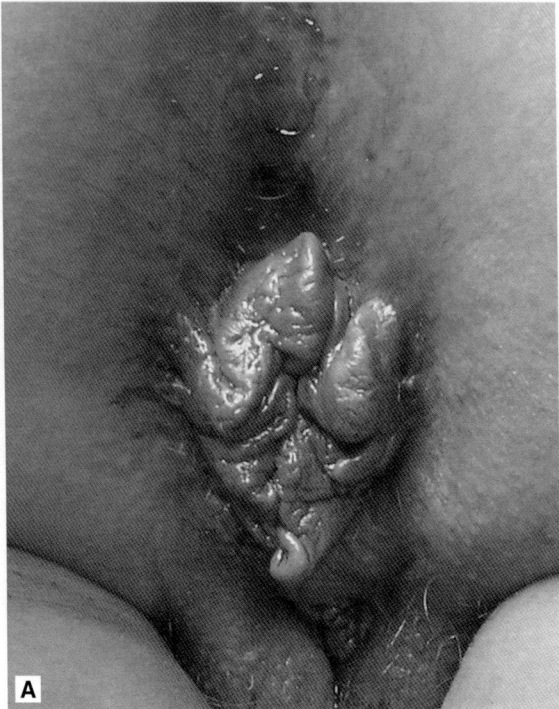

Figure 4–2A. External hemorrhoid component.

Condylomata.

Tumor (malignant, benign).

Hypertrophic anal papilla.

Abscess/fistula.

Proctitis (IBD, infectious, radiation etc).

Rectal varices.

Dieulafoy ulcer of the rectum.

Pathology

Enlarged hemorrhoidal plexus, focal areas of thrombosis. Internal hemorrhoids: proximal to dentate line, covered with columnar/transitional

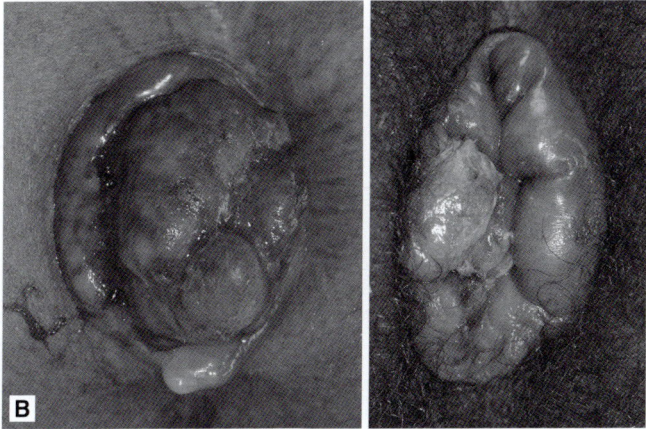

Figure 4–2B. Incarcerated-prolapsed internal hemorrhoids (grade IV).

epithelium. External hemorrhoids: distal to dentate line, covered with squamous-cell anoderm.

Evaluation

Required minimal standard

History: description (presence/absence and extent of prolapse, need for reduction), pattern of occurrence, associated symptoms (bleeding, pain, etc), daily bowel habits, constipation, preexisting incontinence?

Clinical examination: anal configuration (tags, etc)? Visible fissure or local skin pathology? Extent of prolapse (differentiation from rectal prolapse). Axial location with regard to dentate line (internal, external, mixed). Radial location and number of affected hemorrhoidal piles (1–3), presence/absence of complications (thrombosis, necrosis, ulceration, active bleeding). Sphincter tone?

Anoscopy/proctoscopy: tumor, hemorrhoids, proctitis, etc.

Except in emergency: full/partial colonic evaluation as per general screening guidelines and prior to any planned intervention.

Additional tests (optional)

If other diagnoses more likely.

Classification

- Internal hemorrhoid grading: descriptive clinical parameters for hemorrhoids (Table 4–1) should include patient-reported extent of prolapse (grade I–IV), objective axial location with regard to the dentate line (internal, external, mixed), objective radial location and extent in 1–3 of the hemorrhoidal piles, presence or absence of complications such as thrombosis, necrosis/gangrene, ulceration, or active bleeding.
- External hemorrhoid grading available only for thrombosis: ie, acute (< 72 hours post onset), subacute (> 72 hours, still inflammatory changes).

Nonoperative Treatment

Indicated for:

- All grades of internal hemorrhoids, potentially sufficient for grades I/II, occasionally even grade III (and IV).
- Thrombosed external hemorrhoid > 72 hours post onset (individualized exceptions from this rule).
- Coagulopathy.
- HIV infection with manifest AIDS.
- Underlying IBD.
- Pregnancy (relative contraindication for surgical intervention).

→ Dietary/lifestyle modification: fiber-rich diet, sufficient fluid intake, stool softener, decreased time spent on the toilet, Sitz baths for acute symptoms.

→ Topical treatments: short-term (!) use of glycerin suppositories with/ without topical steroids or local anesthetics, numerous over-the-counter preparations with unproven effect.

Operative Treatment

Indication

- General: lack of contraindications; in presence of risk factors (coagulopathy, portal hypertension, pregnancy, etc) → perioperative optimization, possible need for inpatient monitoring.
- Internal hemorrhoids: symptomatic, failure of conservative management, complications (bleeding, anemia, incarceration).
- External hemorrhoid: Acute thrombosis (< 72 hours post onset).

Operative approach

- Office interventions: hemorrhoid banding, sclerosing, infrared coagulation of internal hemorrhoids; excision/enucleation of thrombosed external hemorrhoid.

TABLE 4–1. Grading and Treatment of Hemorrhoids.

Grade of Hemorrhoids	Description (Covered with Mucosa)	Symptoms	Treatment Options
Internal grade I	Bulging into anal canal	Painless bleeding	Diet Local and general drugs Rubber band ligation Infrared coagulation Sclerotherapy
Internal grade II	Protrusion out of anal canal with bowel movements; reduces spontaneously	Painless bleeding, swelling	Rubber band ligation Infrared coagulation Sclerotherapy (PPH/stapled hemorrhoidectomy)
Internal grade III	Protrusion; requires manual reduction	Above + possible strangulation	Rubber band ligation PPH/stapled hemorrhoidectomy Excisional hemorrhoidectomy
Internal grade IV	Constant protrusion; irreducible, or instantaneous reprolapse	Above + high risk of strangulation with pain, necrosis, sepsis	Excisional hemorrhoidectomy (PPH/stapled hemorrhoidectomy)

(Continued)

TABLE 4–1. Grading and Treatment of Hemorrhoids. (*Continued*)

Grade of Hemorrhoids	Description (Covered with Mucosa)	Symptoms	Treatment Options
Mixed hemorrhoids	Internal and external components	According to the predominant component	Treatment according to predominant component: • Excisional hemorrhoidectomy • PPH/stapled hemorrhoidectomy
External hemorrhoids	Skin-covered "protrusions"	Discomfort, itching Severe pain if thrombosed	Symptomatic conservative treatment Incision and enucleation of thrombus Excisional hemorrhoidectomy

PPH, procedure for prolapse and hemorrhoids.

• Surgical procedures: excisional hemorrhoidectomy (Ferguson, Milligan-Morgan, Whitehead), stapled hemorrhoidectomy (PPH), doppler-guided hemorrhoid artery ligation.

Obsolete hemorrhoid procedures: cryoablation → foul-smelling discharge, uncontrolled tissue injury, incontinence.

Outcome

Conservative treatment and office management: 70% chance of success (depending on grade of symptoms). Interventional/operative treatment: 90–95% chance of success. Recurrence rates with PPH unknown.

Complications of surgical management: delayed wound healing, pain, post-operative bleeding, urinary retention, fecal impaction, infection/perineal sepsis, incontinence to stool/gas, stricture formation. Whitehead hemorrhoidectomy: important conventional tool for circumferential hemorrhoids, but risk of ectropion if done improperly.

Follow-up

Recheck patient after 2–4 weeks of initiated or performed treatment. Once hemorrhoidal problem has resolved, no specific follow-up is needed.

Cross-reference

Topic	*Chapter*
Colitis or proctitis	1 (p 7)
Lump or mass	1 (p 30)
Anal fissure	4 (p 161)
Rectal prolapse	4 (p 423)
Hemorrhoid office procedures	5 (p 506)
Excisional hemorrhoidectomy	5 (p 508)
Stapled hemorrhoidectomy/-opexy	5 (p 512)

PERIANAL/-RECTAL ABSCESS *(566)*

Overview

Perirectal abscess is a frequent, commonly not life-threatening but very annoying problem that is associated with pain, risk of recurrence, and fear. Among various causes of an abscess in this area, the most common ones are cryptoglandular in origin.

Pathogenesis of cryptoglandular abscess: 8–12 anal glands entering anal canal in anal crypts at the dentate line → plugging of duct? → retention/entry of bacteria → amplification and expansion along anatomic perirectal spaces → liquefaction (abscess formation). No specific risk factors identified.

Etiologies:

- Local origin: cryptoglandular, Crohn disease, Bartholin cyst, sebaceous glands, anastomotic leak (LAR, IPAA), status post anorectal surgery, locally advanced cancer, tuberculosis, chronic form of LGV, trauma (impalement, foreign body, etc).

- Supralevator origin (very rare): diverticulitis, Crohn disease, malignancy.

Severity of perirectal abscess: varying size of localized abscess, horseshoe abscess (involving postanal space and both ischioanal fossae; caveat: not to be mistaken for supralevator abscess), varying degrees of perifocal phlegmon, Fournier gangrene.

Epidemiology

Population-based epidemiologic data are not available.

Symptoms

Worsening perianal/perirectal or deep rectal pain: constant, not related to bowel activity; increasing local pressure, increasing perianal swelling (may be hidden in ischioanal abscess); positional aggravation (sitting, walking).

Associated symptoms: possible fever, urinary retention; rarely sepsis (maximum: Fournier gangrene, Figure 4–3A).

Symptoms may be masked in immunocompromised patients (neutropenia, leukemia) → pain only, but no abscess formation.

Differential Diagnosis

Pain: anal fissure, thrombosed external hemorrhoid, incarcerated prolapsed internal hemorrhoids, levator ani spasm, anismus, STDs (syphilis, herpes, etc).

Fever: other sources of infection—pelvic, extrapelvic.

Fistula system: hidradenitis suppurativa, Crohn disease, anorectal tuberculosis, actinomycosis, chronic LGV.

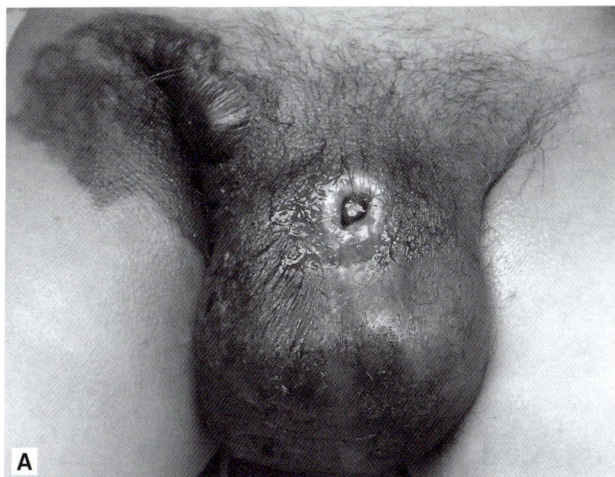

Figure 4–3A. Fournier gangrene.

Pathology

Location within the perirectal spaces:

- Perianal/subcutaneous: 40–65%.
- Intersphincteric/submucosal: 15–25%.
- Ischioanal and deep postanal: 20–35%.
- High intramuscular: 5–10%.
- Supralevator: 5%.

Evaluation

Required minimal standard

History: gradual onset, absence of prolapse as primary symptom, bowel habits, preexisting incontinence, symptoms suggestive of Crohn disease (abdominal pain, diarrhea, bleeding), previous abdominal/pelvic/anorectal surgeries?

Clinical examination:

- External inspection: possible erythema/induration, possible fistula opening, absence of thrombosed external hemorrhoid or fissure.
- Digital rectal exam (only if diagnosis not already obvious): induration/tenderness of perirectal spaces, including ischioanal fossae and/or deep postanal space? Caveat: even large abscesses may never show fluctuance!

Additional tests (optional)
Further tests typically are not indicated in emergency situations (unless patient is under anesthesia):

- Anoscopy/proctoscopy: rule out tumor, proctitis, potential assessment for primary opening (eg, fissure), potential intraluminal bulging of abscess (high intersphincteric/submucosal location).
- Not indicated (unless for special reasons): blood work, imaging studies eg, CT (Figure 4–3B) or ERUS, cultures (unless atypical circumstances/presentation).

Classification

- Cryptoglandular abscess.
- Secondary abscess (anastomotic leak, etc).
- Supralevator abscess.

Nonoperative Treatment

Not indicated.

Antibiotics only for special circumstances: immunosuppressed patient, severe phlegmonous component, valvular heart disease.

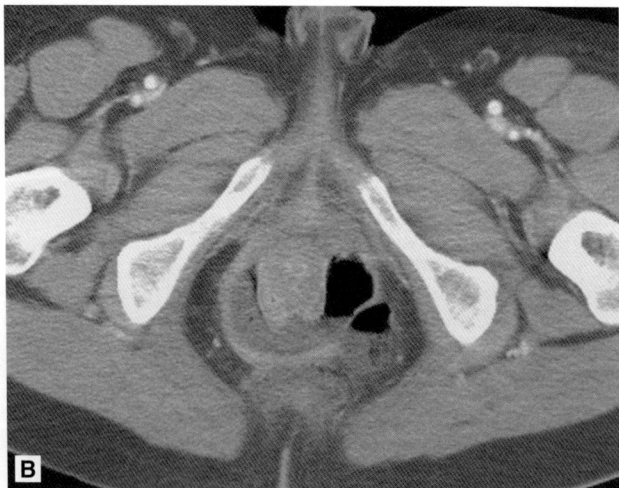

Figure 4–3B. Horseshoe abscess on CT scan.

Operative Treatment

Indication
Any perirectal abscess or suspected abscess (caveat: don't look or wait for "fluctuance").

Operative approach
- Office: incision and drainage of perirectal abscess in local anesthesia, no search for fistula.
- OR: Larger abscess, inability to tolerate local procedure:
  – Incision(s) and possible counter-incisions with placement of drain(s), possible mushroom catheter.
  – Simultaneous evaluation and treatment for fistula (caveat: creation of iatrogenic fistula tract in altered tissue).
- Fournier gangrene: aggressive debridement, possible second look operations, possible ostomy.

Outcome

Adequate drainage results in rapid improvement; ~50% probability of persistent fistula tract after first time I&D.

Follow-up

Recheck patient after 1–2 weeks (resolution of acute inflammation?) and after 4–6 weeks (persistence of fistula?).

Planning of elective fistula surgery.

Full/partial colonic evaluation as per general screening guidelines.

Cross-reference

Topic	*Chapter*
Fistula	1 (p 19)
Lump or mass	1 (p 30)
Pain, perirectal	1 (p 38)
Endorectal ultrasound	2 (p 89)
Perianal/-rectal fistula	4 (p 178)
Pilonidal disease	4 (p 182)
Hidradenitis suppurativa	4 (p 186)
I&D of perirectal abscess	5 (p 477)
Modified Hanley procedure	5 (p 479)

Diseases and Problems

PERIANAL/-RECTAL FISTULA (565.1)

Overview

Perirectal fistula is closely associated with perirectal abscesses. The fistula tract, which connects the primary opening(s) with one or more secondary opening(s), becomes fully manifest upon spontaneous or surgical opening of a perirectal abscess. A significant number of patients do not recall episode of an abscess. In an estimated 50% of drained abscesses (first episode), the inflammatory process may obliterate the fistula tract. Blind-ending sinuses may complicate the picture and become the source of recurrences.

Course of fistula may vary significantly, but some repetitive pattern (Goodsall rule):

- Fistula opening anterior to transverse line and < 3 cm from anal verge → straight radial course to dentate line.
- Fistula opening posterior to transverse line → curved course to the posterior midline.
- Fistula opening anterior to transverse line and > 3 cm from anal verge → curved course to posterior midline.

Epidemiology

Population-based epidemiologic data are limited; one Scandinavian study suggests prevalence of 6–12% per 100,000 people.

Symptoms

Cyclic symptoms: abscess with increasing pain → rupture/surgery with drainage of pus → cooling off with closure of skin ("healing") → beginning of smoldering infection → abscess ...

Persistent symptoms: continued drainage, moisture, itching.

Differential Diagnosis

Cryptoglandular origin: overwhelming majority of fistulae.

Noncryptoglandular origin: Crohn disease, anastomotic leak (LAR, IPAA), status post anorectal surgery/trauma, locally advanced neoplasm, tuberculosis, actinomycosis, chronic form of LGV, hidradenitis suppurativa.

Congenital fistulae.

Pathology

Location defined by anatomic perirectal spaces:

- Subcutaneous/-mucosal fistula.

- Intersphincteric fistula (45–60% of all fistulae): through distal internal sphincter → intersphincteric space → external opening.
- Transsphincteric fistula (25–30%): through both internal and external sphincters.
- Suprasphincteric fistula (< 3%): originates in intersphincteric plane and tracks up and around entire external sphincter complex.
- Extrasphincteric fistula (< 3%): rectal wall above dentate line → around both sphincters: most commonly seen in trauma, Crohn disease, or PID.
- Ischioanal (horseshoe) fistula (20–35%): primary defect most commonly in posterior midline → deep postanal space and extends to bilateral ischioanal fossae with possible multiple secondary openings.

Evaluation

Required minimal standard

History: characterization of symptoms, bowel habits, preexisting incontinence, symptoms suggestive of Crohn disease (abdominal pain, diarrhea, bleeding), previous abdominal/pelvic/anorectal surgeries?

Clinical examination:

- External inspection: identification of possible fistula opening, possibly limited probing, but it is not relevant to preoperatively identify exact course of fistula.
- Anoscopy/proctoscopy: rule out tumor, hemorrhoids, proctitis, etc.

Full/partial colonic evaluation as per general screening guidelines.

Additional tests (optional)

Imaging studies: only for recurrent or more complex appearing fistula—conventional fistulogram, MRI fistulogram, endorectal ultrasound with H_2O_2 injection.

Classification

- Park classification → combinations possible:
  - Intersphincteric fistula.
  - Transsphincteric fistula.
  - Suprasphincteric fistula.
  - Extrasphincteric fistula.
- Simple fistula vs complex fistula (eg, horseshoe fistula, branching fistula, multiple secondary openings etc; Figure 4–4).

Nonoperative Treatment

Asymptomatic fistula.

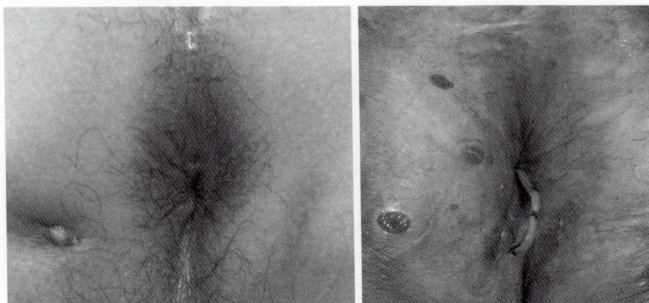

Figure 4–4. Fistula-in-ano: simple (left panel) and horseshoe with inadequate drain (right panel).

Operative Treatment

Indication
Any symptomatic fistula.

Operative approach
General: intraoperative evaluation: insertion of silver probe, injection of peroxide/dye, etc.

Selection of appropriate method based on location and extent of sphincter involvement:

• Fistulotomy, fistulectomy: if < 10–20% of sphincter involvement.
• Seton management: draining vs cutting seton—complex or recurrent fistulae.
• Endorectal advancement flap with/without fistulectomy.
• Plugging of fistula tract (fibrin glue, collagen plug): long, narrow tract, no active suppurations.
• Rerouting of fistula tract.
• External skin advancement flap.

Outcome

Recurrence of fistula: > 10–35% for all methods → no perfect solution.

Risk of incontinence: 0–15% (stool), 0–25% (flatus); even higher in some series!

Follow-up

Recheck patient every 2–4 weeks for outpatient management:

- Open wound: check in regular intervals until healed by secondary intention.
- Draining setons: unless they are intended for long-term use (eg Crohn disease), removal can be considered after 3–4 weeks if inflammation and drainage are decreased.
- Cutting seton: tightening every 3–4 weeks until migrated through the involved muscle.
- Collagen plug: check every 3–4 weeks until fistula opening is dried off.

Cross-reference

PILONIDAL DISEASE *(CYST/SINUS/FISTULA, 685.0/1)*

Overview

Pilonidal disease ("hair nest") is most common in young adults, essentially nonexistent in those > 45–50 years. Males:females = 3:1. Overweight common but not exclusive. Condition is not life-threatening but is annoying and causes significant work/school absences. Range of presentations: asymptomatic pits in the sacrococcygeal region that cause a local infection with acute abscess, recurring abscesses, draining sinus or fistula.

Pathogenesis: hair penetration/development beneath the skin results in foreign body–type infection. Two theories:

1. Congenital: embryologic skin fusion error with resultant entrapment of hair follicles in the sacrococcygeal region.
2. Acquired: external origin (maceration, microtrauma, ingrowth) introduces hair follicles into the subdermal area.

Epidemiology

Prevalence of asymptomatic pilonidal disease unknown. Risk of recurrent abscess: ~30–50% after resolved first episode, 80–90% after two episodes.

Symptoms

Pain (inability to sit down), erythema, swelling, purulent drainage from pits or secondary openings, chronic/intermittent discomfort, chronic/intermittent drainage, secondary skin irritation.

Complications: squamous cell carcinoma (after 20–30 years), sacral osteomyelitis, necrotizing fasciitis, toxic shock syndrome, and meningitis.

Differential Diagnosis

Hidradenitis suppurativa: not uncommonly overlap between and coexistence of both.

Perirectal fistula: cryptoglandular origin.

Presacral tumor.

Meningomyelocele.

Lipoma.

Sebaceous cyst.

Acne inversa.

Pathology

Cystic structure of varying size, containing hairs, debris. Fistulous tracts extending to the skin (midline pits). Varying degrees of acute and chronic inflammatory reaction (neutrophils, lymphocytes). Abscess rupture and/or incision resulting in off-midline openings.

Evaluation

Required minimal standard

Clinical examination: midline pits, off-midline openings, induration, erythema, tenderness.

Digital rectal exam: rule out presacral tumor.

Additional tests (optional)

If presentation not classical → x-ray or CT/MRI to rule out spinal fusion malformation.

Classification

- Asymptomatic/quiescent pilonidal disease.
- Acute pilonidal abscess.
- Recurrent acute pilonidal disease.
- Chronic pilonidal sinus/fistula.

Nonoperative Treatment

Asymptomatic or quiescent pilonidal disease: no treatment needed, prophylaxis impossible.

Mild acute flare-up: suppression with antibiotics (avoid antibiotic abuse).

Operative Treatment

Indication

- Acute pilonidal abscess.
- History of recurrent acute pilonidal disease (two or more episodes).
- Chronic pilonidal sinus/fistula.
- Cancer (→ combined-modality treatment).

Operative approach
Emergency

Acute abscess → incision and drainage (in local anesthesia if possible).

Elective

Treatment parameters = simplicity, associated pain, hospitalization/down time, recurrence rates, wound care, return to normal activity; no surgical approach meets all goals!

Fistulotomy and curettage

Unroofing sinus tracts including pits and secondary openings → conversion to open wound for healing by secondary intention. Advantage: easiness, no limitations to physical activity. Disadvantage: prolonged wound care, requires patient cooperation (meticulous wound care, hair shaving). Time to healing 4–6 weeks; recurrence rates 5–20%.

Lord/Millar/Bascom procedure

Excision of pits, removal of hairs, brushing out the tracts.

Primarily open wide excision (with or without marsupialization of wound edges)

En-bloc excision of cyst, pits, secondary openings, inflammation with creation of shallow funnel-shaped wound, possible marsupialization of skin edges. Advantage: easiness of surgery, easiness of wound care (showers, scrubbing, no packing), no limitations to physical activity, lowest recurrence rates. Disadvantage: prolonged open wound, requires patient cooperation (scrubbing of wound, hair shaving). Time to healing 1–5 months; recurrence rates 1–6%.

Excision with primary closure

- Midline approach: symmetrical excision, primary closure, possibly with deep retention sutures and external compression roll. Advantage: faster overall recovery (if uncomplicated healing). Disadvantage: limitations of physical activity (bed rest, minimal walking) for 2 weeks, 30% risk of wound separation → worse outcome of secondarily opened wound compared to primarily left open wound. Time to healing 2 weeks; recurrence rates 15–25%.

- Lateral approach: lateral incision, unroofing of sinus and fistula tracts, excision of pits with lateral closure. Advantage: faster overall recovery (if uncomplicated healing). Disadvantage: limitations of physical activity (minimal walking) for 2 weeks, risk of separation. Time to healing 2–3 weeks; recurrence rates 10%.

Excision and skin grafting

Complete excision with skin grafting (primarily or after wound conditioning). Advantage: accelerated wound closure. Disadvantage: prolonged down time, risk of graft failure, discomfort/wound care at harvest site. Time to healing 2–4 weeks; recurrence rates 5–10%.

Flap procedures (Z-plasty, Limberg flap, etc)

Complete removal of all sinus tracts and infected cutaneous and subcutaneous tissue with tension-free closure using healthy tissue. Advantage: reduced midline tension, faster overall recovery (if uncomplicated healing). Disadvantage: limitations of physical activity (bed rest, minimal walking) for 2 weeks, risk of separation, worse outcome of secondarily opened wound compared with primarily left open wound. Time to healing 2 weeks; recurrence rates: not confirmed.

Outcome

Factors associated with postsurgical recurrence:

• Primarily open approach: unfavorable wound configuration (deep pockets) with inadequate drainage, hair in the wound, neglected wound care (hair, granulation tissue).

• Closed approach: undebrided devitalized tissue, suture line tension, activity → shearing forces.

Follow-up

Every 2–4 weeks until wound healed.

Cross-reference

HIDRADENITIS SUPPURATIVA *(705.83)*

Overview

Hidradenitis suppurativa is an inflammatory process originating from the apocrine sweat glands with a high chance of chronicity. Combination of acute infection with multifocal suppuration and abscess formation, as well as chronic smoldering, and fistulizing process, may result in progressive disease extension and significant fibroplastic reaction with occasionally grotesque scarring and tissue deformation. Most common locations are buttocks, groins, perineum, and axillae, but the process may extend to the intergluteal cleft (overlap with pilonidal disease) or the perirectal area (overlap with perirectal fistulae).

Pathogenesis: obstruction of apocrine sweat glands (eg, keratin) → retention of secretions → infection within the dermis and subdermis → formation of granulation tissue, tracts, and sinuses. Mixed pathogens, often skin-type origin.

Risk factors include: male gender (2:1), African-American ethnicity, obesity, smoking, hormones, familial history. Age: typically in young adults < 40–45 years. Not proven to be associated with hidradenitis: shaving, depilatory creams, deodorant usage.

Condition is not life-threatening but is annoying and causes significant work/school absences. If untreated, there is a long-term risk of malignant transformation into squamous cell cancer (after 20–30 years).

Epidemiology

Prevalence unknown. Most common in young adults (after puberty to age 45 years, comparable to pilonidal disease). Risk of recurrent abscess: ~30–50% after "successful" treatment.

Symptoms

Pain (inability to sit down), erythema, swelling, purulent drainage from multiple pits or secondary openings, chronic/intermittent discomfort, chronic/intermittent drainage, secondary skin irritation. Relatively rarely: associated lymphadenopathy and systemic signs.

Complications: chronic scarring with deformities, squamous cell carcinoma (after 20–30 years), necrotizing fasciitis, toxic shock syndrome.

Differential Diagnosis

Pilonidal disease.

Cutaneous infections: furuncles, carbuncles, erysipelas, tuberculosis, lymphogranuloma venereum, actinomycosis.

Perirectal fistula/abscess of cryptoglandular origin.

Crohn disease.

Folliculitis.

Sebaceous cyst.

Acne inversa.

Squamous cell carcinoma.

Pathology

Fistulous tracts extending to the skin with varying degrees of acute and chronic inflammatory reaction (neutrophils, lymphocytes) and focal abscess formation. Chronicity with fibrous reaction.

Evaluation

Required minimal standard

Clinical examination (to include all possible locations): multiple openings, diffuse induration, tenderness, areas of erythema. Palpatory pressure $\rightarrow$ multifocal release of purulent secretions.

Digital rectal exam and anoscopy if location close to anus.

Additional tests (optional)

Cultures: Inconsistent, 50% are culture-negative; most common pathogens: *Staphylococcus epidermidis, Streptococcus milleri, E coli,* mixed anaerobes, *Chlamydia trachomatis.*

If presentation is not classical: imaging studies, biopsies.

Classification

- Acute suppurative disease.
- Smoldering hidradenitis.
- Chronic fibroplastic disease.

Nonoperative treatment

Systemic antibiotics (eg, tetracyclines).

Topical antibiotics (eg, clindamycin)

General measures: weight loss, loose-fitting clothes, antiseptic body care.

Uncertain treatments: isotretinoin (retinoic acid derivative), hormone treatment, leuprolide (gonadotropin-releasing hormone agonist), immunosuppressants (cyclosporine, etc).

Operative Treatment

Indication
- Symptomatic disease: (sub-)acute suppurations and abscesses.
- Large disease extent: any but very limited disease unlikely to respond to medical treatment.
- Refractoriness to conservative treatment.
- Cancer → appropriate oncologic management with wide excision and combined-modality treatment.

Operative approach
- Unroofing of multiple tracts (lay-open technique, possible marsupialization) → open wound care.
- Wide local excision → open wound care (reliable).
- Wide local excision with skin grafting.
- Wide local excision with flap reconstruction: particularly in anatomically critical areas.

Outcome

Recurrences or persistent disease very common: perianal < perineal < inguinoperineal. Proactive re-debridements to be anticipated and planned.

Follow-up

Every 2–4 weeks until wound healed.

Cross-reference

FECAL INCONTINENCE *(787.6)*

Overview

Fecal incontinence is the common final pathway of multiple independent etiologies. It is defined as the involuntary loss of rectal contents (feces, gas) through the anal canal and the inability to postpone an evacuation until socially convenient. Consequences of incontinence are significant: (1) secondary medical morbidity (eg, skin maceration, urinary tract infections, decubitus ulcers), (2) substantial direct and indirect financial expenses (to patients, employer, insurance), (3) impact on quality of life (self-esteem, embarrassment, shame, depression, need to organize life around easy access to bathroom, avoidance of enjoyable activities, etc).

Problem: lack of standardization of definitions, lack of correlation between subjective and objective parameters, lack of knowledge about anorectal and continence physiology.

Scoring systems: do not include physiologic components to accurately reflect clinical severity, mostly based on subjective patient-reported assessment of severity and frequency. Easiest and most commonly used score: Cleveland Clinic Florida (Wexner) fecal incontinence score: frequency of incontinence to gas, liquid, solid, of need to wear pad, and of lifestyle changes.

Epidemiology

Very common but difficult to assess (taboo). Estimated prevalence: only known for subsets of population → wide variability depending on method of assessment and target population. International population-based studies: 0.4–18%. US telephone survey: 2.2% (30% > 65 years old, female/male 63%/37%), clinic patients: 5.6% (general outpatients) and 15.9% (urogynecology patients). Disproportionate 45–50% of affected individuals have severe physical and mental disabilities.

Symptoms

Primary symptom: worsening lack of control for different components: solid stool, liquid/semi-formed stool, gas. Descriptive grades: staining < soilage < seepage < accidents.

Daytime/nighttime variation. Reduced sensation for arriving stool, reduced urge-suppressing capacity, shortened maximal deferability.

Associated symptoms: urinary incontinence, vaginal bulging (rectocele, cystocele), prolapse (hemorrhoidal, mucosal, full-thickness rectal), altered bowel habits.

Secondary symptoms: pruritus, perianal skin irritation.

Differential Diagnosis

Typically less doubts about the diagnosis of "fecal incontinence" than its underlying etiology.

Rectovaginal fistula.

Colovaginal fistula.

Perirectal fistula.

Pathology

Plug deficit

- Insufficient outlet resistance (pressure, pressure profile): defect or dysfunction of sphincter muscles (IAS, EAS, puborectalis muscle), anal canal disconfiguration.
- Excessive endoluminal pressure or propulsive force: visceral hyperactivity (diarrhea, IBD, IBS), overflow incontinence (incomplete evacuation, fecal impaction).

Stool alteration

- Decreased consistency (diarrhea): dietary, drug-induced, irritants (bile acids), infectious, IBD, IBS.
- Increased gas formation: IBS, dietary, bacterial overgrowth.

Capacity dysfunction

- Decreased rectal compliance: proctocolitis, rectal scar/anastomosis, radiation-induced.
- Increased rectal compliance: rectocele, megarectum.

Neurologic sensory or motor dysfunction

- Central neurologic deficit: focal (stroke, tumor, trauma, multiple sclerosis); diffuse (dementia, multiple sclerosis, infection, drug-induced)
- Peripheral neuropathy: localized (parity-induced pudendal neuropathy, pelvic radiation), diffuse (diabetes mellitus, drug-induced).
- Functional dysfunction: visceral hypersensitivity (IBS).

Evaluation

Required minimal standard

History: quantitation of complaint and its impact, time of onset, number and type of vaginal deliveries, history of anorectal or spine surgeries, length of interval, underlying diseases (diabetes, stroke, etc), current medications, stool quality, passage of stool/gas through vagina, incomplete evacuation? Prolapse? History of previous colonoscopies? Past treatment failures, current management?

Clinical examination:

- Visual inspection: stool smearing, skin irritation, perineal descent, patulous anus, gapping to lateral traction, preserved anocutaneous sensation and reflex, radial folds, perineal body, keyhole deformity, prolapse or ectropion, etc?
- Digital rectal exam: sphincter integrity, sphincter tone (rest/squeeze), compensatory auxiliary muscle contraction (gluteus muscle), length of anal canal, rectocele, palpable mass?
- Anoscopy/proctoscopy: rule out other pathologies: anorectal cancer, hemorrhoids, proctitis, etc.

Full or at least partial colonic evaluation as per general screening guidelines prior to further investigation or intervention.

Additional tests (optional)

Administration of quality of life instruments: eg, FIQL.

Anorectal ultrasound: method of choice to assess sphincter defect.

Anophysiology studies (highly recommended where available): manometry including sensation/compliance, pudendal nerve terminal latency.

Assessment for suspected associated pelvic floor dysfunction:

- Defecating proctogram.
- Dynamic MRI.
- Urodynamics.
- GYN evaluation.

Classification

- Structural vs functional incontinence.
- Based on etiology of incontinence: see above.
- Based on severity: mild, moderate, severe incontinence.
- Based on onset: acquired vs congenital incontinence.

Nonoperative treatment

Dietary changes:

- Avoidance of foods that cause diarrhea or urgency.
- Supplementary fiber.

Bowel habit training: timing after meals.

Supportive measures:

- Barrier creams (zinc oxide based).
- Rectal washouts, scheduled enemas.

Medications:

- Antidiarrheal medications (loperamide, diphenoxylate, opiates).
- Bile-acid binders (cholestyramine).
- Amitriptyline (antidepressant).
- Caveats: Patients with overflow incontinence (eg, fecal impaction) may rather need routine enemas or laxatives.
- Hormonal replacement therapy? → role not defined.

Physical therapy and biofeedback training: simple, cheap, no adverse physical effects:

- Improve contraction of the external anal sphincter in response to rectal distention.
- Coordination training.
- Sensory training.
- Strength training.

Operative Treatment

Indication

- Treatment-refractory fecal incontinence.
- Incontinence with obvious and correctable deformity: cloaca-like deformity, keyhole deformity.

Operative approach
Restoration of residual sphincter function

- Sphincter repair (sphincteroplasty) where structural defect identifiable → ultrasound = most important diagnostic tool.
- Correction of visible deformities (anus, rectum).
- Sacral nerve stimulation: restimulation of dysfunctional, but anatomically intact anal sphincter muscle.

Replace sphincter or sphincter function

Narrowing of anal canal: → increase of outlet resistance, but no functional element:

- Thiersch, related procedures: anal encirclement (silver wire, silastic band): even if foreign body has to be removed due to infection ~50% improvement (scar-related).
- Secca procedure: radiofrequency ablation to create controlled scar in anal canal.
- Nondynamic graciloplasty: "bio-Thiersch," high risk of complications, lack of functional component.

- Implantation/injection (eg, ultrasound-guided) of implantable microballoons, carbon-coated beads, autologous fat, silicone, collagen.

Dynamic sphincter replacement:

- Implantation of artificial bowel sphincter: functional/dynamic solution, risk of infection/erosion.
- Dynamic graciloplasty: electrical stimulation via an implantable pulse generator → conversion of the fast-twitch, fatigable gracilis muscle to a slow-twitch, fatigue-resistant muscle.

Malone antegrade continence enema (MACE)

→ Reduce fecal load:

- Appendicostomy or continent colostomy (if appendix already gone!).
- Timed washout of the whole colon.
- Problem: leakage of residual colonic fluid during several hours following the irrigation.

Diversion

If other therapies have failed or if comorbidities preclude more aggressive therapy → colostomy: does not restore continence, but allows control of bowel evacuation:

- Fecal diversion = excellent alternative (if done well).
- Permits resumption of a normal personal and social life.
- Caveat: A poorly constructed or located ostomy may even be worse → emphasis to create a well-constructed stoma at an appropriate site.

Outcome

Sphincteroplasty: 60–88% of patients: excellent or good short-term outcome, 15–20%: no change or worsening. Long-term success deteriorating → < 50% continence after 5 years.

Predictors of failure: multilevel fragmentation of anal sphincter muscle, atrophic sphincter muscle during sphincteroplasty, extensive traumatic damage, extensive scaring, neurologic etiologies with intact sphincter muscle, combination of sphincter defect with underlying colorectal disease (IBD, IBS, etc), potential impact of pudendal neuropathy.

Follow-up

Failure after surgical treatment: → biofeedback training → reevaluation and repeat repair after > 6–12 months? → alternative vs repeat strategy?

Cross-reference

PRURITUS ANI *(698.0)*

Overview

Chronic itching in the perianal area which often triggers an irresistible urge to scratch. May be secondary to a true local anorectal pathology or a peri-anal manifestation of systemic disease (eg, dermatoses, leukemia, etc), or may be idiopathic pruritus ani. Most common underlying problem is fecal incontinence, chronic moisture in the area (prolapsing hemorrhoids, rectal prolapse, fistulae, obesity with deep anal cleft, urinary incontinence, vaginal discharge, etc). Idiopathic pruritus is not associated with detectable underlying disease, but most commonly the result of dietary and hygiene habits.

Epidemiology

Very frequent complaint; however, only a minority of individuals will seek medical attention. Male:female ratio = 4:1.

Symptoms

Itching, constant or sporadic, cycles (eg, at nighttime). Look for associated symptoms: moisture, drainage, prolapse, pain/discomfort (particularly after bowel movements).

Differential Diagnosis

Idiopathic pruritus ani: no detectable underlying pathology.

Secondary pruritus ani: result of underlying primary pathology:

- Local diseases: fistula, fissure, incontinence, condylomata and other STDs, prolapse, neoplasm, pinworm infection, etc.
- Dermatoses: psoriasis, lichen sclerosus, allergic/contact dermatitis (often secondary to use of topical medications), radiation injury, etc.
- Systemic diseases: diabetes, lymphoma/leukemia, renal failure, jaundice.

Pathology

Secondary pruritus: depending on underlying pathology.

Idiopathic pruritus: unspecific dermatitis.

Evaluation

Required minimal standard

History: Onset, pattern of occurrence, associated symptoms, daily habits?

Clinical examination: anal configuration? Local skin pathology visible (Figure 4–5) or not visible? Symmetric vs asymmetric, secondary pathology

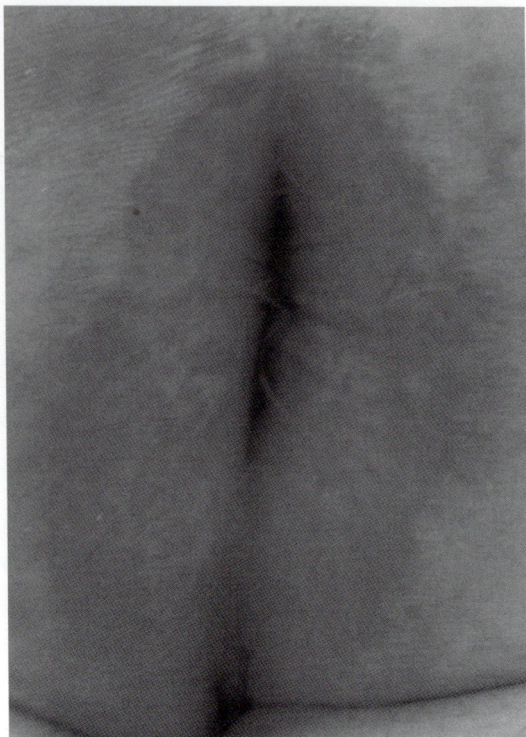

Figure 4–5. Perianal dermatitis.

(eg, scratch excoriations, skin atrophy from chronic steroid use). Signs of chronicity (lichenification)? Evidence of skin pathology in other body areas? Sphincter function?

Anoscopy/proctoscopy: Tumor, hemorrhoids, proctitis, etc.

Full colonic evaluation only necessary if indicated as per general screening guidelines.

Additional tests (optional)

Cultures: fungal, viral (herpes), chlamydia, HPV.

Biopsy: Bowen disease, Paget disease, dermatoses, etc.

Stool cultures, O&P, perianal tape test (pinworms).

Classification

Idiopathic pruritus vs secondary pruritus.

Nonoperative Treatment

Indicated for idiopathic pruritus and for symptomatic improvement in secondary pruritus:

- Elimination of current topical creams/ointments.
- Elimination of soaps, overzealous hygiene, recycled toilet paper, alcohol wipes, deodorants, etc.
- Application of barrier ointment (zinc oxide based, etc), consider $KMnO_7$ sitz baths (2 crystals per bath tub such that water is minimally stained, not purple).
- Corticosteroids creams: only indicated for very short period (< 1 week).
- Weight reduction.
- Elimination of foods: caffeine (including chocolate, tea, etc), spices, alcohol, tomatoes, citrus fruits, nuts.

Operative Treatment

Indication

Only if needed for elimination of underlying pathology (see respective topics). Never indicated for idiopathic pruritus.

Operative approach

Depending on the primary pathology (see respective chapters).

Outcome

Dependent on success of treating underlying pathology. Idiopathic pruritus commonly responds to change of daily habits.

Follow-up

Recheck patient after 4–6 weeks of initiated treatment. Order appropriate tests (eg, cultures/biopsies) if no response. Once resolved, no follow-up needed.

Cross-reference

SOLITARY RECTAL ULCER SYNDROME
(SRUS, 569.41)

Overview

Solitary rectal ulcer syndrome is a distal rectal pathology resulting from recurrent mechanical stress, most commonly rectal prolapse, recurrent digital manipulations, or recurrent autoinstrumentations, etc. The name is misleading: SRUS is not required to be solitary and not even required to include an ulcer; other, hyperplastic/polypoid changes may be present.

Epidemiology

Rare, but prevalence is underestimated. Affects all ages depending on underlying pathology/behavior.

Symptoms

SRUS symptoms: bleeding, mucous discharge, pain, tenesmus, incomplete evacuation, urgency.

Associated symptoms from underlying pathology: eg, recurrent rectal prolapse, incontinence, outlet obstruction (eg, paradoxical puborectalis contraction).

Differential Diagnosis

IBD: ulcerative colitis, Crohn colitis.

Radiation proctitis.

STDs: eg, lymphogranuloma venereum, herpes simplex, HIV-associated ulcers, primary syphilis, chancroid, etc.

Endometriosis.

Adenomatous changes.

Pathology

Characteristic myofibrosis of lamina propria with paucicellular stroma (ie, striking absence of inflammatory cells, particularly neutrophils). In addition, thickened mucosa, distorted crypt architecture.

Evaluation

Required minimal standard

History: symptoms? Evidence of external prolapse (length)? Underlying bowel function (constipation/diarrhea, need for manual support)? Change in bowel habits? Incontinence (fecal/urinary)? Sexual practices? Previous surgeries (eg, prolapse, hysterectomy, etc)? Previous colonic evaluations (flex sigmoidoscopy, colonoscopy, BE)?

Clinical examination: triggerable rectal prolapse? Rectal mass?

Rigid sigmoidoscopy: lead point? Visible mucosal changes (ulcerations, thickening?)

Full/partial colonic evaluation prior to elective surgery.

Defecating proctogram.

Additional tests (optional)
Dynamic MRI.

ERUS: thickening of the mucosa and rectal wall.

Classification

- SRUS with identifiable prolapse.
- SRUS without identifiable prolapse.

Nonoperative Treatment

SRUS without prolapse and manageable symptoms: counseling, dietary changes, fibers, laxatives, abstain from manual or instrument manipulation, possible biofeedback training.

Operative Treatment

Indication
- Any SRUS with identifiable prolapse.
- SRUS without identifiable prolapse, but significant treatment-refractory symptoms.

Operative approach
- Prolapse: abdominal or perineal prolapse repair.
- No prolapse: local transanal excision; in severe cases need for low anterior resection with coloanal anastomosis.

Outcome

Natural course of SRUS not completely documented; some changes are reversible upon correction of cause.

Follow-up

Functional reassessment at regular intervals.

Cross-reference

FOREIGN BODIES *(937, 936/938)*

Overview

Retained or stuck foreign bodies pose a special challenge for defining when surgical intervention is needed. The rate of successful intestinal passage and of spontaneous rectal expulsion is unknown; the problem hence likely is more frequent than reported. Patients only seek medical advice for manifest or pending intestinal obstruction or perforation, pain/discomfort, or if, despite prolonged efforts, they are unable to retrieve the object from the rectum.

Rectal foreign bodies: autoeroticism with lost control because anus/rectum function as a trap that make retrieval difficult: (1) sphincter muscle results in high-pressure closure behind inserted object and causes further proximal dislocation of the object; (2) presacral and puborectalis curvatures result in a change of direction; (3) valves of Houston form additional obstacles. Complications: obstruction, perforation, sphincter injury.

Oral ingestion of foreign bodies (subentity: hair bezoars): young children, underlying psychopathology (Figure 4–6), or intentional body packing. Common GI obstacles: gastroesophageal junction, pylorus, ligament of Treitz, terminal ileum, rectosigmoid, anal canal; in addition, anastomotic sites (recurrent ingestions/explorations), adhesive kinks.

Complications: obstruction, perforation, abscess formation, internal injury, bleeding, corrosion, rupture of body packs with acute intoxication/death.

Epidemiology

Oral ingestion: incidence unknown, spontaneous passage rate unknown.

Rectal insertion: incidence unknown, spontaneous expulsion rate unknown.

Symptoms

Oral ingestion of foreign object: passage dependent on form, size → possible obstruction, possible perforation, possible bleeding, possible complete passage.

Intracorporeal rupture of body packs → acute toxicity and cardiopulmonary collapse.

Rectal insertion of foreign object: pain, discomfort, bleeding, abdominal pain (ominous sign).

Differential diagnosis

Intoxication → other routes of administration, other causes of loss of consciousness.

Obstruction → other causes of SBO/LBO.

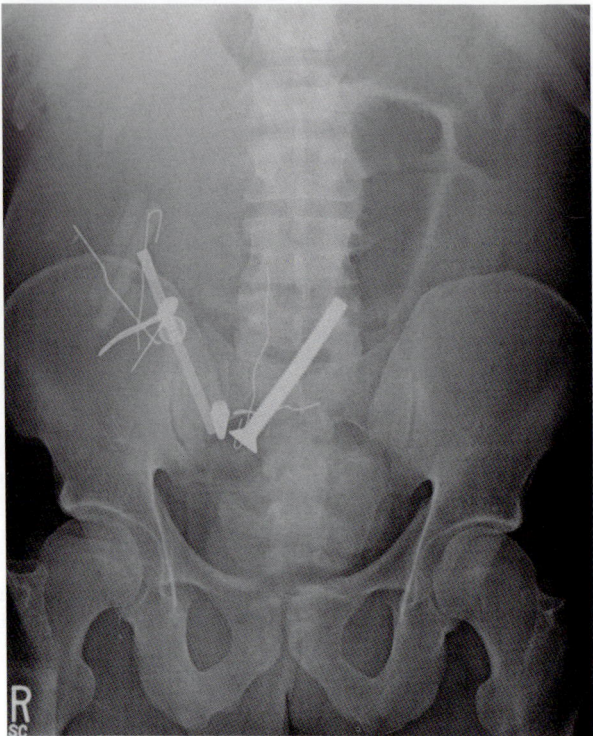

Figure 4–6. Ingested foreign objects in a schizophrenic patient.

Pathology

None.

Evaluation

Required minimal standard
All forms of foreign bodies

History: often not revealing (altered story, denial, psychosis); social and psychological background?

Clinical examination:

• Vital signs: evidence of intoxication?

• Abdominal exam: distention, peritoneal signs?

Initial abdominal and pelvic x-rays: free air, obstructive pattern, identification and characterization of objects (primary and unreported).

Oral foreign body ingestion

Chest-x-ray in two projections: esophageal foreign body, free subdiaphragmatic air, mediastinal air.

Serial abdominal x-rays: change of foreign body position?

Caution with digital rectal exam: potential for sharp objects?

Rectal foreign body

Clinical examination: careful anal (and vaginal) evaluation: risk of laceration, risk to examiner. Gentle digital rectal exam: avoid pushing object more proximally!

Additional tests (optional)

None.

Classification

None.

Nonoperative Treatment

Orally ingested foreign bodies: EGD with attempted endoscopic removal (through protector sheath), or watchful waiting (serial clinical and radiological exam).

Rectal foreign bodies: attempt at bedside extraction (70–75% successful).

Operative Treatment

Indication

• Irretrievable foreign body.

• Foreign body with complication.

Operative approach

• Attempt at extraction under anesthesia.

• Laparotomy with either bimanual expulsion (milking) or enterotomy and retrieval of foreign body.

Outcome

Nonsurgical retrieval or passage of foreign bodies in 75–80%; need for surgical intervention in 20–25%. Unspecified risk of recurrent episodes.

Follow-up

Prevention strategies?

Cross-reference

GAY BOWEL SYNDROME

Overview

Coined in the pre-HIV era, the term "gay bowel syndrome" comprised a rather unselective potpourri of unusual anorectal and GI symptoms experienced by homosexual males: abdominal pain, cramps, bloating, flatulence, nausea, vomiting, diarrhea, enteric infections (bacterial, viral, fungal, parasitic), trauma.

With better understanding of the underlying causes, this term is outdated: the derogatory terminology should be abandoned and more specific entities and terms recognized and used:

- Condylomata acuminata, mollusca contagiosa.
- Hemorrhoids.
- Proctitis (lymphogranuloma venereum, gonorrhea, syphilis, herpes simplex, etc).
- Perirectal abscess/fistula.
- Anorectal ulcer/fissure.
- Acute enteritides (salmonella, shigellosis, *Campylobacter, Clostridium difficile, E coli,* viral pathogens, *Staphylococcus aureus,* etc).
- Chronic diarrhea (*Cryptosporidium, Microsporidium, Cyclospora, Giardia, Isospora, Entamoeba histolytica, Mycobacterium avium* complex [MAC], CMV, HIV enteropathy).
- Benign polyps.
- Lymphoma.
- Viral hepatitis.
- Anorectal trauma and foreign bodies.
- Tuberculosis, atypical mycobacteriosis (MAC).
- Associated symptoms (urethritis, etc).

Cross-reference

HIV-ASSOCIATED ANORECTAL DISEASES *(042)*

Overview

Anorectal disorders are frequent in HIV-positive men who have sex with men (MSM) and may represent the original reason to seek medical attention. Improved treatment options with availability of HAART (highly active antiretroviral therapy) have dramatically changed the previously universally fatal HIV infection as such, and opportunistic infections and HIV-associated tumors (lymphoma, Kaposi sarcoma) have decreased since 1994. Yet, despite HAART, the incidence of anorectal problems has not changed, and anal dysplasia and cancer are on the rise. The original risk constellation (unprotected anorectal intercourse) appears to be primarily responsible for a majority of the problems.

Most common clinical presentations (frequently multiple synchronous problems) are:

- One-third anal condylomata.
- One-third HIV-associated ulcers.
- One-third other problems: abscess and fistula-in-ano, hemorrhoids, STDs, trauma/foreign body, anal dysplasia/neoplasia, molluscum contagiosum, tuberculosis (typical, atypical).

HIV-associated ulcer: painful flat and often eccentric lesion at the anal verge, caused by combination of mechanical trauma, multibacterial and viral infection.

Surgical treatment in HIV-positive patients, which historically (1986) had unacceptably high morbidity/mortality, has become safer: healing time is prolonged and poor outcomes are still possible, but overall symptom relief and eventual healing rate approximates that of HIV-negative patients.

Epidemiology

Anorectal disorders develop in 3–35% of HIV population (particularly MSM).

Symptoms

Depending on pathology → worsening and increasingly constant perianal and/or deep rectal pain, possible fever, possible urinary retention, bleeding/discharge, growth:

- Condylomata: lumps or bumps, itching, bleeding.
- HIV-associated ulcer: pain, purulent discharge, bleeding.
- STDs: perirectal pain (HSV), mucopurulent discharge and urgency/tenesmus (lymphogranuloma venereum), diarrhea, etc.
- Abscess: swelling, pain, inflammatory mass, fevers.

- Anal intraepithelial neoplasia (AIN) → cancer: range between asymptomatic to pain, mass/lesion.
- Hemorrhoids: bleeding, prolapse.

Other HIV-associated symptoms: wasting, fat redistribution syndrome (fat accumulation, lipodystrophy), lymphadenopathy, seborrheic dermatitis, dementia, etc.

Differential Diagnosis

Pain
- Non-HIV related causes: chronic anal fissure, thrombosed external hemorrhoid, abscess, levator ani spasm, anismus.
- HIV-related: HIV-associated ulcer, HSV infection, abscess, STDs, trauma.

Ulceration
- Chronic anal fissure (unlikely in MSM): higher location (anal canal), tight sphincter tone, tags very common.
- Idiopathic HIV-associated ulcer: often also in posterior midline or eccentric/multicentric, low location (anal verge), lax sphincter tone, tags uncommon, possible mucosal bridging.
- Specific infections: HSV, CMV, chancroid, tuberculosis, *Cryptococcus,* actinomycosis.
- Acute trauma (intercourse, foreign bodies).
- Neoplastic: anal cancer, lymphoma.
- IBD (ulcerative colitis/Crohn disease).

Growth/lump
- Condylomata.
- Cancer, lymphoma, Kaposi sarcoma.
- Actinomycosis, chancroid, etc.

Pathology

HIV-associated ulcer: epithelial ulceration, unspecific acute and chronic infiltrates.

Other pathologies: dependent on underlying disease.

Evaluation

Required minimal standard
History: Onset/pattern of symptoms, lumps/bumps, underlying bowel function and habits, preexisting incontinence? HIV test done? Time since HIV infection? Partner diseases? Opportunistic infections and tumors? Weight loss? Current HAART medications?

If not already done: HIV test.

Immune status: CD4 count, viral load.

Clinical examination:

- External inspection (skin tags, thrombosed external hemorrhoid, erythema/induration)? Lateral traction to the buttocks → visible ulcerations.
- If significant pain reported, digital exam or instrumentation at the first presentation not indicated!
- External palpation: normal/reduced sphincter tone?

Rigid/flexible sigmoidoscopy: proctitis, mass, etc.

Further colonic evaluation as per general screening guidelines (if history and findings consistent → may be deferred for 3–4 weeks until acute symptoms improved).

Additional tests (optional)

Cultures (viral, bacterial including for gonococcus, fungal, acid-fast bacilli).

Biopsy of anything unusual.

PPD test.

Possible chest x-ray.

Classification

- HIV-/immunosuppression-driven diseases (causal).
- HIV-associated diseases (linked without direct cause–effect).
- HIV-independent diseases (coincidental).

Nonoperative Treatment

General: assessment of immune status (eg, CD4 < 50) → initiation/adjustment of HAART.

HIV-associated ulcer: empirical medication with metronidazole 3×500 mg PO and acyclovir 3×800 mg PO for 14 days results in 85% resolution; repeat if improved but not resolved.

STDs: antibiotic/antiviral treatment, supportive measures.

Pre-neoplasia: anal canal surveillance.

Hemorrhoids: banding, but contraindicated if evidence for immunosuppression.

Operative Treatment

Indication

- HIV-associated ulcer: failure of empirical treatment.
- Condylomata.

- Lump/mass.
- Persistent cancer after chemoradiation.
- Abscess/fistula.
- Treatment-refractory hemorrhoids.

Operative approach
- Excision of ulcers, potentially with advancement flap → open wound care.
- Hemorrhoids: excisional hemorrhoidectomy. Caveat: stapled hemorrhoidectomy contraindicated in MSM (risk of injury from residual staples).
- Other pathologies: removal of warts, biopsy or excision of lumps, drainage of abscess, etc; persistent cancer after chemoradiation → oncologic resection (see Anal Cancer later in the chapter).

Outcome

HIV-associated ulcer: 85% improvement with conservative treatment; after surgical excision → improvement of pain and discomfort in 90% of patients despite creation of even larger wounds and varying times of wound healing.

CD4 < 50 → poor wound healing.

Follow–up

Monitoring of HAART.

Immediate follow-up every 2 weeks → control and verification of local treatment success.

Long-term follow-up → health management, HAART, at least annual Pap smear, etc.

Cross-reference

SEXUALLY TRANSMITTED DISEASES
(STDS, 091, 098, 099)

Overview

STDs are caused by transmission of pathogens during sexual activity. Affected locations: genital, anorectal, oral. Anorectal STDs are an important health issue in patients engaging in anoreceptive intercourse. Risk behavior of either index patient or partner(s) result in frequently repeated acquisitions of STDs. Multiple simultaneous STDs are common and facilitate acquisition of others (eg, HIV).

- Discharge syndromes: gonorrhea, chlamydia (LGV), HSV.
- Anogenital ulcerations: herpes simplex, HIV-associated ulcers, primary syphilis, chancroid (*Haemophilus ducreyi*), LGV, granuloma inguinale (donovanosis: *Klebsiella/Calymmatobacterium granulomatis*).
- Pain:
  - Yes: HSV, LGV, chancroid.
  - No: syphilis (chancre), granuloma inguinale.
- Proctitis/proctocolitis: gonorrhea, chlamydia (LGV), syphilis, HSV.
- Proliferative syndromes: HPV, HHV-8 (Kaposi sarcoma), lymphoma, syphilis (condylomata lata, gumma).
- Skin rashes: secondary syphilis, disseminated gonorrhea, pediculosis pubis, scabies.

Direct anogenital pathogen infestation: HPV, *Neisseria gonorrhoeae, Chlamydia trachomatis* (including LGV), *Treponema pallidum* (syphilis), HSV.

Indirect pathogen infestation (eg, oral or oral-anal route): *Giardia lamblia, Campylobacter* species, *Shigella* species, *Entamoeba histolytica, C trachomatis,* pediculosis pubis, scabies.

HIV-positive patients: CMV, *Mycobacterium avium intracellulare* complex (MAI/MAC), *Microsporidium, Isospora,* etc.

Epidemiology

US incidence of STDs overall: up to 20 million new infections per year. Active STDs (eg, gonorrhea, syphilis, etc) increase the risk of HIV infection if exposed.

Symptoms

General symptoms

- Proctitis: pruritus, anorectal pain, tenesmus, rectal bleeding, mucus discharge.
- Proctocolitis: same as above; in addition: change in bowel habits (diarrhea), abdominal cramps.

- Enteritis: diarrhea, abdominal cramping without signs of proctocolitis.
- Proliferation: lump, mass, condylomata.

Specific disease features

- Gonorrhea: asymptomatic carrier (reservoir); PID; monoarthritis; skin rash; urethritis; proctitis with thick, cloudy, or bloody discharge; pain.
- Syphilis (Lues):
  - Primary: primary complex (chancre)—small, indurated, clean-based, and painless ulcer; proctitis.
  - Secondary: diffuse, nonitching maculopapular skin rash, possible general symptoms (lymphadenopathy, fever, headache), condylomata lata.
  - Latent: status post infection, but no clinical evidence of disease.
  - Tertiary: no primary manifestation, neurologic symptoms, aortitis, gumma.
- Chancroid: deep, purulent, and painful genital ulcer with tender suppurative inguinal lymphadenopathy.
- Herpes genitalis: multiple and grouped painful vesicular or shallow ulcerative lesions.
- *Chlamydia* serovars D–K: proctitis, urethritis.
- *Chlamydia* serovars L1–L3 (LGV): tender lymphadenopathy, proctocolitis with bloody/mucous discharge, pain/tenesmus, constipation, fever. Long-term sequelae: lymphedema, fistulae, and strictures.
- Granuloma inguinale (donovanosis): progressive, very vascular and friable, painless ulceration without regional lymphadenopathy.

Differential Diagnosis

Other causes of ulceration, bleeding, pain.

Primary neoplasms: anal cancer, Paget disease, Bowen disease, AIN, rectal cancer, melanoma, Kaposi sarcoma, lymphoma.

Other forms of colitis: ulcerative colitis, Crohn disease, *C difficile* colitis, etc.

Pathogens

- Gonorrhea: *N gonorrhoeae,* intracellular gram-negative diplococci $\rightarrow$ selective cultures (Thayer-Martin medium), PCR.
- Syphilis: *T pallidum* (spirochetes) $\rightarrow$ darkfield/immunofluorescence microscopy, serology.

- Chancroid: *H ducreyi,* gram-negative rod → special culture medium (difficult), PCR-diagnosis.
- Herpes genitalis: HSV-1 and HSV-2 (herpes genitalis) → isolation in cell cultures, PCR-based diagnosis.
- *C trachomatis* serovars D–K and L1, L2, L3 (LGV), intracellular pathogen → serology, culture, immunofluorescence test.
- Granuloma inguinale (donovanosis): gram-negative *K granulomatis* (formerly *C granulomatis*) → culture difficult, diagnosis on biopsy: dark-staining Donovan bodies.

Evaluation

Required minimal standard

History: risk behavior, HIV status, specific symptoms.

Clinical examination: inspection → mass/lump, ulcers/blisters, fistulae? Digital exam/palpation of inguinal lymph nodes; anoscopy/sigmoidoscopy → HSV, gonorrhea, LGV, syphilis? Examination of oral cavity.

All patients with STDs → HIV testing (unless known positive).

Cultures:

- Direct cultures: HSV, gonorrhea, chlamydia, *H ducreyi,* tuberculosis.
- Stool cultures, including *Giardia,* cryptosporidiosis, microsporidiosis.

Other examinations:

- Stool WBCs?
- Gram-stained smear of anorectal secretions: gram-negative intracellular diplococci?
- Darkfield light microscopy: *T pallidum*?
- Serologic testing: HSV-2, syphilis, LGV, gonorrhea.

Anogenital ulcers: → syphilis serology + darkfield examination or direct immunofluorescence, HSV culture or antigen test, *H ducreyi* culture.

Reportable diseases: syphilis, gonorrhea, chlamydia, HIV, tuberculosis.

Additional tests (optional)

Chest x-ray or PPD: tuberculosis.

Colonoscopy.

Classification

Based on specific infectious pathogen.

Nonoperative treatment

Proctitis: ceftriaxone + doxycycline.

HSV: one of the following: acyclovir, famciclovir, valacyclovir.

Syphilis: penicillin G → caveat: Jarisch-Herxheimer in first 24 hours: acute febrile reaction, headache, myalgia; alternatives: doxycycline, tetracycline.

Chlamydia/LGV: doxycycline; alternative: erythromycin.

Gonorrhea: ceftriaxone (plus treatment for chlamydia); alternative: spectinomycin → caveat: drug-resistant gonorrhea.

CMV: ganciclovir.

Chancroid: one of the following: azithromycin, ceftriaxone, ciprofloxacin, erythromycin.

Granuloma inguinale: doxycycline; alternatives: azithromycin, ciprofloxacin, erythromycin, or trimethoprim-sulfamethoxazole.

Idiopathic HIV-associated ulcers: empirical treatment with acyclovir + metronidazole.

HPV: see respective chapters.

Operative Treatment

Indications

- Uncertain diagnosis → biopsy and culture of tissue specimen (bacterial, viral, acid-fast bacilli).
- Anogenital condylomata.
- Treatment-refractory HIV-associated ulcer.

Operative approach

See Chapter 5.

Outcome

Higher risk of treatment failure in HIV-positive patients, particularly with low CD4 counts.

Risk factors for recurrent infections: continued risk behavior (promiscuity, unprotected intercourse), untreated partner, uncircumcised individuals.

Follow-up

Assessment of infection clearance → follow-up should be based on specific etiology and severity of clinical symptoms. Difficulty in distinguishing reinfection from treatment failure.

Management of sex partners: evaluation and treatment.

Cross-reference

ANAL CONDYLOMATA *(078.10)*

Overview

Condylomata ("anogenital warts") are hyperkeratotic and often cauliflower-like, solitary or multiple skin lesions that are caused by sexually transmitted infection of squamous epithelia with highly contagious HPV. Before activating proliferative growth mode, HPV may be dormant within the cells for weeks, months, even years: the exact time and "donor" of the infection can therefore not be determined with certainty.

More than 100 HPV serotypes have been identified: ~30 serotypes are sexually transmitted, serotypes 6/11 in > 90% of cases, but coexistence of different serotypes is possible. Currently, routine serotyping is clinically not relevant:

- HPV serotypes with malignant potential: 16, 18, 33, 31, 35, 39, 45, 51, 52 → low- and high-grade squamous intraepithelial lesions (LSIL, HSIL) → invasive cancer.
- HPV serotypes without malignant potential: 6, 11, 42, 43, 44 → genital warts, LSIL

Growth pattern ranging from (1) focal scattered diminutive warts, to (2) large and exophytic warts, (3) carpet-like, often confluent lesions, or (4) inversely growing Buschke-Lowenstein giant condylomata.

Epidemiology

In the US: prevalence of 20 million people with genital HPV infections, annual incidence of 5.5 million people infected every year; 50–75% of sexually active general population have genital HPV infection at some time in their life, 15% with evidence of current infection. Majority of infections are subclinical, ie, not detectable by physical exam or cytology. Anogenital warts: in 1–2% of general population, in 3–25% of HIV-positive population; 13–30% of males with anal warts have penile warts; 70–85% of patients with external warts have also internal warts.

Symptoms

Often asymptomatic.

Presence of indolent palpable/visible grayish or flesh-colored skin lesions (papules, nodules, lumps, masses).

Itching: difficulty with hygiene. With increasing size → bleeding when traumatized.

Caveat: pain is not a symptom of anal warts → differential diagnoses: ulcer, fissure, tumor, abscess.

Differential Diagnosis

Molluscum contagiosum.

Fibroepitheliomata.

Hypertrophic anal papillae.

Seborrheic keratoses.

Sebaceous glands.

Condylomata lata (secondary syphilis).

Bowen disease.

Anal cancer or other tumors.

Paget disease.

Pathology

Papillomatous hyperkeratotic acanthotic lesions. Maintained epithelial maturation toward the surface. Characteristic koilocytosis = perinuclear cytoplasmic vacuolization in conjunction with nuclear irregularity.

Low-grade dysplasia (AIN I) → high-grade dysplasia (AIN III): increasing epithelial disorganization, loss of maturation, increased cellularity to the surface. Podophyllin effect: changes similar to high-grade dysplasia.

Evaluation

Required minimal standard

History: onset, pattern, and sites of occurrence; associated symptoms? HIV status?

Clinical examination: localization and extent of lesions? Confluence of lesions (Figure 4–7)? Estimate of internal and external anoderm involvement. Examination of perineum, penis. GYN exam.

Anoscopy/proctoscopy/sigmoidoscopy: internal involvement, associated STD proctitis, etc.

Full colonic evaluation only necessary if indicated as per general screening guidelines.

Additional tests (optional)

Cultures: if suspicion of other STDs.

Biopsy: if diagnosis in doubt, all excised lesions.

HIV test (recommended).

GYN exam.

Partner examination/treatment.

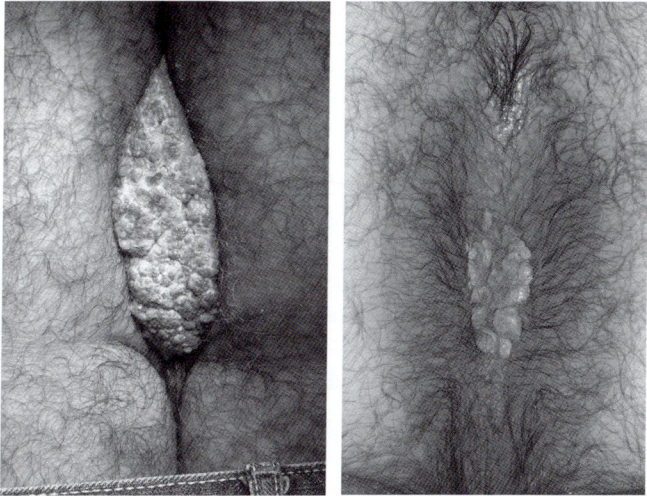

Figure 4–7. Anal condylomata.

Classification

- Condylomata acuminata.
- Condylomata plana.
- Condylomata gigantea (Buschke-Loewenstein).

Nonoperative Treatment

In HIV-infected patients: optimization of immune status (HAART).

Topical treatments for relatively limited and accessible disease, commonly multiple sessions (daily/weekly) needed, recurrence rates > 25%:

1. Patient applied:

   a. Imiquimod 5%: topical ointment, unclear mode of action but multi-level enhancement of local immune response which promotes host suppression of HPV proliferation. Red butt: side effect, often associated with later treatment success. Success rate of 60–70% in HIV-negative, 10–20% in HIV-positive patients.

   b. Podophyllin: 0.5 solution topically twice daily for 8 hours (3–4 days/week), protection of healthy skin recommended; antiproliferative cytotoxic properties (cell cycle arrest in metaphase) → potential risk of carcinogenesis, unsuited for anal canal condylomata. Local side effects: irritation, blistering, ulceration; rare systemic toxicity reported: hepatotoxicity, oncogenicity. Caveat: podophyllin effect on pathology specimen.

   c. 5-FU: 60% eradication after 3–7 days but often associated with intolerable discomfort.

2. Physician applied:

   a. Podophyllin: 25% solution topically once per week (side effects: see above).

   b. Liquid nitrogen: freezing of warts every 1–2 weeks, cheap, discomfort.

   c. Trichloric acid (TCA): chemical burning of warts, once per week.

   d. Intralesional injection of interferon: multiple sessions needed.

3. Unproven treatments: multiple other regimens.

Operative Treatment

Indication

- Larger extent and/or number of external condylomata.
- Internal condylomata.
- Treatment refractoriness.

Operative approach

- Excision of larger lesions at their base, possible combination with injection of interferon alpha.
- Fulguration of smaller/flat lesions, possible combination with injection of interferon alpha.
- Wide excision with flap reconstruction (not commonly indicated).

Outcome

Risk of recurrence dependent on extent of disease, completeness of removal, HIV/immune status. HPV also present in adjacent noncondylomatous epithelium → 30–50% recurrence.

Patient education about safer sex practices (avoidance of reinfection, avoidance of associated STDs), management of sex partner recommended.

Role, indication, timing of HPV vaccination (Gardasil) unclear at this point.

Follow-up

Frequent follow-up in clinic → removal of small recurrences using local anesthesia.

Cross-reference

ANAL INTRAEPITHELIAL NEOPLASIA
(AIN, 235.5)

Overview

Anal dysplasia (like anal cancer) is linked to HPV infection with subtypes HPV16 or HPV18. The concept of AIN in high-risk populations (HIV-positive MSM) is relatively young and still evolving: there is a confusing and nonstandardized overlap between different pathologies and newer vs established terminology:

- AIN (anal intraepithelial neoplasia): neither visible nor palpable, located in anal canal.
- LSIL vs HSIL (low-grade vs high-grade squamous intraepithelial lesion).
- ASCUS (atypical squamous cells of uncertain significance).
- Carcinoma in situ, intraepithelial carcinoma.
- Bowen disease: visible erythematous plaque with an irregular but usually sharp demarcation, located in anal margin area.

AIN terminology and management "borrowed" from cervical cancer prevention/management (ie, CIN), but not entirely applicable:

- Analogies between the two entities:
  - Both are considered STDs: associated with HPV, other HPV manifestations common (condylomata), eradication of HPV difficult (dormant viral genome), identification of precancerous lesions relatively easy.
- Differences:
  - Cervix: common cancer with decreasing incidence (cervical cancer screening programs), precursor lesion treatable without mutilation, early cancers hidden (not in reach of finger), cancer-specific mortality relatively high (except for earliest stages).
  - Anus: rare cancer with increasing incidence (HIV, HAART), precursor lesion difficult to treat (morbidity, risk of mutilation and functional impairment), early cancer readily visible/palpable (in reach of finger), effective treatment available for established cancer, cancer-specific mortality relatively low.
- Problems: the concept of AIN monitoring relies on stepwise progression through different stages. Unfortunately, this concept is not (yet) corroborated by actual data: uncertain whether/when/how AIN can regress or progresses towards cancer or whether therapeutic intervention allows natural course to be changed. Cost-effectiveness of anal screening has not been analyzed.

Epidemiology

HIV-positive MSM found to have AIN of any grade in 81%, AIN II or III in 52%.

Symptoms

Ranging from asymptomatic → mild symptoms (eg, pruritus) → visible/palpable lump/mass or skin changes → increasing pain, possible bleeding, etc.

Differential Diagnosis

Idiopathic pruritus ani.

Perianal skin irritation.

Manifest anal cancer.

Pathology

Cytology from anal Pap smear

Classification according to revised Bethesda system for cervical cytology:

- Normal.
- Atypical squamous cells of uncertain significance (ASCUS).
- Low-grade squamous intraepithelial lesion (LSIL).
- High-grade squamous intraepithelial lesion (HSIL).

Histopathology

Biopsy: nuclear polymorphism with hyperchromasia and mitotic figures; increasing replacement of the stratified squamous epithelium architecture with immature cells similar to basal cells, no signs of invasiveness, ie, no disruption of basement membrane.

Evaluation

Required minimal standard

History: risk stratification → HIV-positive, anal intercourse? Presence/absence of symptoms, lumps/bumps? Time since HIV infection? Current HAART medications? Recent podophyllin applications? Previous Pap smears?

Immune status: CD4 count, viral load.

Clinical examination: external inspection, digital palpation, and anoscopy → skin appearance, condylomata, lumps/bumps, induration?

Additional tests (optional)

Any visible/palpable pathology → biopsy.

No visible pathology but AIN on Pap → high-resolution anoscopy (3% acetic acid or Lugol iodine solution) → biopsy of dysplastic areas to characterize AIN.

Classification

- ASCUS: atypical squamous cells of uncertain significance.
- AIN I: mild dysplasia (LSIL).
- AIN II: moderate dysplasia.
- AIN III: severe dysplasia, intraepithelial carcinoma (HSIL).
- Bowen disease: intraepithelial squamous cell carcinoma in visible anal margin lesion.

Nonoperative Treatment

Expectant approach (watchful waiting) with recurrent clinical and pap monitoring.

Topical imiquimod.

Topical 5-FU (with/without topical imiquimod).

Operative Treatment

Indication

- Any visible or palpable lesion/mass → at least biopsy, or excision if possible.
- AIN III: operative treatment vs watchful waiting?

Operative approach

- Anal mapping → multiple circumferential punch biopsies at defined concentric intervals.
- Wide local excision, potentially with flap reconstruction.

Outcome

Anal Pap screening: sensitivity 65–90% and specificity 30–60% for diagnosing AIN.

Surgical AIN eradication: extensive surgery with significant morbidity (painful recovery, wound care, stricture) → 80% recurrent AIN III within 12 months.

Expectant approach (watchful waiting) → 6–10% invasive cancer.

Topical medications (imiquimod, 5-FU) → > 60% chance of AIN resolution?

Follow-up

Clinical examination and Pap smears: high-grade lesions → every 3 months, low-grade lesions annually.

Cross-reference

BOWEN DISEASE *(235.5)*

Overview

Bowen disease is an intraepithelial squamous cell carcinoma (caveat: Paget disease is an intraepithelial adenocarcinoma). Etiologically, it is frequently associated with chronic/recurrent exposure to arsenic or sunlight (→ location on trunk and extremities) or infection with HPV16 or HPV18 (→ location in genital/perianal region).

Distinction between AIN III and Bowen disease inadequately defined and lacking consensus → varying and inconsistent terminology and possible need to entirely eliminate terms in the future.

Suggested distinction of clinical entities (Table 4–2): in contrast to invisible AIN I–III (located in nonkeratinizing anal canal anoderm), Bowen disease is located inside or outside anal margin (distal to anal verge in

TABLE 4–2. Comparison of Intraepithelial Neoplasias.

	AIN	*Bowen Disease*	*Paget Disease*
Visible/ palpable lesion	No	Yes	Yes
Pap smear	Yes	No	No
Histology	Squamous cell dysplasia	Intraepithelial squamous cell carcinoma	Intraepithelial adenocarcinoma
Location	Anal canal	Anal margin genital area extragenital locations	Anal canal to anal margin
HPV-related	+	+ (extra-anogenital: arsenic, sunlight)	–
Multifocal	100%	10–20%	?
Malignant potential	6–10%	6–10%	30–50%
Association with internal malignancies	–	–	20–50%

AIN, anal intraepithelial neoplasia; HPV, human papillomavirus; +, positive; –, negative; ?, uncertain.

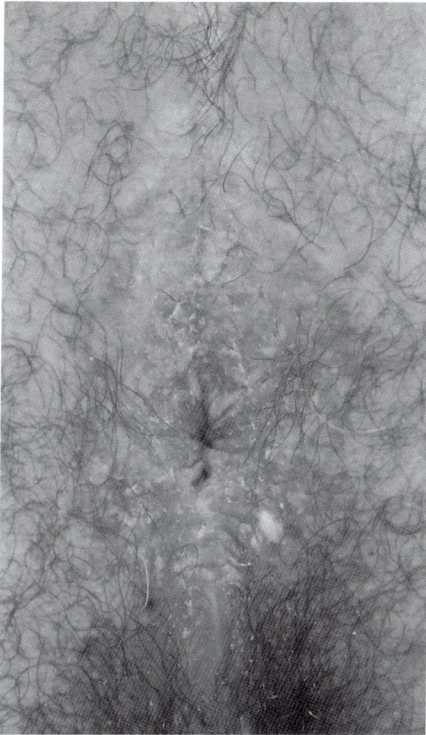

Figure 4–8. Bowen disease.

keratinizing squamous epithelium) → presenting as macroscopically visible/palpable skin lesion in form of a scaly or thickened erythematous plaque with an irregular but usually sharp demarcation (Figure 4–8).

Bowen disease is not associated with internal GI malignancies (in contrast to Paget disease → 20–50% internal malignancy!).

Epidemiology

Incidence: 14–120 new cases per 100,000 per year.

Symptoms

Range: asymptomatic → mild symptoms (eg, pruritus) → enlarging skin changes → increasing irritation, possible bleeding, etc.

Differential Diagnosis

Idiopathic pruritus ani.

Perianal skin irritation.

Candidiasis.

Manifest anal cancer.

Bowenoid papulosis.

AIN I–III.

Paget disease.

Pathology

Macropathology

Scaly or thickened erythematous skin alteration with irregular but usually sharp demarcation.

Histopathology

Epithelium with nuclear polymorphism with hyperchromasia and mitotic figures → replacement of the stratified squamous epithelium architecture with immature cells similar to basal cells up to the surface, no signs of invasiveness, ie, no disruption of basement membrane.

Evaluation

Required minimal standard
See discussion of AIN, earlier.

Additional tests (optional)
Any visible/palpable pathology: biopsy.

Classification

Bowen disease: intraepithelial squamous cell carcinoma in visible lesion.

Nonoperative Treatment

Expectant approach (watchful waiting).

Topical imiquimod.

Topical 5-FU (with/without topical imiquimod).

Topical photodynamic therapy.

Operative Treatment

Indication
Any visible or palpable lesion/mass: at least biopsy, excision if possible.

Operative approach
- Anal mapping: multiple circumferential punch biopsies at defined concentric intervals.
- Wide local excision with negative margins, potentially with flap reconstruction.

Outcome

Surgical treatment: high risk of local recurrence. Associated morbidity: discomfort, wound dehiscence, anal stenosis, incontinence.

Expectant approach (watchful waiting): < 6–10% developing invasive cancer → watchful waiting and selective treatment justifiable.

Follow-up

Clinical examination every 3 months; biopsy or excision if progression.

Cross-reference

Topic	*Chapter*
Skin rash	1 (p 48)
HIV-associated anorectal diseases	4 (p 206)
Anal condylomata	4 (p 215)
AIN	4 (p 220)
Anal cancer	4 (p 230)
Medications against viral pathogens	App I (p 724)

BUSCHKE-LOWENSTEIN GIANT CONDYLOMATA
(078.10, 235.5)

Overview

Buschke-Lowenstein giant condylomata represent large and expansive verrucous growth with invasive squamous cell carcinoma (verrucous carcinoma): locally destructive growth pattern with high risk for local recurrence but low tendency to metastasize.

The condition (like other condylomata and anal cancer) is an STD ($\rightarrow$ located on penis, anus, vulva) related to HPV infection, but other as of yet unknown factors result in this characteristic growth pattern. Aggravated progression is observed during pregnancy and in immunosuppressed patients.

Epidemiology

Rare $\rightarrow$ anecdotal series only.

Symptoms

Visible/palpable mass.

Differential Diagnosis

Extensive anal condylomata.

Pathology

Macroscopic
Visible exophytic and verrucous mass.

Microscopic
Epidermal hyperplasia with hyper-/parakeratosis, koilocytosis, lack of horn pearls; invasion of dermis, but no vascular or lymphovascular invasion; inflammatory reaction.

Evaluation

Required minimal standard
HIV testing, pregnancy test. Generous and deep biopsy.

Otherwise as for anal cancer.

Additional tests (optional)
As for anal cancer.

Classification

- Buschke-Lowenstein giant condylomata.
- Verrucous carcinoma.

Nonoperative Treatment

Immunomodulation: antiretroviral therapy (HAART) in HIV-positive patients.

Topical imiquimod.

Injection of interferon or bleomycin?

Chemoradiation (Nigro protocol): Caveat: the verrucous carcinoma and Buschke-Lowenstein giant condylomata are the one exception to the otherwise primarily nonsurgical approach to anal cancer.

Operative Treatment

Indications
Large bulky tumor.

Operative approach
Depending on location:
- Wide local excision if possible (anal margin).
- Cautery ablation of tumor bulk ($\rightarrow$ chemoradiation).
- Rarely: abdominoperineal resection.

Outcome

Anecdotal data only.

Follow-up

Oncologic follow-up with regular clinical examination every 3–6 months.

Cross-reference

ANAL CANCER *(154.2, 154.3)*

Overview

Anal cancer historically was relatively rare (1.5–2% of all GI tumors) and a disease affecting persons of middle to advanced age, predominantly women. The HIV epidemic and prolonged survival due to highly active anti-retroviral therapy (HAART) have resulted in a dramatic increase in the incidence of anal cancer among HIV-positive patients, predominantly men who have sex with men (MSM) and at a younger age, along with an associated risk of cervical, vaginal, and vulvar cancer in women, and other STDs.

Anal cancer is considered an STD: transmission of HPV occurring through repetitive anal intercourse with serotype 16, but also 18, 33, (31, 35) represents the highest risk. Other risk factors: immunosuppression (HIV, drug-induced, etc), smoking, chronic trauma/wounds.

Numerous pathologic subtypes, wide spectrum of special manifestations, and precursor diseases: AIN I–III, Bowen disease, verrucous cancer, anal cancer in fistula, perianal cancer. Although cancer screening is expanding (anal Pap smears), its role is not precisely defined.

An overwhelming percentage of new anal cancers are misdiagnosed by non-colorectal specialists as a benign condition. Staging is based on tumor size, not on depth of penetration (see Appendix II: tumor staging).

For treatment decisions, anatomic location is crucial:

• Anal canal involved: primary location or secondary involvement from large perianal tumor.

• Anal canal not involved: perianal (anal margin) cancer.

Treatment in the past: primary radical surgery with wide local excision (anal margin) or APR (anal canal). Modern strategy for anal canal has shifted to highly effective and sphincter-saving chemoradiation (Nigro protocol) as the first-line approach, with radical surgery reserved for patients with incomplete response (large tumors more likely) or recurrences. Nonetheless a substantial fraction of patients (> 25%) ultimately require colostomy for various reasons.

Epidemiology

Classical form (before HIV): women in their 50s–60s, 0.7 new cases per 100,000 men overall, 25–37 new cases per 100,000 MSM.

New epidemic (since advent of HIV): younger HIV-positive males (MSM) → relative increased risk ratio compared with pre-HIV era: 84.1 in homosexual and 37.7 in nonhomosexual patients. Epidemic rise in annual incidence in US: from 3400 new cases in 1997 to 4700 new cases and 700 cancer-related deaths in 2007.

Symptoms

Bleeding (55–60%), anal pain and tenesmus (40–50%), visible or palpable mass (25–40%), change in bowel habits (eg, pencil-like stools, incontinence), constipation, diarrhea, mucous discharge, pruritus. Completely asymptomatic (20%).

Associated benign anorectal pathology in > 25% of patients: hemorrhoids, condylomata acuminata (> 50% in MSM), Bowen disease, fissure, fistula, leukoplakia, pruritus → symptoms frequently ignored or misallocated for > 3 months before diagnosis of cancer is established.

Differential Diagnosis

Perianal (anal margin) tumors: distal to transition of hairless anal canal to hair-containing perianal skin, but < 5 cm away from anal verge.

Skin cancer: > 5 cm away from anal verge.

Rectal cancer (→ adenocarcinoma): above dentate line.

Infiltration from extensive cancer of the bladder, cervix, vagina, vulva, etc.

Other rare (pre-)malignant anorectal tumors: Paget disease, Bowen disease, carcinoid, lymphoma, GIST, melanoma, small cell cancer, Kaposi sarcoma.

Benign lesions: anal condylomata, Buschke-Lowenstein giant condylomata, fistula with chronic perifistular induration, fissure with sentinel skin tag, thrombosed external hemorrhoid.

Pathology

Macroscopic
Visible or palpable mass, ulcerative lesion, asymmetric "fissure" → primarily locally destructive growth pattern (Figure 4–9). Inguinal lymph node involvement at time of diagnosis: 10–25%.

Microscopic
Several histopathologic subtypes (little impact on clinical decision-making process and outcome):

- Squamous cell (cloacogenic) carcinoma (SCC, large cell keratinizing, 70–80%): with subtypes, transitional (large cell nonkeratinizing) and basaloid.
- Adenocarcinoma (10–15%): arising from anal glands or apocrine skin glands.
- Other histologies (2–10%): eg, small cell carcinoma.

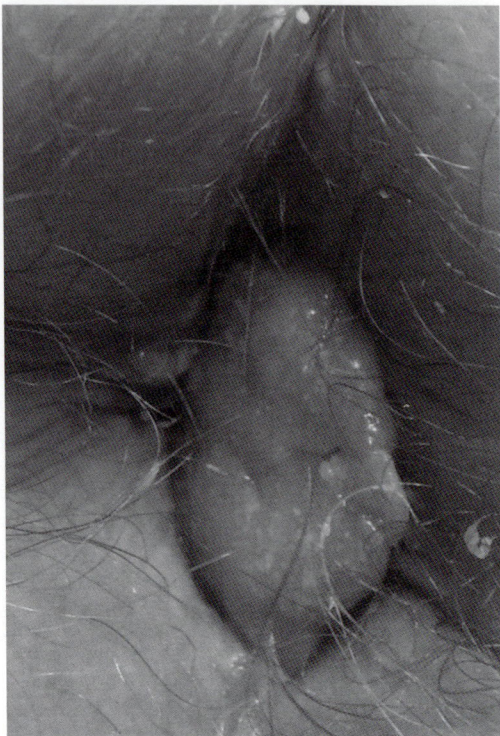

Figure 4–9. Anal cancer.

Evaluation

Required minimal standard

History: bleeding, change in bowel habits, obstructive symptoms, weight loss? Any nonhealing anorectal condition? HIV status?

Clinical examination:

- Inspection: visible skin changes (symmetric, asymmetric), lumps/bumps, eccentric ulcerations, secondary fistula openings, discoloration? Anything unusual? Concomitant pathology (eg, condylomata, hemorrhoids, tags, etc)?
- Digital exam: perirectal induration, exact anatomic location, size, and internal extension of tumor? Sphincter tone?
- Palpation of inguinal lymph nodes.

Biopsy (forceps, incisional): histologic confirmation of malignancy and subtype → most notably distinction between SCC and adenocarcinoma (rectum, anal glands).

HIV testing.

Anoscopy/proctoscopy: assessment of rectum for concomitant diseases (eg, STD proctitis)?

Females: GYN exam and assessment for concomitant cervical/vaginal pathology.

Staging: CT scan of abdomen and pelvis with inclusion of chest, or separate chest x-ray.

Full/partial colonic evaluation as per general screening guidelines and prior to any planned intervention (Note: anal cancer is not associated with an increased risk of colorectal cancer).

Additional tests (optional)

Blood work: CBC (anemia?), liver function (albumin, PTT, PT), kidney function.

Anorectal ultrasound: role not completely defined → evaluation of tumor size, depth of penetration, sphincter involvement, mesorectal lymph nodes.

Fine-needle aspiration or core biopsy of enlarged inguinal lymph nodes.

MRI, PET, PET-CT: role not yet defined in primary assessment unless tumor locally advanced.

Classification

• Anal cancer: involvement of anal canal.

• Anal margin cancer → staged and treated as "skin cancer."

Nonoperative Treatment

Anal cancer:

• Nigro protocol (some variation of protocols): chemoradiation with 45–59 Gy in conjunction with 5-FU and mitomycin C.

• Alternative: chemoradiation combined with 5-FU and cisplatin: particularly in HIV-positive parients.

Incidental carcinoma or carcinoma in situ pathology specimen (eg, excision of condylomata, hemorrhoidectomy) with clinically no residual tumor:

• Watchful waiting with frequent clinical examination (vs reexcision of scar).

• Alternative: Nigro protocol (as above).

Operative Treatment

Indications

Local tumor:

- Anal SCC (including subtypes):
  - Residual tumor after completion of Nigro protocol.
  - Inability to tolerate chemoradiation (including noncompliance).
  - Recurrent tumor after initial complete clinical response.
  - Treatment-refractory, inoperable but highly symptomatic tumor.
- Adenocarcinoma: after neoadjuvant chemoradiation.
- Perianal (anal margin) SCC: treatment as for skin cancer.
- Buschke-Lowenstein tumor.

Regional lymph node manifestation: lymph node dissection not routinely performed, only for isolated inguinal nodal disease.

Long-term sequelae of tumor or tumor treatment:

- Stricture.
- Radiation proctitis.
- Nonmanageable fistula.
- Incontinence.
- Tumor infiltration with pain.

Operative approach

Curative intent:

- Abdominoperineal resection, if necessary with en-bloc resection of involved organs (vagina, bladder).
- Same as above, but with inguinal lymphadenectomy (involvement = poor prognostic sign): radical lymphadenectomy or excision of enlarged nodes only ("cherry picking").
- Inguinal lymphadenectomy alone: regional lymph node recurrence with primary tumor in remission.
- Perianal (anal margin) cancer: local excision with negative margins.

Diagnostic intent:

- Not established diagnosis: incisional (rarely excisional) biopsy.
- Exam under anesthesia, incisional/excisional or TruCut biopsies → distinction between residual tissue induration vs persistent tumor.

Palliation: creation of colostomy.

Outcome

Complete clinical response to combined modality treatment (80–90%): 5-year survival 65–75%.

Residual disease after CMT (10–15%): 5-year survival 45–60%.

Locally recurrent disease (10–30%): 5-year survival 0–35%.

Probability of colostomy (due to persistent/recurrent disease or treatment sequelae: anorectal dysfunction, stenosis): 25–40%.

HIV-positive patients: worse outcome, lower tolerance to chemoradiation, increased treatment-related toxicity (80% vs 30%), fewer complete response (62% vs 85%), shorter time to death (1.4 vs 5.3 years).

Follow-up

Oncologic follow-up:

• Clinical examination and blood work: every 3–6 months.

• Imaging (CT abdomen/pelvis, chest x-ray/-CT): at least every 12 months.

Surgical reintervention for metastatic disease: benefit-risk analysis of surgery as opposed to more chemotherapy with/without radiation dependent on individual circumstances.

Cross-reference

POLYPS *(211.3)*

Overview

Polyp represents a descriptive term for any mucosal elevation. Characterization of polyps is based on:

• Degree of attachment to bowel wall (eg, pedunculated, sessile, flat).
• Pathologic nature (eg, hyperplastic, hamartomas or adenomas).
• Histologic appearance (eg, tubular, tubulovillous, villous).
• Neoplastic dignity (ie, benign, malignant).

Adenomatous and large serrated form of hyperplastic polyps are potentially malignant, whereas nonadenomatous polyps (eg, hyperplastic, hamartomatous, or inflammatory polyps) are benign. The adenomatous transition from benign to cancerous to some degree is paralleled by the increase in size (advanced adenoma: > 1 cm) and varying degrees of dysplasia: once dysplastic cells cross the boundaries of the mucosa (basement membrane) and start to invade the submucosa, a true cancer (carcinoma) with the potential to metastasize is established.

Nonepithelial polyps include lipoma and other mesenchymal lesions.

Epidemiology

Incidence: at least 1 polyp in 25–40% of average-risk persons $\geq$ 50 years. Distal polyps = indicators $\rightarrow$ 5 times higher risk for more proximal lesions; > 50% of proximal advanced adenomas do not have distal polyps.

Presence of adenomatous polyps $\rightarrow$ 2–4 times higher risk of metachronous polyps (compared with absence of polyps). Repeat colonoscopy after 1–3 years $\rightarrow$ 3–5% advanced adenomas.

Symptoms

Polyps (regardless of pathology) most commonly asymptomatic; larger polyps $\rightarrow$ bleeding, anemia, lead point for intussusception, obstructive symptoms; large villous adenoma $\rightarrow$ mucus drainage, electrolyte imbalances.

Differential Risk Assessment

Adenomatous polyps $\rightarrow$ cancer risk: villous > tubulovillous > tubular; size: < 1 cm $\rightarrow$ 3–9%, 1–2 cm $\rightarrow$ 10%, > 2 cm $\rightarrow$ 30–50%.

Hyperplastic polyps: no increased cancer risk, except for large serrated polyps.

Serrated adenoma: intermediate pathology between hyperplastic and adenomatous polyp $\rightarrow$ dysplasia and risk of cancer.

Hamartomatous polyps: no increased risk from the polyp itself, but potentially an indicator for otherwise increased risk → polyposis syndromes.

Inflammatory polyps: no increased risk of the polyp itself, but chronic inflammation (ulcerative colitis, Crohn disease) → increased cancer risk (often without polypoid mass).

Pathology

Adenomatous polyps

At least low-grade dysplasia (by definition) → high-grade dysplasia if presence of irregular branching, back-to-back glandular and cribriform structures, loss of polarity, frequent mitosis:

- Tubular adenoma: packed epithelial tubules with largely preserved basoapical cell differentiation and narrow stroma → some distortion, hyperchromic nuclei, mitotic figures rare.
- Tubulovillous adenoma: combination of tubular and villous components.
- Villous adenoma: > 80% long finger-like projections.

Nonadenomatous polyps

- Hyperplastic polyps: 2–5 mm, most frequently in rectosigmoid, often multiple; crypt elongation, loss of columnar and goblet cell regularity → papillary or serrated appearance, moderate chronic inflammatory cells.
- Hamartomatous polyps: non-neoplastic, incorrect combination of tissue components → "Swiss cheese" pathology: mucus-filled cystic spaces, connective tissue with acute and chronic inflammatory cells.
- Inflammatory polyps (pseudopolyps).

Evaluation

Required minimal standard

Colorectal cancer screening and surveillance (per guidelines).

Diagnostic colonic evaluation for symptomatic patients.

Histopathology of resected/biopsied polyps → guidance for repeat testing.

Additional tests (optional)

Genetic counseling/testing if familial clustering or patient at young age.

Classification

Haggitt classification for cancerous polyps → description of tumor invasion in pedunculated or sessile polyp:

- Pedunculated polyps:
  - Level 1: invasion limited to the head.
  - Level 2: invasion to the neck.
  - Level 3: invasion into the stalk.
  - Level 4: invasion to the base, ie, submucosa at the level of the bowel wall → 10% risk for lymph node metastases (like other T1 cancers).
- Sessile polyps → all lesions are level 4 (as above), additional level of submucosal invasion (Kudo classification: levels Sm1, Sm2, Sm3).

Nonoperative Treatment

Endoscopic polypectomy and surveillance.

Chemoprevention: COX inhibitors, calcium, ASA → up to 35–45% reduction of metachronous polyps.

No benefit of oncologic resection: complete removal (snared in one piece) of cancerous polyp Haggitt levels 1, 2, and 3, well differentiated, no lymphovascular invasion, > 2 mm margin.

Operative Treatment

Indications

- Any polyp that is not amenable to endoscopic removal (unless prohibitive contraindications).
- Cancerous polyp with invasion into submucosa (Haggitt level 4, deep invasion into level Sm3), < 2 mm margin or piecemeal excision, unfavorable histology (poor differentiation, lymphovascular invasion).

Operative approach

- Colon polyp: colonoscopic tattooing of target site → laparoscopic vs. open segmental resection (satisfying oncologic criteria) with primary anastomosis.
- Rectal polyp:
  - Transanal excision or transanal endoscopic microsurgery (TEM).
  - Low anterior resection (LAR).

Outcome

Colonoscopic polypectomies: reduction of cancer incidence by 76–90% (compared with expected historic rates). Risk of complications from polypectomy: perforation 0.1–0.3%, bleeding 0.5–3%.

Follow-up

Schedule for follow-up colonoscopies per guidelines.

Cross-reference

POLYPOSIS SYNDROMES *(211.3, 235.2)*

Overview

Polyposis syndromes are characterized by the presence/development of numerous polyps in various parts of the GI tract, but frequently involve other manifestations. Some invariably lead to malignant transformation of the polyps and the development of cancer (eg, FAP, AFAP); other syndromes have polyps that remain benign and do not pose a direct cancer risk but may be an indicator of an increased risk for other intestinal or extraintestinal tumors.

Familial adenomatous polyposis (FAP, AFAP)

- Phenotype: multiple adenomatous polyps throughout the colon, periampullary duodenal polyps, gastric polyps, extracolonic manifestations (desmoids, etc).
- Genetics: autosomal dominant, near complete penetrance.
- Gene location: adenomatous polyposis coli (*APC*) gene on chromosome 5q21.
- Natural course: nearly 100% colon cancer by age 40–45, 3–12% periampullary carcinoma.
- Associated malignancies: colon cancer, pouch cancer, periampullary adenocarcinoma, desmoid, thyroid cancer.
- Variants:
  - Gardener syndrome: osteomas, desmoid tumors, thyroid neoplasms, congenital hypertrophy of the retinal pigment epithelium.
  - Turcot syndrome: brain tumors.
  - Attenuated FAP (AFAP): later presentation, more proximal polyp distribution.

MYH-associated Polyposis (MAP)

- Phenotype: often indistinguishable from FAP, except for slightly lower number of adenomatous polyps throughout the colon; extracolonic manifestations are present but less frequent than FAP: upper GI tract polyps (→ periampullary cancer), osteomas, dental abnormalities, CHRPE, etc.
- Genetics: autosomal recessive, near complete penetrance.
- Gene location: base excision repair gene *MYH,* chromosome 1p34-32.
- Natural course: diagnosis of MAP around age 50, nearly 100% colon cancer by age 65.
- Associated malignancies: colon cancer, periampullary adenocarcinoma, breast cancer, thyroid cancer.
- Counseling: both parents and all children are gene carriers.

Peutz-Jeghers syndrome
- Phenotype: hamartomatous polyps of the GI tract, particularly upper GI tract, cutaneous melanin deposits (eg, perioral, buccal mucosa, etc).
- Genetics: autosomal dominant, variable penetrance.
- Gene location: *LKB1/STK* (chromosome 19p13), and other genes.
- Natural course: majority of patients asymptomatic, rarely obstructive symptoms or bleeding.
- Associated malignancies: moderately increased risk of GI and extraintestinal malignancies.

Juvenile polyposis syndrome
- Phenotype: hamartomatous polyps, 15% associated with congenital birth defects.
- Genetics: autosomal dominant.
- Gene location: *BMPR1A* or *SMAD-4* gene (chromosome 18q21), and other genes.
- Natural course: average age of onset 18 years, polyps most frequently in rectosigmoid region; variable symptoms: GI bleeding, intussusception, rectal prolapse, protein-losing enteropathy.
- Associated malignancies: significant risk of colorectal cancer.
- Diagnostic criteria: ≥ three juvenile polyps, polyposis involving entire GI tract, or any number of polyps but known family history of juvenile polyps.
- Caveat: isolated juvenile polyps without malignant potential.

Cowden syndrome
- Phenotype: multiple hamartoma-neoplasia syndrome from ectodermal and less from endodermal elements: tricholemmoma 80%, macrocephaly 40%, GI polyposis only in 35%, benign thyroid or breast disease.
- Genetics: autosomal dominant, nearly complete penetrance.
- Gene location: *PTEN* tumor suppressor gene, chromosome 10q23.
- Natural course: symptomatic by age 20 years.
- Associated malignancies: no increased risk of GI malignancy, 10% thyroid cancer, 30–50% breast cancer.

Bannayan-Riley-Ruvalcaba syndrome (formerly Ruvalcaba-Myhre-Smith syndrome)
- Phenotype: excessive growth before/after birth, macrocephaly, mental and psychomotor retardation, and other abnormalities; multiple hamartomatous polyps in GI tract; lipomas; genital pigmented macules.
- Genetics: autosomal dominant, nearly complete penetrance.

- Gene location: *PTEN* tumor suppressor gene, chromosome 10q23.
- Natural course: pediatric counterpart to Cowden syndrome.
- Associated malignancies: no increased risk of colorectal cancer, or any other GI or extraintestinal malignancy.

Cronkhite-Canada syndrome
- Phenotype: diffuse polyposis throughout entire GI tract (except esophageal sparing), ectodermal abnormalities (eg, alopecia, onychodystrophy, skin hyperpigmentations).
- Genetics: autosomal dominant.
- Gene location: *PTEN* tumor suppressor gene, chromosome 10q23.
- Natural course: diarrhea, protein-loosing enteropathy, weight loss, nausea, vomiting, anorexia, paresthesias, seizures and tetany related to electrolyte abnormalities.
- Associated malignancies: increased risk for cancer of stomach, colon, and rectum (15% with malignant tumor at time of diagnosis).

Hyperplastic polyposis syndrome
- Phenotype: multiple hyperplastic polyps throughout entire colon and rectum, including large polyps (> 1 cm) and location proximal to sigmoid colon.
- Genetics: unknown.
- Gene location: unknown.
- Natural course: average age 50–70 years, no specific symptoms.
- Associated malignancies: increased risk for colorectal cancer, proximal > distal.

Nodular lymphoid hyperplasia
- Phenotype: multiple lymphoid polyps throughout entire colon and rectum.
- Genetics: unknown.
- Gene location: unknown.
- Natural course: children and adults, no specific symptoms, occasionally associated with immunodeficiency disorders.
- Associated malignancies: no increased risk for colorectal cancer.

Additional tests
Genetic counseling and testing → individual and family risk assessment.

Cross-reference

FAMILIAL ADENOMATOUS POLYPOSIS
(FAP; 211.3, 235.2, V84.09)

Overview

FAP is an autosomal dominant inherited syndrome with near complete penetrance in forming benign and malignant colonic and extracolonic tumors. Caused by a germline mutation in the adenomatous polyposis coli (*APC*) gene on chromosome 5q21 which results in transcription of truncated/nonfunctional protein instead of tumor-suppressing APC protein. Phenotype varies depending on exact location of *APC* mutation. Affected patients develop > 100, often several thousand, adenomatous intestinal polyps, starting at young age (early teens to early 20s), with nearly 100% probability of developing colorectal cancer (CRC) by age 40–45 years unless prophylactic surgery is performed. Attenuated variant of FAP (AFAP) with lower number of polyps, later onset of resulting cancer, often rectal sparing.

Extracolonic manifestations:

- Duodenal adenomas in > 80% of FAP patients; periampullary adenocarcinoma in 3–12% of FAP patients = second most frequent cancer in FAP, main cause of cancer-related death (since colorectal cancer [CRC] risk is eliminated by prophylactic surgery).

- Desmoids: locally invasive/expansive proliferation of fibromatous tumors affecting 10–15% of FAP patients (majority after surgical trauma); familial pattern → leading cause of death in FAP patients (ureteral and SBO, inability to perform other necessary surgeries); specific sites of *APC* mutations associated with increased desmoid risk.

- Gastric fundic gland polyps: in 30–60% of FAP patients, nonadenomatous nature, no malignant potential.

- Congenital hypertrophy of the retinal pigmented epithelium (CHRPE): most common extracolonic manifestation of FAP (60–85% of patients with FAP): bilateral benign pigmented hamartomas; no clinical significance; 95% specific as cheap, noninvasive screening test in families with FAP.

- Papillary thyroid cancer: 1–2%, especially in younger women.

- Hepatoblastoma: uncommon tumor in children with FAP.

Epidemiology

Less than 1% of all CRC, 1 in 7000–10,000 live births; 70–80% are truly inherited (even if positive family history not always evident), 20–30% are new germline mutations.

Symptoms

Negative family history: symptoms from growing and increasingly numerous polyps/cancer: bleeding, urgency, colorectal cancer at young age, potentially extracolonic manifestations (osteomas, dental malformation, retinal hyperpigmentation).

Positive family history: diagnosis and prophylactic treatment before symptoms!

Differential Diagnosis

Other types of hereditary cancers: HNPCC (autosomal dominant), MAP (homozygous recessive).

Familial CRC without identifiable gene mutation.

Nonadenomatous polyposis, eg, hyperplastic polyposis.

Diffuse lymphoid hyperplasia.

Pathology

Macroscopic: > 100 polyps throughout the colon, starting as small sessile polyps, increasing in size.

Microscopic: adenomatous polyps.

Evaluation

Required minimal standard
All patients

Identification/management of family members at risk: chart documentation that patient was counseled and informed about this aspect (caveat: litigation!).

Biopsy confirmation of adenomatous nature of polyps.

EGD: baseline endoscopy in early 20s, subsequent frequency depending on findings.

Asymptomatic patient/family members with positive family history

Family history, genetic counseling/testing (unless already done).

Annual colonoscopy starting at age 12–14 years, removal of larger polyps.

Screening for other extracolonic cancers: EGD (bi-)annually.

At age 15–25 years or if already diagnosed with cancer or large/high-grade polyps → surgery.

Patients with CRC and multiple synchronous polyps

Diagnosis: rigid sigmoidoscopy or flexible endoscopy + biopsy → multiple adenomatous polyps.

EGD: upper GI involvement?

Family history.

Genetic counseling/testing.

Individual workup as for sporadic CRC → surgery.

Additional tests (optional)

Same as for CRC.

Genetic testing.

Thyroid ultrasound.

Classification

Variants of the adenomatous polyposis syndrome classified as:

- Gardener syndrome (*APC* mutation at the 3′ end of exon 15): osteomas, dental anomalies (form/number), epidermal cysts, desmoid tumors, thyroid neoplasms, CHRPE.
- Turcot syndrome: brain tumors (medulloblastoma, glioblastoma).
- AFAP (attenuated FAP): lower number and later onset of both the polyps and the resulting cancer, rectum often spared.

Nonoperative Treatment

Caveat: currently, nonoperative management can only be considered supportive, but not with the intent to replace surgery.

Chemoprevention: role not defined. NSAID-derivatives with inhibition unselectively for COX-1/COX-2 or selectively for COX-2 (eg, sulindac, celecoxib): reduction of colonic polyps, but uncertain whether cancer reduced or delayed; no effect on duodenal adenomas. Potential benefit for desmoid tumors: overall only a supportive but never a definitive treatment for FAP.

Annual colonoscopy and polypectomy (does not replace need for prophylactic surgery).

Depending on tumor stage: adjuvant chemotherapy (colon cancer), chemoradiation (proven rectal cancer): always in neoadjuvant setting if ileal J-pouch planned to avoid radiating the pouch.

Operative Treatment

Indications

- Asymptomatic affected member of FAP family: plan surgery at age between 15–25 years.
- Symptomatic patients (incidental FAP diagnosis): any cancer, advanced adenoma (large size or high-grade dysplasia), or increasing number of

polyps, unless diffuse metastases or prohibitive contraindications. Caveat: neoadjuvant chemoradiation for all rectal cancers!

Operative approach

- Proctocolectomy with ileal J-pouch anal anastomosis (IPAA): double-stapling technique (routine), or mucosectomy and handsewn anastomosis (rectal cancer/dysplasia/very distal polyps).
- Colectomy and ileorectal anastomosis (IRA): if < 20 rectal polyps, no cancer.
- Proctocolectomy and ileostomy: if contraindication for J-pouch.

Outcome

Prophylactic surgery → elimination of CRC, elimination of ampullary cancer, but persistent risk for desmoids, small bowel, and pouch cancer.

Outcome of therapeutic surgery for CRC, ampullary cancer, and thyroid cancer is dependent on tumor stage.

Follow-up

Continued annual surveillance/screening of residual rectal mucosa and/or pouch.

Frequency of EGD is dependent on upper GI involvement.

Participation in registry for inherited CRC is recommended.

Cross-reference

Topic	*Chapter*
Carcinogenesis	3 (p 156)
Polyps	4 (p 236)
Polyposis syndromes	4 (p 240)
Colorectal cancer	4 (pp 252–265)
(Sub-)Total colectomy	5 (p 553)
Proctocolectomy/IPAA	5 (p 560)
Chemoprevention	6 (p 636)

HEREDITARY NONPOLYPOSIS COLON CANCER
(HNPCC, 153.8, V84.09)

Overview

HNPCC (Lynch syndrome I/II, syndrome X) is the most common form of inherited colorectal cancer (CRC). Underlying autosomal dominant mutations in DNA mismatch repair genes: *hMLH1* and *hMSH2* (90% of the mutations in HNPCC families), *hMSH6* (7–10%), *PMS1,* and *PMS2* (5%).

Caveat: despite "nonpolyposis" label, cancer arises within polyp precursor lesion, but there are not hundreds of polyps.

Epidemiology

Constitutes 3–5% of all CRC. HNPCC: autosomal dominant disorder, penetrance ~80%. Accelerated adenoma-carcinoma sequence (2–3 years). Lifetime risk of developing colon cancer ~80%, endometrial cancer 40–60%, urinary tract cancer 18–20%, ovarian cancer 9–12%. Risk of metachronous colorectal cancer 45% (after segmental resection, 10–15% after total colectomy/ileorectostomy); 70% of colon tumors are proximal to splenic flexures.

Symptoms

Development of colorectal (and associated) cancer at young age. Symptoms often absent, otherwise not principally different from sporadic CRC.

Differential Diagnosis

Other types of hereditary cancers: FAP, MAP.

Familial CRC without identifiable gene mutation.

Pathology

Macroscopic: limited number of (often flat) polyps, predominantly right-sided (ie, proximal to splenic flexure).

Microscopic: cancers often poorly differentiated adenocarcinoma; medullary growth pattern, signet ring, and mucinous differentiation.

Microsatellite instability (MSI): 90–95% of HNPCC tumors are MSI+, high frequency of MSI (changes in ≥ two of the five panels) compared with 15–20% MSI+ in sporadic CRC.

Evaluation

Required minimal standard
All patients
Identification/management of family members at risk: chart documentation that patient was counseled and informed about this aspect (caveat: litigation!).

Asymptomatic patient/family members with positive family history
Family history, genetic counseling/testing (unless already done).

Annual colonoscopy starting age of 25 years (no later than 10–15 years prior to cancer onset in youngest family member).

Women: $\rightarrow$ annual endometrial aspiration.

Screening for other extracolonic cancers: lack of clear guidelines $\rightarrow$ according to family patterns. If cancer, high-grade polyps, or increasing number of polyps $\rightarrow$ surgery.

Patient < 50 years of age with CRC
Family history: Amsterdam criteria? In ~50% of proven HNPCC, families do not meet criteria.

Genetic testing: Bethesda criteria?

Identification/management of family members at risk: chart documentation that patient was informed about this aspect (caveat: litigation!)

Individual workup as for sporadic CRC prior to surgery.

Additional tests (optional)
Same as for CRC.

Classification

- Amsterdam II criteria: ~50% of families who meet criteria have HNPCC.
- Bethesda criteria $\rightarrow$ MSI+, MSI–.
- Lynch I: CRC only.
- Lynch II: CRC and extracolonic malignancies.
- Muir-Torre syndrome: inherited CRC with sebaceous tumors of the skin.
- Syndrome X: familial CRC of undetermined type; strong family history of CRC only (Amsterdam-positive, MSI-negative, normal *MMR* genes), more common on the left side, nonmucinous, not multifocal, average age of onset: 50th decade.

Nonoperative Treatment

Chemoprevention: role not defined.

Annual colonoscopy and polypectomy.

Depending on tumor stage: adjuvant chemotherapy (colon), or (neo-)adjuvant chemoradiation (rectum).

Operative Treatment

Indications

Any cancer, advanced adenoma (large size or high-grade dysplasia), or increasing number of polyps, unless diffuse metastases or prohibitive contraindications.

Operative approach

- Subtotal colectomy (therapeutic + prophylactic): recommended for all tumors proximal to sigmoid colon, unless rejected by patient or patient-specific medical contraindication to extensive colon shortening).
- Segmental colorectal resection: therapeutic only (following oncologic principles).
- Rectal cancer in HNPCC: low anterior resection (with/without neoadjuvant chemoradiation), prophylactic proctocolectomy typically not recommended because of its significant functional impact.
- Women (particularly if uterine cancer in family, or mutations in *hMSH6*, or in *hMSH2* and *hMLH1*): consideration/discussion of hysterectomy/oophorectomy (when childbearing completed, beginning of menopause, or during any other abdominal surgery).

Outcome

Controversial whether in a stage-by-stage comparison MSI is associated with better outcome and better response to chemotherapy than sporadic CRC despite poor histopathologic features.

Follow-up

Continued surveillance/screening for CRC and extracolonic tumors → annual complete endoscopy of colorectal mucosa: colonoscopy (presurgery), flexible sigmoidoscopy (after surgery), endometrial aspiration.

Cross-reference

Topic	Chapter
Carcinogenesis	3 (p 156)
Polyps	4 (p 236)

COLORECTAL CANCER—COLON CANCER *(153.X)*

Overview

Colorectal cancer (CRC) is the most frequent malignancy in the realm of the colorectal surgery specialty, the third most frequent cancer overall, and the second leading cause of cancer death. Cancer therefore in the differential diagnosis of almost any symptom.

Intrinsic risk factors: family history, polyps, genetic mutations (FAP, HNPCC), IBD (eg, ulcerative colitis), African American ethnicity.

Extrinsic risk factors: sedentary lifestyle, smoking, radiation colitis, status post ureterosigmoidostomy; diet high in fat/calories/protein and alcohol, low in fiber (more recently questioned again); lack of vitamin D, sun exposure, calcium, folate.

Population risk categories (Table 4–3):

- Low or average risk (65–75%): asymptomatic—no risk factors, no CRC in any first-degree relatives.
- Moderate risk (20–30%): CRC in one first-degree relative aged ≤ 55 years, or ≥ two first-degree relatives of any ages (Table 4–4), personal history of curative resection of colorectal malignancy or large polyp (> 1 cm) or multiple colorectal polyps of any size.
- High risk (6–8%): FAP, HNPCC, IBD.

Evolution from normal colon to established cancer: 10 years (average population), 3–5 years (HNPCC). Slow evolution, carcinogenesis through visible precursor stage (polyp), and ability to completely visualize the colon make CRC theoretically completely preventable. Screening guidelines established but not even close to full implementation.

Choice of optimal treatment depends on stage and tumor location, complications of disease, presentation (ie, emergency vs elective), presence of underlying colonic disease, presence of comorbidities. Distinction of colon cancer (eg, sigmoid cancer) from rectal cancer very important for treatment planning to define the role of (neo-)adjuvant radiation.

Epidemiology

Annual incidence in US: 145,000 new cases of CRC, 55,000 CRC deaths (9–10% of all cancer deaths). Average lifetime risk: 1:18 Americans (5–6%). Peak incidence during 7th decade, but 5% of patients are < 40 years old, 10% < 50 years old. In 90% of patients tumors are sporadic, 10% have positive family history, 1% FAP. CRC is 90% curable if detected early.

Stage at presentation: stage I = 25%, stage II = 30%, stage III = 35%, stage IV = 20%.

TABLE 4-3. Comparison of Major Risk Categories.

	Sporadic Colorectal Cancer	FAP	HNPCC	IBD
Variants		AFAP, Gardner, Turcot	Lynch I/II	Ulcerative colitis Crohn disease
Genetics	–	+ Autosomal-dominant	+ Autosomal-dominant	?
Genes	Chromosomal deletions, k-ras, DCC, p53, APC	APC	MSH2, MLH1, PMS1/2, MSH6	?
Age of onset	> 40 years; average 70–75 years	Polyps start after age 10–20 years, cancer in nearly 100% by age 40 years; later onset in AFAP	< 50 years	Any, often young patients
Number of polyps	Variable, < 10	> 100	< 10	Inflammatory pseudopolyps
Risk	5–6% of population	100%	> 80%	Depending on age at onset, duration of disease, extent of active disease

(Continued)

TABLE 4–3. Comparison of Major Risk Categories. (Continued)

	Sporadic Colorectal Cancer	FAP	HNPCC	IBD
Location	Left > right colon	Any location	Right colon > left	Active disease
Chemoprevention	NSAID? Vitamins? Calcium?	NSAID	?	IBD suppression?
Screening	> 50 years; > 45 years in African-Americans	> 10–15 years Genetic counseling	> 25 or 10–15 years before cancer onset in youngest family member Genetic counseling	7 years post onset, annually
Associated risks	?	Ampullary cancer, desmoids, thyroid cancer, other abnormalities	Endometrial and other cancers	Extracolonic disease

AFAP, attenuated FAP; FAP, familial polyposis syndromes; HNPCC, hereditary nonpolyposis colon cancer; IBD, inflammatory bowel disease.

TABLE 4–4.   Impact of Family History on Risk for Colorectal Cancer.

Affected Family Members	Estimated Risk Compared to 6–7% Lifetime Risk in General Population
1 FDR with CRC	2–3×
2 FDR with CRC	3–4×
1 FDR ≤40 years with CRC	3–4×
1 FDR with adenomatous polyp	2×
1 SDR (grandparents, aunt/uncle) with CRC	1.5×
2 TDR (cousins etc) with CRC	1.5×

CRC, colorectal cancer; FDR, first-degree relative; SDR, second-degree relative; TDR, third-degree relative.

Symptoms

Most commonly asymptomatic → symptoms are always late signs of the cancer!

Incidental detection during colonoscopy.

Symptoms: bleeding, unexplained anemia, altered bowel habits, constipation, narrowed stools, complete obstruction, abdominal pain, perforation, abdominal mass, weight loss.

Complications: massive bleeding, large bowel obstruction, perforation, liver failure.

Differential Diagnosis

Symptoms: any other cause for bleeding or obstruction—IBD, particularly Crohn disease, other forms of colitis (ischemic, infectious including pseudomembranous *C difficile* colitis, radiation), diverticulitis, IBS.

Secondary colon involvement from other malignancies: stomach, pancreas, OB/GYN, kidney, lobular invasive breast cancer, leukemic infiltrates.

Rare tumors: carcinoid, lymphoma, GIST, melanoma.

Premalignant polyps: particularly villous polyps may involve large and circumferential area.

Nonmalignant: endometriosis, prolapse/intussusception, benign tumors (eg, lipoma), pseudoobstruction (Ogilvie syndrome).

Pathology

Macroscopic

- Polypoid friable mass vs ulcerating crater with elevated edges, variable size, and involvement of the circumference (Figures 4–10A and 4–10B). IBD: cancer growth often flat, diffusely growing into wall.

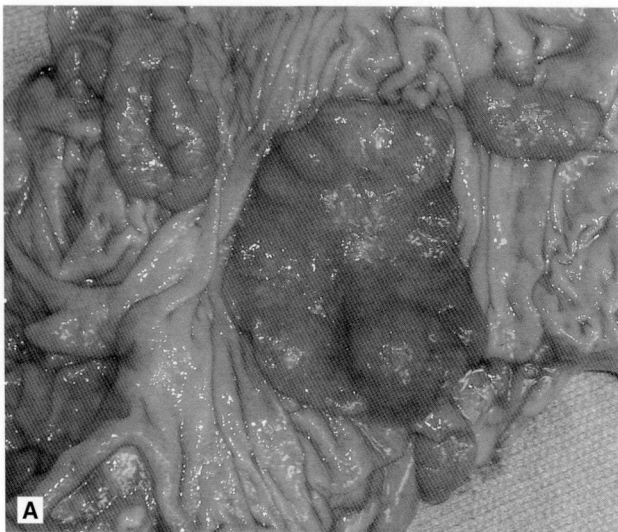

Figure 4–10A. Colorectal cancer specimen with additional polyps.

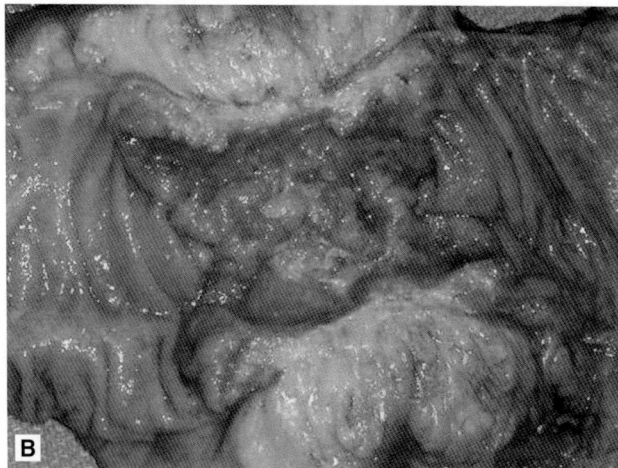

Figure 4–10B. Colorectal cancer specimen with circumferential tumor.

• Pattern of metastatic dissemination: lymphovascular → lymph nodes, hematogenous → portal system → liver metastases → lung metastases.

Microscopic

• Adenocarcinoma in the overwhelming majority of cases (> 95%). Rare subforms: mucinous or signet ring cell carcinoma, adenosquamous carcinoma.
• Intramucosal carcinoma (T_{is}) = carcinoma in situ = high-grade dysplasia: cancer not penetrating through muscularis mucosa. Invasive cancer: invasion of muscularis propria and beyond.
• Negative prognostic growth patterns: lymphovascular invasion, perineural invasion, extranodal tumor deposits.
• Minimum of 12–15 lymph nodes necessary for adequate oncologic staging of specimen.

Evaluation

Required minimal standard

History: bleeding, change in bowel habits, obstructive symptoms, weight loss?

Clinical examination: palpable tumor, abdominal distention, local tenderness or peritoneal signs, organomegaly, digital rectal exam → palpable tumor, blood on stool, or melena?

Distinction between sigmoid cancer and rectal cancer: 15 cm from anal verge by means of rigid sigmoidoscopy.

Colonoscopy: gold standard to establish diagnosis, full colonic evaluation always needed prior to elective surgery to rule out synchronous cancer or polyps to determine extent of resection, low threshold for tattooing of tumor site or most distal/proximal polyp → facilitation of intraoperative localization, particularly for laparoscopic approach.

Abdominal imaging study (sonography, CT scan): evaluation of involvement of liver or urinary system (Figure 4–10C), evidence for carcinomatosis?

Tumor marker: CEA.

Chest x-ray (or chest CT): metastatic disease, free air, cardiopulmonary operability?

Additional tests (optional)

Contrast studies (barium or Gastrografin enema): incomplete colonoscopy, nearly obstructing tumor, suspected perforation (→ water-soluble contrast).

Virtual colonoscopy: role not defined, risk of perforation.

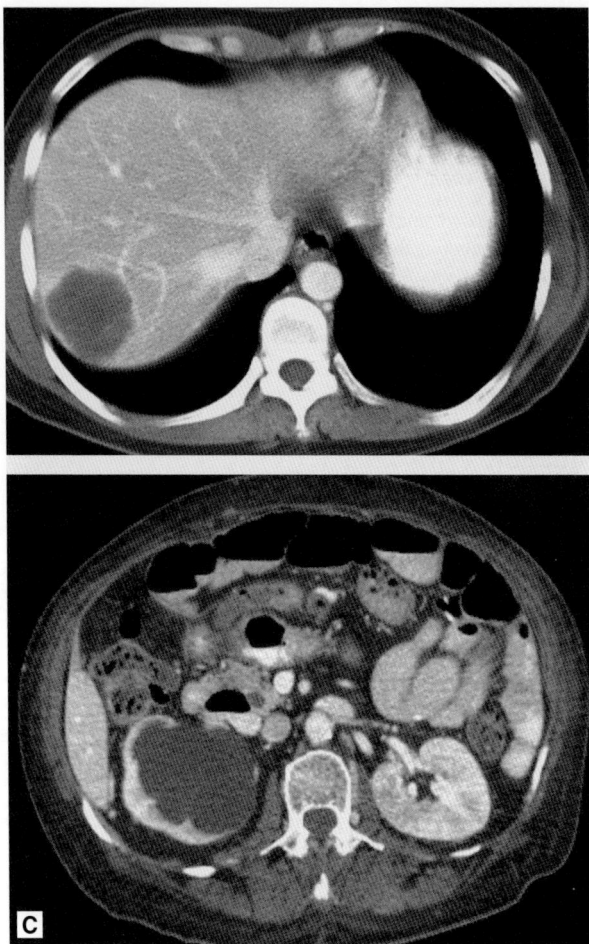

Figure 4–10C. Advanced colorectal cancer with liver metastases or hydronephrosis.

MRI, PET, PET-CT: role not yet defined in primary assessment.

Blood work: anemia, liver function (albumin, PTT, PT), kidney function.

Classification

- Based on location in colon.
- Based on stage: localized, locally advanced (size, infiltration of other structures), metastatic.
- Based on TNM stage.

Nonoperative Treatment

Inoperable patients due to comorbidities

Inoperable/incurable due to extent of abdominal tumor (eg, carcinomatosis) → symptom control, possible stenting.

Metastatic disease with liver replacement > 50% → palliative chemotherapy.

Operative Treatment

Indications

- Any colon cancer (unless prohibitive contraindications).
- Even in presence of systemic tumor manifestations, achieving local tumor control still desirable, potentially simultaneous or staged metastasectomy in curative intent still possible.

Operative approach
Curative intent

- Oncologic resection with lymphadenectomy: > 5 cm safety margin, exact extent of resection depends on site of tumor and lymphovascular drainage (Figure 4–10D):

  – Cecum/ascending: right hemicolectomy with right branch of middle colic artery.

  – Hepatic flexure/transverse colon: extended right hemicolectomy including full middle colic artery.

  – Splenic flexure: (1) extended left hemicolectomy including middle colic artery, (2) extended right hemicolectomy/subtotal colectomy.

  – Descending colon: (1) left hemicolectomy with left branch of middle colic artery to IMA/left colic artery, (2) subtotal colectomy.

  – Sigmoid colon: sigmoid resection with superior hemorrhoidal artery or IMA.

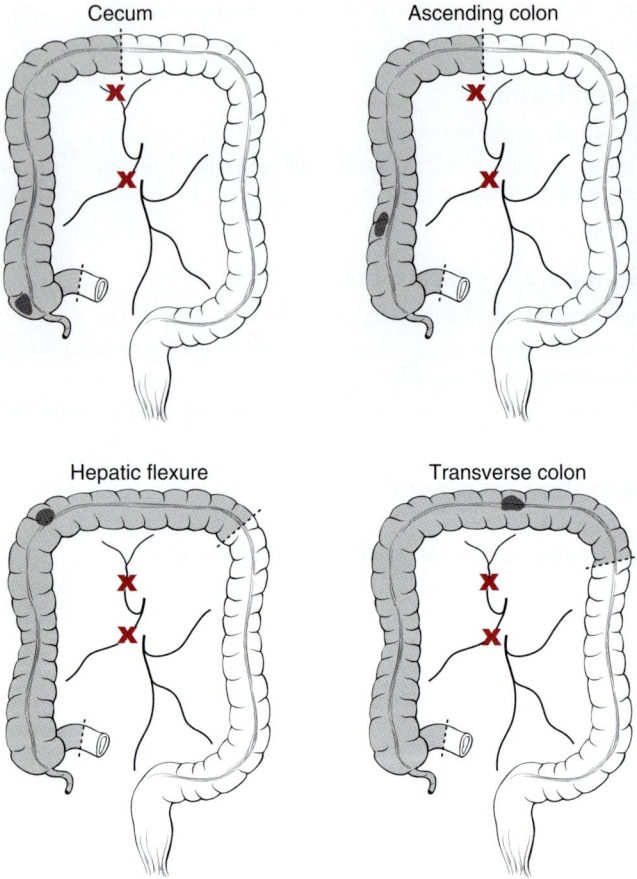

D

Figure 4–10D. Oncologic resections.

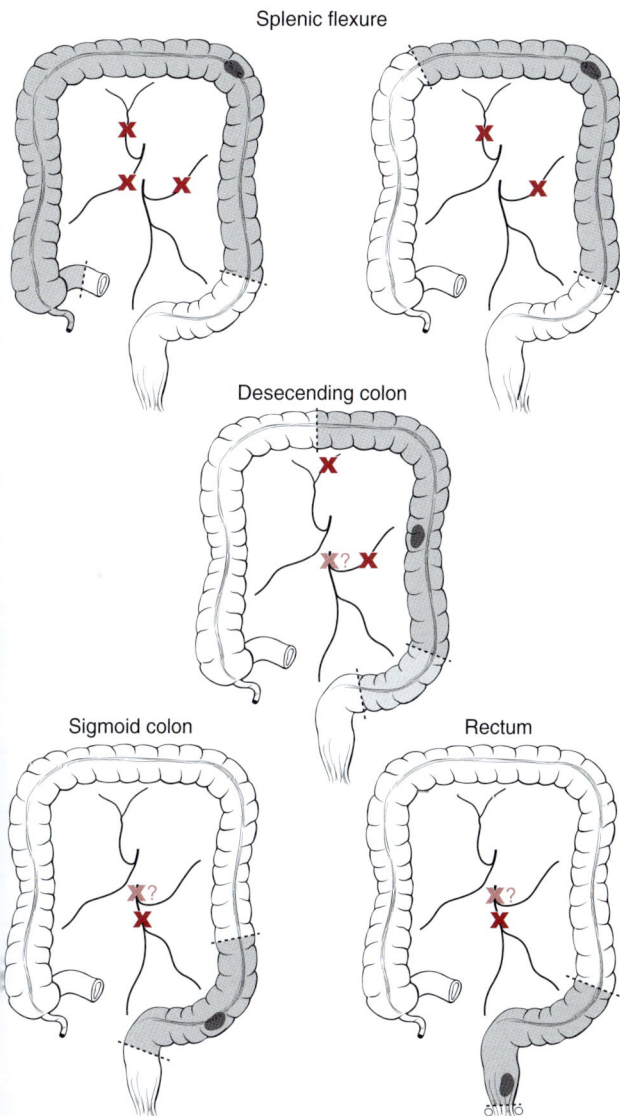

Splenic flexure

Desecending colon

Sigmoid colon

Rectum

D

Figure 4–10D. *(continued)*

- Special considerations:
  - Synchronous cancers: (1) two separate resections, (2) subtotal colectomy.
  - Cancers adhering to other structures: en-bloc resection.
  - Liver metastases: simultaneous resection reasonable if feasible and tolerated (vs staged resection).
  - Prophylactic oophorectomy not indicated but recommended when one or both ovaries grossly abnormal.
  - Carcinomatosis: resection of primary tumor, no routine role for intraperitoneal catheter.
  - Laparoscopic approach equivalent in skilled hands.
- Patient < 50 years/HNPCC: (1) (sub-)total colectomy with ileosigmoidal/-rectal anastomosis, (2) segmental resection (as above)
- FAP: (1) proctocolectomy, (2) total abdominal colectomy with ileorectal anastomosis if no rectal cancer and number of rectal polyps < 20.
- Sentinel lymph node mapping: concerns about high false-negative rate, role not defined.

Emergency
- Right-sided tumor: definitive surgical treatment as above, primary ileo-colonic anastomosis.
- Left-sided tumor:
  - Resection with on-table lavage and primary anastomosis.
  - Stent placement for decompression of LBO → bridging to (semi-)elective resection with primary anastomosis.
  - More extensive resection to allow ileocolonic anastomosis: subtotal colectomy with primary ileosigmoidal or ileorectal anastomosis.
  - Two-stage procedure: (a) Hartmann type resection (→ elective Hartmann reversal), (b) primary anastomosis with proximal diversion (→ elective ostomy takedown), (c) proximal diversion (→ elective resection and ostomy takedown)
  - Three-stage procedure (largely abandoned): proximal diversion (transverse colostomy) → elective resection and anastomosis (with maintained diversion) → elective ostomy takedown.

Palliation
- Segmental wedge resection.
- Proximal diversion only.
- Internal bypassing of obstructed segment.
- Stenting.

Outcome

Five-year survival: all stages 65%; stage I 90–93%, stage II 80–85%, stage III 60–65%, stage IV 5–8%. Prognostic factors: see Table 4–5.

Mortality of elective oncologic resection: 1–3%.

Rate of permanent stoma: minimal in specialized colorectal centers, higher in nonspecialized units: 20–40% of "temporary" stomas (eg, Hartmann resection) never reversed.

Complications: bleeding, wound infections (5–10% elective, 15–40% fecal peritonitis), anastomotic leak (1–2%), abscess formation, enterocutaneous fistula, splenic injury, pancreas injury, ureteral injury.

Follow-up

Emergency intervention: planning of necessary subsequent surgeries after adequate physical/nutritional recovery.

Adjuvant chemotherapy: for all stage III tumors and for selected stage II tumors.

Palliative chemotherapy: for stage IV tumors.

TABLE 4–5.   Prognostic Factors for Resected Colorectal Cancer.

Category	Parameter
Stage	Tumor penetration through the bowel wall (T4 tumor stage)
	Regional lymph node involvement (N1, N2)
	≥4 positive regional lymph nodes (N2)
Surgeon/pathologist	Tumor involvement of surgical margins
	≤12 lymph nodes removed (surgeon) or examined/reported (pathologist)
Tumor complication	Bowel obstruction
	Bowel perforation (particularly if perforation at tumor site)
Histopathology	Poorly differentiated histology
	Lymphovascular invasion
	Perineural invasion
Marker	Preoperative CEA > 5.0
	Microsatellite-stable tumors
	Specific chromosomal deletions (eg, chromosome18q loss of heterozygosity)

CEA, carcinoembryonic antigen.

Oncologic follow-up: colonoscopy after 1 year, subsequently depending on findings. Clinical examination and blood work (including CEA) every 3–6 months. Imaging (CT abdomen/pelvis, chest x-ray/-CT annually).

Surgical reintervention:

- Metastatic disease: sandwich approach (resection of primary tumor, chemotherapy, resection of metastases).
- Recurrent disease: re-resection if localized.
- Carcinomatosis: one exploration often justified, subsequently individualized.

Cross-reference

COLORECTAL CANCER—RECTAL CANCER *(154.1)*

Overview

Colon and rectal cancer share the majority of baseline features (eg, etiopathogenesis, symptoms, pathology). However, rectal cancer—unlike colon cancer—is more complex and carries an increased risk of local recurrences. Higher complexity is related to intricate rectal anatomy with bony pelvic confinement, proximity to other organs, proximity to sphincter and pelvic floor muscles; various levels of blood supply; multidirectional lymphovascular drainage within a defined fascial compartment.

Treatment of rectal cancer has therefore evolved from a surgery-only to a multi-modality approach. While spectrum of treatment options continue to expand (radical vs local, sphincter-preserving vs APR, open vs laparoscopic, etc), the surgeon's experience and surgical technique as well as pretreatment assessment of tumor extension are of utmost importance for outcome.

Except for very early stages of rectal cancer, preoperative or postoperative radiotherapy, generally in combination with chemotherapy, is indicated per NCI guidelines to improve local tumor control, even though overall survival is not necessarily prolonged. Quality-of-life issues (eg, sphincter preservation, ostomy, urogenital function) are much more relevant in the decision-making process for rectal than for colon cancer.

Definition of proximal beginning of rectum:

1. Anatomic/intraoperative: confluence of tenia.
2. Endoscopic (most relevant because of neoadjuvant treatment): 15 cm above anal verge as measured by rigid sigmoidoscope.

Obsolete definitions (because too variable): peritoneal reflection, sacral promontory.

Epidemiology

Annual incidence in US: 42,000 new rectal cancers, 15,000 rectal cancer deaths. Increasing incidence after age 50, peak in the 7th decade, but 5–10% of patients are younger than 50 years.

Symptoms

Asymptomatic → detection during routine exam.

Bleeding (most common), change in bowel habits (frequency, consistency, diameter), constipation, abdominal pain, tenesmus. Rectal/pelvic pain is uncommon and an ominous sign.

Complications: massive bleeding, obstruction, invasion of other organs, perforation, formation of fistula (rectovaginal, perirectal, rectourinary).

Differential Diagnosis

Anal cancer: based on location, most commonly squamous cell cancer (caveat: adenocarcinoma arising from anal canal glands).

Adenocarcinoma of other primary origin: prostate cancer, ovarian and endometrial cancer. Tumor (also adenocarcinoma) may invade through rectal wall → overall presentation, histology, and immunohistochemistry needed for differentiation.

Rare anorectal tumors: carcinoid, lymphoma, GIST, melanoma, presacral mass (chordoma, teratoma, etc).

Premalignant polyps: particularly villous polyps may involve large and circumferential area.

Benign conditions: rectal prolapse/intussusception, solitary rectal ulcer syndrome, endometriosis, inflammatory conditions (radiation proctitis, IBD, etc).

Pathology

Macroscopic
- Polypoid friable mass vs ulcerating crater with elevated edges, variable size, and involvement of the circumference.
- Pattern of metastatic dissemination: (1) lymphovascular → lymph nodes: perirectal (mesorectum), lateral pelvic sidewall, retroperitoneal; (2) hematogenous → portal system → liver metastases → lung metastases. (3) hematogenous → vena cava → lung metastases.

Microscopic
- Adenocarcinoma in the overwhelming majority of cases (> 95%). Rare subforms: mucinous or signet ring cell carcinoma, adenosquamous carcinoma. Small cell carcinoma (1%): dismal prognosis!
- Intramucosal carcinoma (T_{is}) = carcinoma in situ = high-grade dysplasia: cancer not penetrating through muscularis mucosa. Invasive cancer: invasion of muscularis propria and beyond.
- Negative prognostic growth patterns: lymphovascular invasion, perineural invasion, extranodal tumor deposits.
- Minimum of 12–15 lymph nodes necessary for adequate oncologic staging of the specimen, but decreased number after radiation.
- Additional secondary postchemoradiation changes include tissue fibrosis, residual mucinous lakes, endangitis obliterans of arterioles.

Evaluation

Required minimal standard

History: specific symptoms—bleeding, constipation, change in bowel habits, pain, weight loss, urinary/vaginal symptoms, preexisting sexual or anal sphincter dysfunction; family history; comorbidities.

Clinical examination:

1. Digital rectal exam:
   a. Exact description of tumor location:
      (1) Radial: anterior, posterior, lateral, or circumferential.
      (2) Axial: distance of most distal tumor edge from anal verge and from puborectalis muscle, relation to level of the prostate, proximal end reachable? For very distal tumors: assessment of distance to intersphincteric groove, assessment of baseline sphincter strength.
   b. Clinical impression of stage: mobile, tethered, fixed tumor, nearly obstructing.

2. Rigid sigmoidoscopy/proctoscopy: sufficient to establish diagnosis (and perform biopsy), should be repeated prior to elective surgery, particularly after neoadjuvant treatment → assessment of distance from anal verge to bottom of tumor, location, circumferential extent, length and patency of tumor-involved segment, condition of noninvolved rectum.

3. Abdominal exam: habitus, organomegaly, etc.

4. Inguinal lymph node palpation: mandatory for very low rectal and anal tumors; ominous sign if found to be enlarged.

Biopsy: histologic confirmation of clinical suspicion, basis for treatment planning.

Full colonic evaluation (preferably colonoscopy) mandatory prior to elective surgery: → rule out synchronous cancers or polyps, rule out underlying colonic disease.

Evaluation of local extension and tumor staging:

• Local evaluation:
  – ERUS: assessment of T stage (80–95% accuracy), N stage (65–81% accuracy), not reliable for circumferential/lateral margins (fascia propria of the rectum).
  – MRI: evaluation of circumferential margins (60–90% accuracy), but less reliable for T stage (75–85%).

• Systemic evaluation:
  – CT scan of abdomen/pelvis: evaluation of distant metastases (liver, retroperitoneal lymph nodes), evidence of urinary tract involvement (hydronephrosis/-ureter? blurring of rectoprostatic plane?).
  – Chest x-ray (or chest CT): metastatic disease, operability?

Additional tests (optional)
Tumor marker: CEA.
Blood work: anemia, liver function (albumin, PTT, PT), kidney function.
PET (?): if suspicion of distant tumor manifestations.
CT scan of chest: not routinely, required by some study protocols.
Urologic exam, GYN exam: if specific symptoms or findings.

Classification

• Based on location: low (0–5 cm), mid (5–10 cm), or upper rectum (10–15 cm).
• Based on stage: localized, locally advanced (size, infiltration of other structures), metastatic.
• Based on TNM stage.
• Early favorable tumor: uT1-2N0, < 40% of circumference involved, < 3–4 cm, well-differentiated adenocarcinoma, absence of lymphovascular or perineural invasion.

Nonoperative Treatment

Inoperable patients due to comorbidities or metastatic liver replacement > 50%.

Inoperable/incurable due to extent of local tumor → symptom control.

Neoadjuvant chemoradiation (combined modality treatment) to achieve local tumor control:

• 2500 cGy short-term radiation over 1 week, followed by radical surgery after 1 week.
• 5040 cGy radiation over 6 weeks, followed by radical surgery after 6–12 week interval.
• 15–25% complete clinical and endosonographic response: → while surgery is still considered standard of care, nonoperative/ expectant approach to be offered to patient → clinical, endoscopic, and endosonographic reevaluation within short intervals, salvage surgery if evidence of recurrence.

Small cell cancer: systemic disease, dismal prognosis → chemoradiation, but most commonly no role for surgery.

Operative Treatment

Indications
• Any rectal cancer (unless prohibitive contraindications), with/without neoadjuvant chemoradiation.

• Even in presence of systemic tumor manifestations, achieving local tumor control still desirable, potentially later metastasectomy in curative intent possible.

Operative approach
Curative intent (local tumor control, overall intent to cure)
• Local excision: option for early and favorable tumors → transanal local excision or transanal microscopic excision (TEM).
• Radical excision (oncologic resection with lymphadenectomy): total/partial mesorectal excision (TME), abdominoperineal resection (APR) vs sphincter-salvaging operation with primary anastomosis (one/two stage).
• Pelvic exenteration.
• Rare approaches: Kraske (posterior proctotomy), York-Mason (posterior anoproctotomy).

Emergency
• Temporizing measures: stent placement vs proximal diversion.
• Definitive surgical treatment: as above for elective, or Hartmann-type resection.

Palliation
• Proximal diversion.
• Stenting.
• Local destruction: electrocoagulation, laser, endocavitary radiation therapy.

Outcome

Benchmark of radical surgical technique: local recurrence rate < 10% without neo-/adjuvant treatment.

Local recurrence rates for transanal excision: 20–30%.

Five-year survival: all stages 65%, stages I 90–93%, stage II 80–85%, stage III 60–65%, stage IV 5–8%.

Mortality of elective oncologic resection: 3–5%.

Rate of permanent stoma: 5% in specialized colorectal centers, 20–25% in nonspecialized units.

Complications: bleeding 4–10% (presacral veins), wound infections 5–10%, leak with/without pelvic sepsis 5–15% (particularly after neoadjuvant radiation), abscess formation, fistula (perirectal, rectovaginal), ileostomy-related complications, SBO. Sexual and urinary dysfunction.

Follow-up

Emergency surgery: planning of subsequent surgeries after complete physical/nutritional recovery, and potential chemoradiation treatment.

Elective surgery:

• Ileostomy takedown > 6 weeks if clinically and radiologically no evidence for leak, often delayed until full course of adjuvant chemotherapy delivered (eg, 6 months).

• Local excision: final pathology T1 → surgery only, T2 → chemoradiation or radical surgery, T3 → radical surgery.

Long-term: oncologic follow-up, possible complemented with ERUS. Management of recurrent rectal cancer.

Cross-reference

RECURRENT RECTAL CANCER *(789.3, 154.1)*

Overview

Recurrent rectal cancer is a challenge to management and surgical skills. Nihilistic approach is counterproductive, as there is a good chance for cancer cure or at least best local palliation. Local tumor recurrence is the endpoint of failure in primary treatment of rectal cancer. The most effective way to manage recurrent disease is to avoid it.

Several factors contribute to primary local tumor control:

- Primary prevention.
- Tumor-related: tumor stage, localization of the primary tumor and/or its lymph node metastases, pathologic and molecular features.
- Treatment-related: surgical technique, neo-/adjuvant chemoradiation.
- Secondary prevention: follow-up and surveillance → detection of locoregional or distant recurrence, or metachronous lesions.

Natural course of locally advanced, unresectable rectal cancer: shortened median survival time (7–8 months without any treatment), accumulation of severe disabling local problems.

Recurrent rectal cancer remains confined to pelvis in ~25–50% and hence justifies an aggressive surgical approach. Even in the presence of distant metastases, an aggressive local approach may achieve the best and fastest palliation, but other treatment options have to be considered.

Epidemiology

Benchmark: local recurrence rate to be < 10% without chemoradiation, but reports indicate recurrence rates between 3% and 50%. Transanal local excision: alarming incidence of local recurrences of 18–37% in even early tumor stages (T1, T2). Greater than sixty percent of recurrences occur during the first 2 years after surgery.

Symptoms

Asymptomatic: detected through follow-up studies: imaging, blood work.

Symptomatic: increasing and potentially severe pain, bleeding, bowel and urinary obstruction, fecal and urinary leakage, vaginal symptoms, fistula/abscess formation.

Differential Diagnosis

Pelvic scaring.

Inflammatory process (chronic leak, fistula, abscess, organizing hematoma, etc).

Other pelvic malignancy (eg, prostate, GYN).

Pathology

Should be consistent with primary tumor.

Evaluation

Required minimal standard

Patient history and follow-up data, previous surgery, current symptoms (rectal, pelvic, urinary, GYN), performance status.

Clinical examination: general appearance, abdominal exam (mass, organomegaly, etc), digital rectal exam (palpable anastomosis, palpable lesion, involvement of pelvic floor and sphincter complex, involvement of prostate).

Colonoscopy: evidence for endoluminal recurrence or metachronous primary colorectal cancer.

Imaging:

- ERUS (for lower lesions).
- CT/MRI abdomen/pelvis: invasion of adjacent organs?
- PET or PET-CT: pelvic activity, evidence for extrapelvic disease?

Verification of recurrence: biopsy (endoscopic, CT- or ultrasound-guided) vs time-dependent change on imaging and blood work, consistent only with recurrence.

Additional tests (optional)

Contrast studies: assessment of residual colon length.

Urology/GYN consultation: if potential tumor invasion cannot be ruled out.

Assessment of general operability.

Classification

Location of the recurrence:

- Central pelvis.
- Lateral pelvic sidewall.
- Presacral.

Nonoperative Treatment

Chemotherapy: indicated for all patients who tolerate it except for immediate perioperative period.

Radiation therapy:

- Tumors not previously radiated: first-line treatment option, potentially followed by a later resection.

– Previously radiated tumors: consideration for intraoperative radiation therapy (IORT), high-dose brachytherapy, or IMRT if status post previous radiotherapy.

Best palliative care: if nonresectable tumor or nonoperable patient.

Operative Treatment

Indications

For aggressive resection:

– Resectable-appearing local recurrence without extrapelvic disease.

– Highly symptomatic, resectable-appearing local recurrence with extrapelvic disease.

For palliative surgery: highly symptomatic, but nonresectable recurrence.

Operative approach

• Re-resection of posterior compartment: redo-LAR with coloanal anastomosis, redo-APR (intraoperative ureteral stents!), potential defect closure with myocutaneous flap.

• Re-resection of posterior compartment (as above), with extension to middle/anterior compartments:

– Male: pelvic exenteration with/without fecal/urinary reconstruction.

– Female: vaginectomy/hysterectomy vs pelvic exenteration, with/without fecal/urinary reconstruction.

Comment: No continence preservation (1) if the anal sphincter complex/pelvic floor muscles tumor-involved and have to be resected, (2) if proximal bowel not reaching pelvic floor, (3) if preoperative fecal incontinence documented, or (4) if the sphincters have been resected in previous procedure.

• Major resection (as above), with inclusion of distal sacrum, etc: high morbidity!

• Nonresective palliation: creation of colostomy/urostomy, stenting.

Outcome

Survival: estimated 30–35% long-term cure.

Symptom control: except for the first 3 months, surgical approach achieves better symptomatic relief than nonsurgical options.

Follow-up

Functional and cancer follow-up with repeated imaging at regular intervals.
Continuation of chemotherapy.

Cross-reference

COLORECTAL CANCER—LIVER METASTASES
(197.7)

Overview

Liver is the most common site for metastatic dissemination of GI malignancies (Figure 4–11). An aggressive workup and management approach is justified in fit patients to improve short- and long-term survival. Systemic chemotherapy generally is indicated if tolerated. Hepatic arterial infusion chemotherapy offers no benefit. Surgical resection carries potential of cure and long-term survival in 30–50% of selected patients (vs 1% 5-year survival if untreated).

Poor prognostic parameters:

- Multiple metastases (> 4).
- Bilateral liver metastases.
- Short interval after primary resection.
- Hilar lymph node metastases ("metastases from metastases").
- Insufficient volume and quality of remnant liver tissue.
- Ascites.

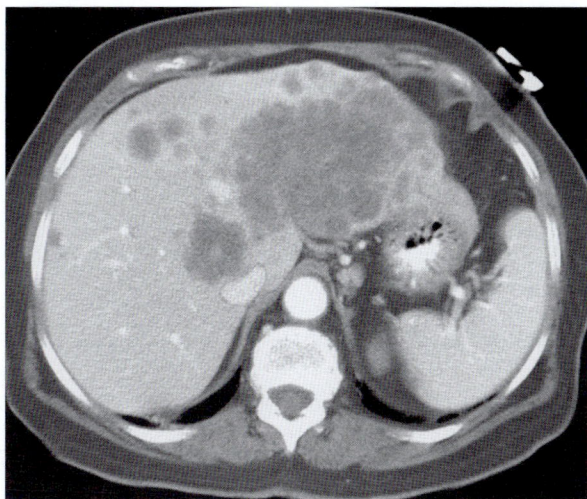

Figure 4–11. Extensive liver metastases.

Timing of liver resection:

- One-stage approach: simultaneous resection (with primary tumor) if both procedures relatively simple.
- Two-stage approach: liver resection after 8–12 weeks of interval chemotherapy. Advantages: assessment of tumor responsiveness to chemotherapy regimen, tumor downsizing with better resectability, elimination of rapidly progressive disease patients.
- Reversed two-stage approach (uncertain rational and benefit): liver resection first, resection of primary tumor after interval chemotherapy.

Epidemiology

Affects 40–50% of patients with colorectal cancer (CRC): 20% of CRC patients → synchronous metastatic disease at time of cancer diagnosis; 20–30% → metachronous metastases after resection of the primary tumor.

Symptoms

Most commonly asymptomatic: detection intraoperatively during primary resection, or through imaging studies and CEA/liver parameters during primary workup and/or follow-up.

Complications: liver failure (particularly after surgery) if > 50% of liver replaced by tumor; rarely: rupture of metastasis → intraperitoneal bleeding → hemorrhagic shock, peritonitis, cancer seeding.

Differential Diagnosis

Nonmalignant liver lesions: cysts, hemangioma, *Echinococcus,* liver adenoma, focal nodular hyperplasia.

Hepatocellular carcinoma.

Metastases from noncolorectal primary tumor.

Pathology

Same as primary tumor.

Evaluation

Required minimal standard

History: patient's overall condition, performance status, comorbidities, operability.

Clinical examination: palpable tumor, jaundice, abdominal distention, cardiopulmonary assessment.

Blood work: anemia, liver function (albumin, PTT, PT), kidney function. Tumor marker: CEA.

Imaging studies for liver assessment and to rule out extrahepatic tumor disease:

– CT chest/abdomen/pelvis: hypodense focal lesions, 70–90% sensitivity.
– MRI (contrast-enhanced): 65–90% sensitivity.
– PET-CT: most accurate for staging and patient selection, > 90% sensitivity if performed before chemotherapy administered.

Additional tests (optional)

Biopsy: tissue confirmation.
Biopsy of perifocal liver tissue: rule out liver cirrhosis.

Classification

- Resectable liver metastases.
- Potentially resectable metastases.
- Nonresectable (based on number, distribution, proximity to vital structures).

Nonoperative Treatment

Inoperable patients due to comorbidities and poor performance status.

Extrahepatic tumor manifestations (of uncurable extent).

Hepatic-only metastases that are:

- Nonresectable.
- Only potentially resectable.

→ palliative chemotherapy, reassessment for future resectability if chemoresponsive.

→ radiofrequency or cryoablation.

→ no benefit from: hepatic arterial infusion chemotherapy, ethanol injection, radiation, transplant.

Operative Treatment

Indications

- Resectable metastases (unless prohibitive contraindications: comorbidities, extrahepatic tumor dissemination).
- Resectability: R0 resection feasible, sparing of two adjacent liver segments possible, preservation of vascular in-/outflow and biliary drainage possible, remnant liver of normal structure and > 20% of total liver volume.

Operative approach

Intraoperative management of preoperatively known metastases

Diagnostic laparoscopy with laparoscopic intraoperative ultrasonography should be considered (particularly in absence of top-quality preoperative

imaging) as unnecessary laparotomy may be avoided in up to 25% of patients.
- Intraoperative ultrasonography → change or guidance of surgical procedure.
- R0 resection: with goal of 1 cm safety margin, minimum margin of > 1 mm less ideal.
  - Anatomic resection: hemihepatectomy, trisegmentectomy.
  - Nonanatomic resection: metastasectomy, segmentectomy.
  - Combinations: eg, hemihepatectomy + radiofrequency ablation of contralateral focus.

Intraoperative management of preoperatively unknown metastases
- Resection if feasible (as above).
- At least: Tru-cut biopsy for tissue confirmation.
- Portal vein ligation: not commonly indicated.

Outcome

Five-year survival after resection of liver metastases: 30–50% (caveat: highly selected patients). Elective mortality of liver resection: decreased from 20% to currently 1%.

Complications: bleeding, wound infections 5%, biliary leak, biloma, liver failure.

Follow-up

Continuation of adjuvant/palliative chemotherapy indicated for:
- All patients after metastasectomy.
- Patients ineligible for surgical resection as long as benefit > side effects.

Oncologic follow-up:
- Colonoscopy: depending on overall prognosis and colonic condition.
- Clinical examination and blood work (including CEA) as clinically indicated, at least every 3 months.
- Imaging (CT chest/abdomen/pelvis, PET): depending on clinical course and treatment protocols.

Surgical reintervention:
- Re-resection for recurrent liver metastases in highly selected candidates.
- Resection of pulmonary metastases in selected patients.

Cross-reference

COLORECTAL CANCER—LUNG METASTASES
(197.3)

Overview

Lung is the third most common site (after liver and peritoneal carcinomatosis) for metastatic dissemination of GI malignancies including colorectal cancer. Pulmonary metastases most frequently represent surgically incurable tumor extent. Systemic chemotherapy therefore is the principle treatment option and is indicated if tolerated.

Poor prognostic parameters:

• Multiple metastases (> 4).

• Bilateral lung metastases.

• Short or no interval to primary tumor.

• Insufficient residual lung function.

Surgical resection may play role in highly selected individuals who are fit and have a limited number of metastases with relatively slow progression and no residual extrapulmonary tumor manifestations. Potential of cure and long-term survival averages 38% (range 30–70%) of these highly selected patients (vs 5-year survival of < 1% in the whole group with lung metastases).

Timing of lung resection: generally not indicated at the time of abdominal resection but rather 2-stage approach: lung resection after 12–16 weeks of interval chemotherapy. Advantages: assessment of tumor response to chemotherapy, tumor downsizing with better resectability, elimination of nonbeneficial surgery in patients with unfavorable disease with rapid extrapulmonary or intrapulmonary progression.

Epidemiology

Affects 10–15% of patients with colorectal cancer (CRC) → metachronous metastases after resection of the primary tumor.

Symptoms

Most commonly asymptomatic → detection during primary workup or follow-up.

Differential Diagnosis

Primary lung cancer.

Nonmalignant pulmonary nodule.

Pathology

Should be consistent with the primary tumor.

Evaluation

Required minimal standard

History: patient's overall condition, performance status, comorbidities (particularly cardiopulmonary, smoking, and other risk factors for lung cancer), operability.

Clinical examination:

- Abdominopelvic: rule locally recurrent tumor, jaundice, ascites, etc.
- Cardiopulmonary assessment and pulmonary function tests: operability, decreased lung function, emphysema, COPD, right ventricular congestion, etc.

Blood work: arterial blood gas analysis, anemia, liver function (albumin, PTT, PT), kidney function, tumor marker (CEA).

CT chest/abdomen/pelvis and/or PET-CT: rule out extrapulmonary tumor disease.

Additional tests (optional)

Bronchoscopy: if primary lung cancer more likely.

Biopsy (eg, CT-guided): tissue confirmation.

Classification

- Resectable lung metastases.
- Nonresectable (based on number, distribution, proximity to vital structures).

Nonoperative Treatment

Nonresectable pulmonary metastases (disseminated tumor disease, extrapulmonary tumor).

Inoperable patients due to comorbidities and poor performance status.

Operative Treatment

Indications

Resectable metastases.

Operative approach

Metastasectomy (rarely more extensive resection):

- Video-assisted thoracoscopic surgery (VATS): faster recovery, higher miss rate.
- Open resection: higher morbidity, lower miss rate (allows for palpation of lung tissue).

Outcome

Five-year survival after resection of lung metastases: 30–70% (caveat: highly selected patients).

Complications: bleeding, wound infections, air leak, respiratory failure.

Follow-up

Continuation of adjuvant/palliative chemotherapy indicated for:

• All patients after metastasectomy.

• Patients ineligible for surgical resection as long as benefit > side effects.

Cross-reference

Topic	*Chapter*
CT scan	2 (p 117)
PET	2 (p 126)
Recurrent rectal cancer	4 (p 271)
Colorectal cancer—liver metastases	4 (p 275)
Chemotherapy protocols—curative intent	6 (p 645)
Chemotherapy—metastatic colorectal cancer	6 (p 649)
Follow-up for colorectal cancer	6 (p 660)
CEA monitoring for colorectal cancer	6 (p 663)

GASTROINTESTINAL STROMAL TUMOR
(GIST; 171.9)

Overview

GIST is the most common mesenchymal tumor of the GI tracts and origi-nates from the intestinal pacemaker cells, the interstitial cells of Cajal. Dis-tinguished from other mesenchymal tumors (eg, leiomyoma, schwannoma) through immunohistochemistry identifying markers of GIST, which are equally expressed in interstitial cells of Cajal:

- CD117 (KIT): gene product of stem cell factor receptor proto-oncogene c-kit.
- CD34: hematopoietic progenitor cell antigen.
- PDGF receptor alpha (PDGFRA): alternative and mutually exclusive oncogenic mechanisms to c-kit pathway.

Malignant potential of GISTs is difficult to assess:

- Favorable prognostic factors: gastric location, < 5 cm in diameter, mitotic index ≤ 5 mitoses per 10 HPFs, absence of necrosis, low proliferating cell nuclear antigen, Ki-67 analogue index < 10%, confined tumor, lack of metastasis to other sites.
- Unfavorable prognostic factors: esophageal/colonic/rectal location, > 10 cm in diameter, mitotic index ≥ 10 mitoses per 10 HPFs, presence of coagu-lative necrosis, invasion of adjacent organs, evidence of peritoneal seed-ing or distant metastases.

GIST is highly resistant to conventional chemotherapy. Treatment is pri-marily surgical resection of localized GIST if tumor is resectable without mutilation. Recurrent and locally advanced or metastatic tumors are increas-ingly treated with imatinib (Gleevec) in palliative, adjuvant, or neoadjuvant setting. Tumor response imatinib (Gleevec, KIT kinase activity inhibitor) correlates with expression of CD117.

Epidemiology

Constitutes 0.1–3% of all GI neoplasms. Estimated annual incidence: 10–15 new cases per 1 million people, ie, every year approximately 3000–5000 new cases in the US. Median age: 50–60 years, no gender pre-dominance.

GIST locations: stomach 50–60%, small intestine 25–30%, colon/rec-tum/rectovaginal septum 2–10%, esophagus 9%. Other locations: retroperi-toneal, pancreas, etc. Up to 50% of GISTs are metastatic/multifocal at the time of presentation.

Symptoms

Unspecific symptoms: pain, obstruction, bleeding, or visible/palpable mass. Incidental finding on imaging or endoscopy studies.

Differential Diagnosis

Other benign mesenchymal tumors: leiomyoma, lipoma, neurofibroma (schwannoma).

Other malignant mesenchymal tumors: leiomyosarcoma, neurofibrosarcoma, etc.

Epithelial neoplasms.

Pathology

Macroscopic

- Solid or focally cystic mass of varying size: 1–20 cm.
- Hemorrhage.
- Focal necrosis.
- Pattern of tumor dissemination: lymph node involvement comparably rare (< 25%); metastases to liver and peritoneal cavity, less frequently to lung and bones.

Microscopic

Spindle cell, epithelioid, or pleomorphic (mixed) tumors → ultrastructural and immunohistochemical distinction from leiomyoma, leiomyosarcoma, or schwannoma.

Immunohistochemical positivity

- CD117 (KIT): 75–80% (cytoplasm).
- CD34 (hematopoietic progenitor cell antigen): 60–70%.
- PDGFRA: 5–10%.

Conventional prognostic parameters: (1) tumor size, (2) mitotic rate (mitoses/number of HPFs). KIT positivity correlating with imatinib response.

Evaluation

Required minimal standard

Full colonic evaluation (preferably colonoscopy) mandatory prior to elective surgery to rule out multifocal tumors, synchronous cancers or polyps, rule out underlying colonic disease.

Imaging studies: CT, PET, MRI for assessment of local tumor extension and to rule out distant metastases.

Additional tests (optional)
Same as for CRC.
EGD.

Classification
- Immunocharacterization: KIT-positive (GIST 85–95%) vs KIT-negative GIST (5–15%).
- Tumor behavior: benign GIST vs malignant GIST.
- Operable GIST vs inoperable or multifocal/metastatic GIST.

Nonoperative Treatment
Depending on tumor extent at presentation:
- Potentially adjuvant treatment in all resected cases?
- (Neo-)adjuvant therapy with imatinib (Gleevec, tyrosine kinase inhibitor) for borderline-resectable GIST.
- Recurrent, locally advanced, and unresectable or metastatic GIST: palliative Gleevec treatment, results in 45–80% initial response.

No defined role for radiation therapy.

Operative Treatment
Indications
- Any localized GIST that allows complete resection without mutilation unless diffuse metastases or prohibitive contraindications.
- Multifocal GIST only in highly selected cases (after neoadjuvant imatinib treatment).

Operative approach
En-bloc resection of tumor-involved organ with inclusion of intact pseudo-capsule; radical lymphadenectomy not routinely indicated.

Outcome
Data evolving in the literature:
- Localized GIST: disease-specific 1-year survival 80–90%, 5-year survival approximately 50% after complete surgical resection.
- Metastatic GIST: median survival about 20 months, but 80% of patients show initial benefit from imatinib.

Follow-up

Overall clinical follow-up not yet clearly defined:

→ imaging studies: CT, PET in regular intervals.

→ continued endoscopy (colonoscopy, EGD) in at least 6–12 months intervals.

→ depending on location: endorectal ultrasound.

Cross-reference

Topic	*Chapter*
CT scan	2 (p 117)
PET	2 (p 126)
Imatinib (Gleevec)	6 (p 670)

CARCINOID TUMORS *(235.2)*

Overview

Carcinoids are of neuroendocrine origin and represent the most frequent endocrine tumor of the GI tract but comprise only < 1% of GI tumors overall: biologically/morphologically heterogeneous, size-dependent potential to metastasize (liver, lung, bone, etc), frequently multicentric.

Modern nomenclature: carcinoids are classified as neuroendocrine tumors. Historically: labeled as APUDomas based on neuroectodermal cell origin with common biochemical steps of amine precursor (5-hydrotryptophan) uptake and decarboxylation to produce several biologically active amines (serotonin, bradykinins, histamine, vasoactive intestinal peptide [VIP], ACTH, prostaglandins, substance P, etc). Circulating serotonin and other active peptides metabolized during first-pass effect in the liver (eg, serotonin → urinary metabolite 5-hydroxyindolacetic acid [5-HIAA]): therefore, carcinoid syndrome generally only manifests once liver or other systemic metastases are present.

Tumor characteristics vary depending on location. Definition of malignancy is based on invasion or presence of metastases, not on histologic picture. Growth pattern: slow progression with development of metastases after 7–14 years; metastatic potential dependent on depth of invasion and size:

  < 1 cm: low probability.

  1–2 cm: gray zone: uncertain behavior (< 3% metastases).

  > 2 cm: high probability of metastases (30–60%).

Epidemiology

Prevalence in US: 50,000 cases; incidence in US: estimated at 1.5–5.5 new cases per 100,000 people. Slight female preponderance. Peak age: 50–70 years. Constitutes 12–35% of all small bowel tumors, 15–45% of all small bowel malignancies.

Distribution pattern of GI carcinoids (caveat: difference between clinical vs autopsy series!): small intestine 40–45% (particularly ileum >> jejunum >> duodenum), rectum 12–20%, appendix 15–20%, colon 7–10%, stomach 5–10%. Historical data: appendix 40% > rectum 12–15% > small bowel 10–14%.

Multicentricity: ileal 25–30%, colon 3–5%.

Symptoms

Early (most frequently): asymptomatic → incidental discovery on colonoscopy or surgery for other abdominal conditions.

Intermediate size: intermittent vague abdominal pain (partial/intermittent obstruction, postprandial intestinal angina).

Metastatic disease:

– Carcinoid syndrome (in < 10% of midgut carcinoids): flushing (80–85%), GI hypermotility with diarrhea (~70%), carcinoid heart disease (30–40%, right heart disease), bronchial constriction/wheezing (15–20%), myopathy (5–10%), pellagra-like skin pathology (5%), weight loss, arthralgia, peptic ulcers.

– Peritumoral fibrosis: → intestinal obstruction 50–75%

Associated symptoms: from associated tumors in multiple endocrine neoplasia type I (MEN-I) syndrome (foregut carcinoids).

Differential Diagnosis

IBS or spastic colon.

Noncarcinoid GI malignancies: large intestine cancer, small intestine cancer (proximal > distal), stomach/pancreas, OB/GYN, carcinomatosis, GIST, lymphoma, melanoma (melanotic, amelanotic), mesothelioma, etc.

Benign extramucosal tumors: lipoma, leiomyoma, etc.

Pathology

Macroscopic

• Yellow-gray to pink-tan submucosal nodule/thickening up to sessile/pedunculated polyp; with increasing size → ulcerated, annular, obstructive, peritoneal/mesenteric fibrosis.

• Tumor extent at presentation: locally advanced/metastatic spread in 3–5% of rectal carcinoids, 13–38% of midgut carcinoids → liver, peritoneal, omentum, lung, bone, lymph node involvement (~80%), simultaneous satellite lesions > 25–30%.

• Secondary pathology: carcinoid heart disease (plaque-like fibrous endocardial and valvular thickening in the right heart).

• Associated neoplasms: colonic malignancy in 2–5% of colonic and in 30–60% of ileal carcinoids; other associated malignancies: lymphoma, breast.

Microscopic

• Submucosal nests of round/polygonal cells with prominent nucleoli and eosinophilic cytoplasmic granules.

• Five histologic patterns: insular, trabecular, glandular, undifferentiated, mixed. Limited value of traditional morphologic criteria to assess malignant potential.

Immunohistochemistry

Chromogranin A (CgA) and synaptophysin positive; in addition:

- Foregut carcinoids: argentaffin-negative, argyrophil-positive, produce 5-hydroxytryptophan.
- Midgut carcinoids (duodenum to midtransverse colon): argentaffin-positive, argyrophil-positive, frequently multicentric, produce several vasoactive compounds → carcinoid syndrome.
- Hindgut carcinoids (distal transverse colon to rectum): rarely argentaffin- or argyrophil-positive, typically solitary; carcinoid syndrome < 5% of colonic carcinoids, almost never for rectal carcinoid (do not produce serotonin).

Evaluation

Required minimal standard

Suggestive symptoms → screening tests:

- Chromogranin A (plasma): positive 75–90% of foregut, midgut, and hindgut carcinoids.
- 5-HIAA levels (random urine sample or 24-hour urine): positive 70–85% of foregut and midgut carcinoids, but negative in hindgut carcinoids.

Positive screening test, positive incidental biopsy, suspicious incidental imaging finding:

- Endoscopy: small bowel: capsule endoscopy; colon: colonoscopy; rectum: colonoscopy plus endorectal ultrasound.
- Imaging:
  - CT/MRI: liver and lymph node metastases (→ CT-guided biopsy), "spoke wheel" desmoplastic mesenteric masses.
  - Octreotide scintigraphic scan (^{111}In-labeled octreotide): 80–90% sensitivity.

Evidence of metastatic disease: echocardiogram.

Additional tests (optional)

PET, PET-CT: uncertain value because of slow progression and low metabolic rate of tumor.

Blood work: anemia, liver function (albumin, PTT, PT), kidney function.

Classification

- Based on site of origin: foregut, midgut, hindgut.
- Based on specific location: small bowel, appendix, colon, rectum.
- Based on stage: localized, locally advanced (size, infiltration of other structures), loco-regional metastatic, distant metastatic.
- Based on secretory activity: functional vs nonfunctional.

Nonoperative Treatment

For palliation (patient not operable or not curable extent of tumor):

- Carcinoid syndrome (flushing, diarrhea, wheezing): somatostatin-analogues (octreotide).
- Tumor control/reduction: no benefit from conventional chemotherapy or radiation → intra-arterial 5-FU? Streptozotocin? Systemic fluorodeoxyuridine (FUDR) + doxorubicin? Interferon? Radioactively labeled somatostatin analogues.

Preoperatively in preparation for surgery: octreotide → prevent carcinoid crisis.

Supportive measures: eg, for diarrhea—loperamide, cholestyramine, etc.

Operative Treatment

Indication

- Curative intent: standard oncologic resection = treatment of choice for any operable patient and amenable tumor extent → avert local complications, decrease hormone secretion, limit secondary pathology.
- Palliative intent: debulking, cytoreduction, wedge resection → obviate mechanical bowel obstruction, decrease of endocrine symptomatology.

Operative approach

Appendiceal carcinoid:

- < 1 cm and not at base (70–80%): appendectomy.
- 1–2 cm or mesoappendiceal extension or subserosal lymphatic invasion (→ 0–3% metastatic): right hemicolectomy.
- > 2 cm, appendiceal base, mucin production (30% metastatic): right hemicolectomy.

Small bowel and colon: standard oncologic resection.

Rectum:

- < 2 cm, no invasion of muscularis mucosa: transanal excision.
- > 2 cm or invasion of muscularis mucosa: oncologic resection.

Hepatic metastases: liver resection (formal vs metastasectomies), radiofrequency ablation, chemoembolization; occasionally orthotopic liver transplantation.

Prophylactic cholecystectomy (in case of a palliative resection) to mitigate biliary toxicity of octreotide treatment.

Outcome

Five-year survival rates: 65–75% overall → survival based on location and tumor extent:

- Small bowel carcinoid: overall 70–80%, local disease 90–95%, lymph node involvement 75–85%, distant metastases 40–50%.
- Appendiceal carcinoid: overall 70–80%, local disease 90–95%, lymph node involvement 75–85%, distant metastases 35–45%.
- Rectal carcinoid: overall 85–90%, local disease 90–95%, lymph node involvement 45–55%, distant metastases 5–15%.
- Colon carcinoid: local disease 45–95%, lymph node involvement 25–75%, distant metastases 10–30%.

Follow-up

Hepatic carcinoid metastases: resection, chemotherapeutic embolization, cryotherapy, hepatic arterial infusion chemotherapy.

Octreotide scan and blood tests at regular intervals.

Cytoreductive surgeries as needed.

Cross-reference

PRESACRAL TUMORS *(789.3)*

Overview

Presacral tumors—located in the space between sacrum and rectum—comprise a relatively rare variety of pathologies of benign, potentially malignant, or malignant character. The complex embryology of that region predisposes to errors. Hence, two-thirds of lesions are congenital. Risk for malignancy increases with age, reaching 25–40% overall.

• Congenital lesions: epidermoid cyst, dermoid cyst, enteric cyst (tailgut, duplication), teratoma, teratocarcinoma.

• Neurogenic lesions: chordoma, neurofibroma/sarcoma, neurilemmoma, ependymoma, neuroblastoma, anterior sacral meningocele.

• Osseous: osteoma/chondroma/sarcoma, simple bone cyst, giant cell tumor, Ewing sarcoma, chondromyxosarcoma.

• Miscellaneous: metastatic disease, GIST, sarcoma, hemangioma, lymphoma, desmoid, carcinoid, inflammation (abscess, chronic leak, hematoma).

Epidemiology

Rare, ~0.01% of annual admissions.

Two age peaks: neonate to early childhood (most frequent: teratoma), adults > 40–50 years of age (most frequent: epidermoid cyst, chordoma).

Symptoms

Children: obvious mass.

Adults:

– Frequently asymptomatic: incidental finding on digital rectal exam or imaging studies.

– Most frequent symptoms: pain (30–40%), pelvic fullness, constipation (25–30%), abscess/ discharge (15–20%), urinary retention (15%), buttock mass (5–10%).

– Suspicious symptoms: recurring deep postanal abscess, recurring anal fistulae without cryptoglandular pathology, tailbone infection otherwise consistent with pilonidal cyst but in atypical patient, known spinal or anal congenital deformity.

– Complications: malignant transformation, fistula formation, infection.

– Malignant lesions → high risk of metastatic disease.

Differential Diagnosis

Benign cyst.

True presacral tumor: chordoma, giant cell tumor, congenital tumors.

Postsurgical changes: presacral abscess/sinus (anastomotic leak), hematoma.

Recurrent or metastatic cancer.

Postradiation changes (pelvic fibrosis).

Deep postanal abscess (ischioanal abscess).

Meningocele.

Osteomyelitis, pilonidal sinus, tuberculosis, etc.

Pathology

Epidermoid, tailgut, enterogenous cysts (benign, malignant potential if untreated): simple epithelium, no skin appendages.

Sacrococcygeal teratoma (benign with malignant potential): tumor derived from pluripotent stem cell with presence of more than one germ-cell layer → potential transformation into malignant tumor:

– Common structures: hair, salivary gland, smooth muscle, cartilage, bone, neural tissue, retina, pancreas, thyroid, teeth, bronchus, fat.

– Rare structures: skeletal muscle, cardiac muscle, kidney, liver tissue.

Dermoid cyst (benign): structural elements derived from ectodermal layer.

Chordoma (malignant): derived from remnants of notochord, locally aggressive malignant tumor with size-dependent sacral destruction.

Evaluation

Required minimal standard

History: specific symptoms: bleeding, constipation, change in bowel habits, pain, weight loss, urinary/vaginal symptoms, preexisting sexual or anal sphincter dysfunction; family history; comorbidities.

Clinical examination:

• Digital rectal exam: presacral mass, anterior surface of sacrum/coccyx not palpable.

• Rigid sigmoidoscopy: mucosal lesion? Extraluminal compression?

Imaging studies:

• Plain x-ray: bony destruction = scimitar sign (caveat: not to be mistaken for thoracic scimitar sign in anomalous pulmonary venous drainage).

- MRI or CT abdomen/pelvis: delineation of soft tissue structures and relation to bone.

Colonic evaluation prior to elective surgery.

Additional tests (optional)

ERUS: involvement of rectal wall?

Tumor marker: alpha-fetoprotein (AFP), human chorionic gonadotropin (HCG): little value in differentiating between benign/malignant.

Aspiration or biopsy: controversial, not routinely recommended or even contraindicated because:

- – Risk of seeding → planning such that tract would be excised during surgical resection.
- – Risk of meningitis (meningomyelocele).
- – Lack of negative predictive value, lack of impact on need for surgery.

Classification

- Congenital vs acquired.
- Benign vs malignant.
- Low vs high location.

Nonoperative Treatment

Inoperable patients due to comorbidities.

Inoperable/incurable due to extent of local tumor → symptom control.

Chordoma or other malignant tumors → role of (neo-)adjuvant chemoradiation?

Operative Treatment

Indications

Any presacral lesion (unless prohibitive contraindications).

Operative approach

- Low lesion: access through York-Mason or Kraske approach, resection of coccyx, sacral resection required for local control of chordoma.
- High lesion: combined abdominosacral approach—abdominal mobilization of rectum, posterior resection of sacrum, possible flap closure.

Outcome

Sacral resection relatively safe: pelvic stability → preserve S1; sphincter/bladder function → preserve S2/S3.

Malignant presacral tumors: intact resection of nonmetastatic chordoma has best prognosis (50% 5-year survival); prognosis for other malignancies dismal.

Complications: bleeding (presacral veins), wound infections, osteomyelitis, sexual and urinary dysfunction, recurrence.

Follow-up

Optimization of defecation/fecal control and urinary control.

Surveillance for recurrence.

Role of adjuvant chemoradiation?

Cross-reference

Topic	*Chapter*
CT scan	2 (p 117)
MRI	2 (p 124)
Kraske approach	5 (p 628)
Resection of presacral lesion	5 (p 631)

RARE TUMORS

Overview

Although colorectal cancer and anal squamous cell cancer account for the overwhelming majority of tumors encountered in the colorectal specialty, there are a number of known entities that may never be seen but remain important differential diagnoses to other conditions.

Malignant melanoma

- Incidence: ~1% of anorectal malignancies, 2% of all melanomas, third most common melanoma site (after skin, eye).
- Cause: arises from melanocytes in ATZ.
- Associated disease: none.
- Presentation: polypoid masses of varying size, 60% are black, 40% amelanotic, often mistaken for hemorrhoids.
- Treatment options: wide local excision vs abdominoperineal resection. Immunotherapy.
- Prognosis: poor (regardless of surgical approach).

Kaposi sarcoma

- Incidence: overall ~0.5–0.6% of organ transplant recipients; most commonly involving skin etc; extremely rarely involving anorectum or intestines.
- Cause: human herpesvirus-8 (HHV-8) infection in conjunction with immunosuppression (eg, HIV/AIDS, chronic steroid or immunosuppressant medication, etc).
- Associated disease: HIV, immunosuppression (eg, IBD, transplantation).
- Presentation: bluish-purple nodules.
- Treatment options: improvement of immune status if possible: HIV → HAART; IBD → proctocolectomy to eliminate need for immunosuppression. Chemotherapy/potentially radiotherapy, or interferon in patients in whom immune status cannot be improved.
- Prognosis: good if immunosuppression can be improved.

Lymphoma

- Incidence: GI tract is the most common site of extranodal non-Hodgkin-lymphoma; 1–4% of all GI malignancies (mostly in stomach and small bowel), only 0.2–0.5% in the colon (cecum) or rectum; male/female ratio 2:1.
- Cause: often unknown; viral infection more common, eg, Epstein-Barr virus (EBV) infection in conjunction with immunosuppression (eg, HIV/AIDS, chronic steroid use, etc).

- Associated disease: HIV, immunosuppression (eg, IBD, transplantation).
- Presentation: diffuse infiltrative mass, varying degrees of ulcerations, varying size, stricturing, bowel wall thickening → GI symptoms (pain, bleeding, obstruction, mass, etc), B-symptoms (fever, weight loss, sweating). Rare form: multiple lymphomatous polyposis.
- Subtypes: B-cell lymphomas (85%): mucosa-associated lymphoid tissue (MALT) lymphoma, mantle cell lymphoma, Burkitt B-cell lymphoma; T-cell lymphoma (15%).
- Treatment options: if confined lymphoma and resection possible without mutilation → surgical resection; all others → chemo- and immunotherapy. MALT lymphoma → trial of anti-infectious treatment.
- Prognosis: good; 5% risk of perforation with induction chemotherapy.

Desmoid
- Incidence: 3.5–13% of FAP patients, < 0.01% in patients without FAP.
- Cause: gene mutation in 3′ region of *APC* gene between codons 1445 and 1578 → benign fibroblastic tumors arising from mesenchymal primordial germ layer.
- Associated disease: FAP with other extracolonic manifestations.
- Presentation: usually slow growing (10% grow rapidly) mesenteric, abdominal wall, and retroperitoneal/pelvic soft tissue mass, often without defined margin; multicentricity but not metastasizing → pain (50%, typically due to bowel or ureteral obstruction, ischemia), painless mass, or incidental finding.
- Treatment options: radical surgical resection. Chemotherapy, imatinib, hormone ablation therapy (eg, tamoxifen), immunotherapy.
- Prognosis: most frequent non–cancer-related cause of death in FAP patients: (1) direct tumor effects (eg, ischemic bowel, intestinal obstruction, urinary obstruction, fistula, sepsis, etc); (2) surgical mortality. Recurrence rate 65–85% after resection.

Other rare tumors
Small-cell neuroendocrine carcinoma.

Metastases from other primary cancers (eg, lobular breast cancer, lung cancer, etc).

Leukemic or plasmocytoma infiltrates.

Sarcomas (including gastrointestinal stroma tumor).

Vascular tumors: cavernous hemangioma, angiomas, etc.

Cross-reference

RADIATION PROCTITIS/ENTERITIS *(558.1)*

Overview

Acute or chronic side effect from radiation exposure to the pelvis (most commonly for GYN and prostate malignancies). Typical examples: prostate cancer 6400–7200 cGy, cervical cancer 4500 cGy, endometrial cancer 4500–5000 cGy, rectal cancer 2500–5040 cGy, bladder cancer 6400 cGy. Very focal rectal injury can result from brachytherapy: seeds (eg, prostate) or cervical cap. Radiation damage may occur in sites outside of primary therapeutic field: eg, stray radiation may result in diffuse radiation enteritis!

Injury dependent on total dose (typically > 4000 cGy), beam energy and percentage depth dose, fractionation size, field size, duration of delivery, tissue proliferation, tissue oxygenation.

Radiation damage occurs in two phases:

1. Acute: typically self-limited cytotoxicity from radicals and induced DNA damage to high-turnover cell populations (intestinal epithelia, bone marrow, skin annexes, etc).

2. Chronic: permanent and irreversible damage through microischemic pathway resulting from obliterative endarteritis, endothelial degeneration, neovascularization, interstitial fibrosis, epithelial distortion.

Preventive strategies during administration of radiation remain controversial: balsalazide, misoprostol, sucralfate, etc.

Epidemiology

Early injury: in 30–70% of patients undergoing pelvic radiation treatment, < 3–6 weeks of treatment.

Chronic injury: 1–20 years after radiation exposure. Older series: 20–25% incidence; newer series: 3–8% (likely the result of improved radiation calculation/simulation techniques).

Symptoms

Acute proctitis: diarrhea, passage of mucus and blood per rectum, urgency/incontinence, tenesmus, pain, perianal dermatitis. Systemic effects uncommon and more likely related to general treatment side effects: anemia, anorexia, malnutrition/weight loss. Resolution of acute symptoms after 6–12 weeks.

Chronic radiation proctitis: bleeding (ulcerations, telangiectasias), diarrhea, mucous discharge per rectum, urgency/incontinence (decreased reservoir volume and compliance), tenesmus, perianal dermatitis. Complications include: hemorrhage, obstructive symptoms (stricture formation), fistula formation (eg, rectovaginal fistula), incontinence (nerve damage, sphincter damage, loss of reservoir). Increased risk of secondary malignancy.

Differential Diagnosis

Tumor recurrence, IBD (ulcerative colitis, Crohn disease, indeterminate colitis), ischemic colitis, infectious colitis (including pseudomembranous *C difficile* colitis), STD proctitis (eg, lymphogranuloma venereum, gonorrhea), IBS.

Caveat: avoid fast-track "hemorrhoid" diagnosis/treatment in previously radiated rectum!

Pathology

Macroscopic
Congested/edematous mucosa, necrosis, ulcerations/fistula opening, telangiectasias, strictures, bowel foreshortening.

Microscopic
• Acute injury: epithelial ulcerations, meganucleosis, inflammation in the lamina propria, lack of mitotic activity.
• Chronic injury: subintimal arteriolar fibrosis (endangitis obliterans), endothelial degeneration, fibrosis of the lamina propria, crypt distortion, hypertrophy of myenteric plexus of Auerbach.

Evaluation

Required minimal standard
Rigid or flexible sigmoidoscopy: usually sufficient to establish diagnosis, full colonic evaluation generally indicated.

Caveat: no biopsy of anterior ulcers/pathology—risk of iatrogenic rectovaginal/rectourinary fistula.

Additional tests (optional)
Contrast studies (barium or Gastrografin enema): only if colonoscopy unfeasible (eg, stricture) or road map needed (eg, fistula).

Virtual colonoscopy: role not defined, risk of perforation.

MRI, PET, PET-CT: role not defined.

Anophysiology studies: evaluation of anorectal functionality (eg, rectal compliance, etc).

Lab work: nutritional status.

Small bowel follow-through: evidence for short bowel (foreshortening)?

Classification

- Radiation proctitis: acute vs chronic, localized vs diffuse.
- Radiation enteritis: acute vs chronic, localized vs diffuse.
- Secondary radiation-induced complications (stricture, fistula, etc).

Nonoperative Treatment

Acute radiation injury: temporizing measures (stool management, antidiarrheal medication, perianal skin care) and patience; topical medications (sucralfate, steroid, or 5-ASA enemas), fecal diversion if symptoms severe and poorly tolerated.

Chronic radiation injury: no cure, poor tissue quality → control symptoms:

- Antidiarrheals/antispasmodics as needed.
- Topical anti-inflammatory medications: suppositories/enemas with steroids, 5-ASA, sucralfate, misoprostol.
- Oral antibiotics: metronidazole.
- Vitamin supplements: vitamin C and vitamin E.
- Possible benefit from home TPN.
- Colonic mucosal integrity: short-chain fatty acid enemas (chemically unstable, therefore not practical for use).
- Laser ablation: multiple sessions needed.
- Formalin instillation: proctoscope/endoscope 50-mL aliquots of 4% formalin → 2–3 minutes contact with area of interest, followed by copious washout with saline. Usually quickly effective, may need repeat treatment if relapse.

Operative Treatment

Indications

- Significant and treatment-refractory symptoms: hemorrhage, tenesmus, discharge, incontinence.
- Obstruction: stricture formation.
- Fistula formation.
- Uncertainty about possible tumor recurrence.

Operative approach

- Excision of area with radiation injury, with or without reconstruction (may be very challenging).
- Palliation of symptoms without resection of injured tissue: fecal and/or urinary diversion.

Outcome

Acute radiation injury: self-limited, resolution typically within 6–12 weeks.

Chronic radiation injury: frequently responding adequately to nonoperative management, repeated sessions needed. Severe injuries expected to decrease in the future (more sophisticated radiation techniques).

Anastomosis in radiated area: increased leak rate → temporary fecal diversion recommended.

Diversion alone: some symptoms may persist (mucus discharge, bleeding, pain).

Follow-up

Frequent clinic visits until symptoms under control, per routine guidelines thereafter.

Cross-reference

Topic	*Chapter*
Ulceration	1 (p 50)
Ulcerative colitis	4 (p 320)
Rectovaginal fistula	4 (p 385)
Complications—leak	4 (p 466)

ISCHEMIC COLITIS *(557.X)*

Overview

Ischemic colitis—caused by inadequate blood flow—is the most common form of intestinal ischemia (~60%). Various degrees of severity depending on location and extent, acuity of onset, presence of collaterals, and level of occlusion: commonly, splenic flexure, rectosigmoid junction, and right colon most vulnerable. Numerous different etiologies result in a final common pathway:

• Occlusive disease:

  – Major vascular occlusion: infrarenal aortic bypass, SMA thrombosis/embolism, portal vein/SMV thrombosis, trauma, acute pancreatitis, aortic dissection.

  – Microvascular (peripheral vessels): diabetic vasculopathy, thrombosis, embolism, vasculitis, amyloidosis, rheumatoid arthritis, radiation injury, trauma, interventional radiology embolization (for lower GI bleeding), hypercoagulable states (protein C and S deficiency, antithrombin III deficiency, sickle cell disease).

• Nonocclusive disease:

  – Shock, sepsis, and low flow state (eg, atrial fibrillation, myocardial infarction, cardiopulmonary bypass machine), steal phenomenon, abdominal compartment syndrome.

  – Colonic obstruction, volvulus, hernia.

  – Toxic: cocaine, medications (NSAIDS, vasopressors, digoxin, diuretics, chemotherapy, gold compounds).

Caveat: patients may have other relevant colonic pathology (eg, cancer) in affected or unaffected segments.

Treatment ranging from conservative management (milder to moderate forms) to a segmental or even total abdominal colectomy (severe and life-threatening form).

Epidemiology

Incidence peak between 6th and 9th decades. Females > males. Results in 1:2000 acute admissions to the hospital. True incidence unknown: under- or misdiagnosis. Historically: up to 10% ischemic colitis after infrarenal aortic replacement, less frequent with interventional radiology procedures. Location: 80% on the left side (between splenic flexure and sigmoid), 10–20% in ascending to transverse colon, < 3% in rectum.

Symptoms

Acute ischemia

- Initial stage: acute ischemia → sudden onset of abdominal pain, potentially crampy, hyperperistalsis, potentially associated with diarrhea or urge to defecate.
- Second stage: beginning tissue necrosis (after 12–24 hours) → ileus, paradoxical decrease of pain level, bleeding (hematochezia), subtle peritoneal signs.
- Third stage: peritonitis, sepsis—increasing peritoneal signs, signs of toxicity (fever, elevated WBC with left shift, tachycardia); complete ileus, nausea and vomiting, hemodynamic instability, septic shock.
- Complications:
  - Colonic dilation and structural weakening → perforation, sepsis, oliguria, multiorgan failure, death.
  - Sepsis → bacterial seeding to ischemia-associated implants (eg, valves, aortic graft etc).

Chronic ischemia

- Angina abdominalis: postprandial pain as result of inadequate increase of intestinal blood flow.
- Ischemic colonic stricture → obstructive signs.

Differential Diagnosis

IBD: ulcerative colitis, Crohn disease.

Infectious colitis: shigella, enterohemorrhagic *E coli,* salmonella, *Campylobacter,* etc.

Colorectal cancer.

Diverticulosis, diverticulitis.

Radiation proctocolitis.

Other causes of acute abdominal pain and/or lower GI bleeding.

Pathology

Macroscopic

- Acute: bowel and mucosal edema → geographic areas of ulcerations or necrosis, segmental full-thickness necrosis → segmental gangrene.
- Chronic: chronic fibrotic stricture, mucosal surface intact.

Microscopic

- Acute: superficial mucosal necrosis, crypts initially intact → hemorrhage and pseudomembranes → full-thickness wall necrosis (loss of nuclei, ghost cells, inflammatory reaction, increasing architectural distortion); potentially visible thrombus, embolus, cholesterol embolus.

• Chronic: largely intact mucosa, but crypt atrophy and focal erosions, thickened/hyalinized lamina propria, crypt atrophy, diffuse fibrosis.

Evaluation

Required minimal standard

History:

– Recent cardiovascular surgery, history of embolic disease, "angina abdominalis," history of vasculitis, medications (including warfarin, ASA).

– Current symptom triad: acute abdominal pain, rectal bleeding, diarrhea.

Clinical examination:

– Vital signs: absolute arrhythmia (atrial fibrillation), hemodynamic stability?

– Abdominal distention, disproportionate abdominal pain, hyperperistalsis vs ileus, peritoneal signs?

– Femoral or distal extremity pulses: maintained? Evidence of diffuse arteriosclerosis?

Blood work: CBC → elevated WBC/anemia/thrombocytopenia?, lactate, acidosis, creatine kinase-BB (CK-BB), hypophosphatemia, coagulopathy, hypoproteinemia?

Imaging:

– Abdominal x-ray, chest-x-ray: free peritoneal air, thumb printing, loss of haustrations, dilation of loops.

– CT scan with oral/IV contrast if possible (kidney function!): most practical test if pain is the primary symptom → free peritoneal air, segmental wall thickening, thumb printing, pneumatosis, loss of haustrations, dilation of loops, pneumatosis coli, double halo sign, portal vein gas? Other causes of abdominal pain? Assessment of main vascular run-offs: thrombus?

Colonoscopy: gold standard: most sensitive test, contraindicated in presence of peritoneal signs: normal rectum (unless complete aortic occlusion); segmental mucosal changes → hemorrhage, necrosis, ulcers, friability? Stricture?

Additional tests (optional)

Contrast enema: not typically indicated in acute setting (would show: thumbprinting, colonic wall edema, loss of haustration, ulcers); chronic ischemia → colonic road map, stricture?

Visceral angiography (with intervention: eg, thrombolysis): role relatively limited in acute setting unless realistic probability for successful thrombolysis; evaluation of chronic ischemic symptoms → vascular road map.

Classification

Based on etiology: occlusive vs nonocclusive ischemia.

Based on pathology:

- Gangrenous ischemic colitis (15–20%):
- Nongangrenous ischemic colitis (80–85%):
  - Transient, reversible (60–70%).
  - Chronic, irreversible → chronic segmental colitis (20–25%) → stricture (10–15%).

Nonoperative Treatment

Hemodynamic resuscitation: volume rather than vasopressors.

Broad spectrum antibiotics, temporary bowel rest → serial clinical exams.

Heparinization if tolerated.

Possible interventional radiology.

Repeat colonoscopy: as needed to monitor progress, reevaluate colon for other pathology under more optimal conditions.

Operative Treatment

Indications

- Acute ischemia: peritonitis, disproportionate pain (contrast with clinical exam), evidence of gangrene, treatment-refractory sepsis, pneumoperitoneum; failure to improve, persistent protein-losing colopathy (arbitrary > 14 days' duration).
- Chronic ischemia: recurring sepsis, symptomatic colonic stricture, any stricture for which neoplasia cannot be ruled out.

Operative approach
Acute ischemia

- Surgical bowel resection of affected segments → intraoperative assessment of colonic viability: bleeding mucosal edges, venous thrombi, presence of palpable pulse?
  - Primary anastomosis vs ostomy (eg, double barrel).
  - Questionable viability: planned second look operation vs more extensive primary resection.
- Exploratory laparotomy: "open-close"—if extent of ischemia too large to be compatible with life.

Chronic ischemia
• Resection and primary anastomosis of affected segment.
• Angina abdominalis: possible vascular intervention and reconstruction.

Outcome

Transient ischemia: relatively good prognosis, largely dependent on prognosis of other organ systems; 50% reversible: clinical resolution in 48–72 hours, endoscopic resolution in 2 weeks; more severe forms: time healing to healing much longer (up to 6 months) → stricture?

Gangrenous ischemia: 50–60% mortality—less favorable patient population (comorbidities) with more severe disease!

Chronic ischemia: morbidity and mortality similar to colon resection for other reasons, but higher cardiovascular risk.

Follow-up

Full colonic evaluation after 6 weeks (if condition permits).

Emergency surgery: → planning of subsequent surgery, ie, elective restoration of intestinal continuity, after complete physical/nutritional recovery.

Definition of type and duration of anticoagulation.

Cross-reference

Topic	*Chapter*
MRI	2 (p 124)
Angiography with possible embolization	2 (p 128)
Vascular anatomy	3 (p 138)

PSEUDOMEMBRANOUS/*CLOSTRIDIUM DIFFICILE* COLITIS *(008.45)*

Overview

Pseudomembranous or *C difficile* colitis presents a wide clinical spectrum ranging from mild diarrhea to fulminant and potentially fatal colitis. Pseudomembranous colitis in the preantibiotic era was caused by various bacteria (eg, *Staphylococcus*); nowadays it is most commonly associated with antibiotic use and resulting overgrowth of commensal anaerobe *C difficile*.

Pathophysiology: antibiotic-related disruption of normal colonic bacteria (few days to 10 weeks post antibiotic use) allows for colonization with toxin-producing *C difficile* by oral-fecal route. Release of toxins A and B causes mucosal damage and inflammation. Basis for variable disease expression likely related to (1) host immune factors and (2) virulence factors of the organism.

Antibiotics associated with *C difficile* colitis: any antibiotic (with few exceptions: eg, vancomycin), frequency largely reflecting overall use of the respective agents: penicillins, cephalosporins, quinolones, clindamycin, even metronidazole (despite being used in treatment of *C difficile* colitis).

Treatment ranges from conservative management (milder to moderate forms) to total abdominal colectomy (severe and life-threatening form), which is potentially lifesaving if performed before point of no return.

Epidemiology

C difficile is the most common nosocomial infection of the GI tract. Epidemically rising incidence from 6–7 per 1000 admissions in 1990 to 23 per 1000 admissions in 2004; > 3 million cases per year in the US, > 60 per 100,000 short-stay discharges with *C difficile* as primary diagnosis.

Clusters of particularly virulent strains (6% of isolates) with increasing severity of *C difficile*–associated disease: toxinotype III, CD binary toxin, ribotype 027.

Asymptomatic colonization with *C difficile:*

• > 50% of healthy neonates.

• 1–3% of healthy adults.

• 25% of adults recently treated with antibiotics → important hidden reservoir of *C difficile.*

• 20–25% of inpatients become colonized with *C difficile* during hospital stay.

Symptoms

Variations in severity and dynamics of the disease: asymptomatic, self-limited/intestinal only, progressive/systemic, chronic smoldering/systemic, fulminant/multiorgan failure:

• Asymptomatic carrier status.

• Simple antibiotic-associated diarrhea: diarrhea mild, no macroscopic colitis, systemic symptoms absent: *C difficile* accounts for only 20% of this category.

• *C difficile*–associated diarrhea/colitis (without pseudomembrane formation): more serious illness, watery diarrhea, some malaise, some abdominal pain, nausea, anorexia, low-grade fever, peripheral leukocytosis. Endoscopy: nonspecific diffuse or patchy erythematous colitis without pseudomembranes.

• Pseudomembranous *C difficile* colitis: more profound symptoms, more systemic impact. Endoscopy: classic pseudomembranes present, but in 10–20% of patients not in reach of flexible sigmoidoscopy.

• Chronic smoldering *C difficile* colitis: persistent diarrhea, persistent colonic inflammation with colonic thickening (CT), varying but rather mild systemic impact, leukocytosis (leukemoid reaction: massive WBC increase up to 50,000).

• Fulminant, life-threatening colitis: 3% of patients with *C difficile* infection, acutely ill, lethargy, mental status change, fever, tachycardia, abdominal pain, oliguria. Symptom sequence: diarrhea → paralytic ileus and colonic dilation → paradoxical decrease in diarrhea, but increasing abdominal distention and marked tenderness; loss of colonic muscular tone → toxic dilation/megacolon. Rebound tenderness: suspicious for colonic perforation and peritonitis?

Complications: colonic dilation (initial presentation as Ogilvie syndrome) → toxic megacolon, perforation, sepsis, oliguria, multiorgan failure, death.

Rare presentations:

• *C difficile* enteritis or pouchitis after proctocolectomy with ileostomy or ileoanal pouch.

• Superinfection/exacerbation of active ulcerative colitis.

Differential Diagnosis

Antibiotic-associated diarrhea not caused by *C difficile* (80%): unspecific diarrhea, other pathogens (*Staphylococcus, Clostridium perfringens, Candida albicans,* etc).

Diarrhea not associated with antibiotics: eg, secretory, dietary, medications (eg, NSAIDS, prokinetics), neuroendocrine tumors, etc.

Post–*C difficile* colonic dysfunction: may last for weeks to months after clearing of *C difficile.*

IBD: exacerbation of ulcerative colitis with *C difficile* superinfection.

Infectious colitis: *Shigella,* enterohemorrhagic *E coli, Salmonella, Campylobacter,* etc.

Ischemic colitis.

Diverticulitis.

Pathology

Microbiology

- *C difficile:* ubiquitous anaerobic gram-positive bacillus, forming heat-resistant spores able to persist in environment for months or years → differentiation between nonpathogenic strains (do not produce toxins) vs pathogenic strains (produce toxins that cause diarrhea and colitis).

- Infection from oral ingestion of spores, which can survive the acidic stomach environment → conversion to vegetative forms in colon.

- Environmental *C difficile* particularly common in hospitals/long-term care facilities:
  - Hospital floors, toilets, bedpans, bedding, mops, scales, furniture.
  - Increased risk after recent treatment of patients with diarrhea from *C difficile* infection.
  - Health care personnel acting as carriers: hands, ties, rings, stethoscopes.

- Pathogens:
  - Toxin A (308-kD enterotoxin): fluid secretion, mucosal damage, and intestinal inflammation.
  - Toxin B (250-to-270-kD cytotoxin): in tissue culture 1000 times more cytotoxic than toxin A but not enterotoxic in animals. Causes disintegration of filamentous actin → collapse of the microfilament cytoskeleton → cell rounding and cell death.

Macroscopic/microscopic (Figure 4–12A)

Characteristic yellow-white pseudomembranous plaques that bleed when scraped:

- Type I (earliest lesion): patchy epithelial necrosis, exudation of fibrin and neutrophils into colonic lumen → discrete yellow-white plaques of < 10 mm separated by normal or mildly hyperemic and friable mucosa.

- Type II lesion: "volcano" or "summit" lesions with focal intercrypt necrosis and ballooned crypts → rise of pseudomembrane (fibrin, neutrophils, mucin); intact or mildly hyperemic/friable surrounding mucosa.

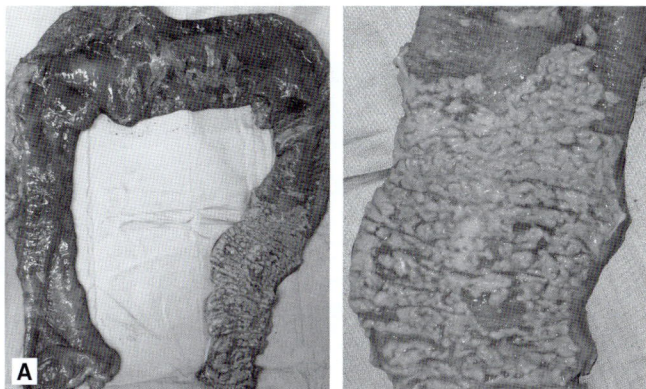

Figure 4–12A. *Clostridium difficile* colitis specimen.

• Type III lesion: diffuse epithelial necrosis and ulceration, overlaid by pseudomembrane consisting of mucin, fibrin, leukocytes, and cellular debris.

After resolution of *C difficile* infection: normalization of mucosa, residual glandular irregularity, often persistent dysfunction for months.

Evaluation

Required minimal standard
Diarrhea only
Stool analysis for *C difficile* toxins A and B (cultures for *C difficile* are not indicated!):

 – Stool cytotoxin test: 95% sensitivity, 99% specificity, result in 2–3 days.
 – ELISA for toxin: 70–90% sensitivity, 99% specificity, result in 4–6 hours.
 – PCR of toxin B gene: sensitivity 96%, specificity 100%, result within hours.

Diarrhea and abdominal/systemic or uncertain symptoms
Rigid or flexible sigmoidoscopy: sufficient to establish diagnosis in 75–80% of patients: characteristic adherent yellow plaques, diameter 2–10 mm.

Plain abdominal x-ray: mucosal edema (thumbprinting) and abnormal haustral pattern, ileus pattern (28% of patients) → toxic megacolon or perforation?

CT scan: distention and diffuse segmental or pan-colonic thickening of colon wall, pericolonic inflammation (Figure 4–12B). In that situation, CT

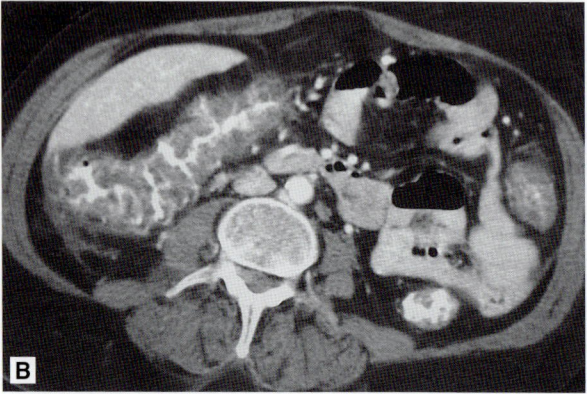

Figure 4–12B. CT diagnosis of *C difficile* colitis.

alone is often diagnostic when pain, fever, leukocytosis is present, but diarrhea is absent.

Colonoscopy (potentially with decompression): diagnostic in 90% of the patients, including the 20% of the cases with disease only proximal to splenic flexure. Perforation hazard in patients with colonic dilation.

Blood work: CBC (leukocytosis with WBC varying from 10,000–50,000/mL), creatinine, albumin.

Additional tests (optional)
Fecal leukocytes: positive test with > 3–5 leukocytes/HPF → excludes benign diarrhea; but negative result does not exclude colitis.

Classification
• Antibiotic-associated diarrhea (ABAD).
• *C difficile*–associated diarrhea (CDAD).
• Pseudomembranous *C difficile* colitis (PMC).
• Chronic smoldering *C difficile* colitis.
• Fulminant/toxic *C difficile* colitis with/without megacolon.

Nonoperative Treatment
Outpatient or inpatient with mild symptoms
• Discontinuation of offending antibiotic.
• Correction of underlying process.

- Perianal skin care: barrier ointments.
- Single antibiotic treatment for at least 10 days with one of the following:
  - Metronidazole $3 \times 250–500$ mg PO (cheap).
  - Vancomycin $4 \times 125–250$ mg PO (expensive).
  - Rifaximin 3×200 mg PO.

Inpatient with significant comorbidities/ICU patient
- Discontinuation of offending antibiotics (if possible)
- Correction of underlying disease process
- Perianal skin care: barrier ointments.
- Combined antibiotic treatment (dual coverage) for at least 10 days with:
  - Metronidazole 3×500 mg PO or IV (cheap).
  - Vancomycin $4 \times 125–250$ mg PO or via NGT (expensive).
  - Rifaximin 3×200 mg PO.
- Refractory/recurrent colitis: combination of vancomycin and rifaximin for 10 days, pulse dose thereafter.

Alternatives
- Binding agents: cholestyramine $3–4 \times 4$ g PO (will also bind oral antibiotics!), colestipol
- Other antibiotics: Bacitracin.
- Antidiarrheal agents: to be used with caution, contraindicated as long as infectious component uncontrolled.
- Steroids?
- Probiotics: eg, *Saccharomyces boulardii* (nonpathogenic yeast, except risk in ICU patients with central lines), *Lactobacillus* GG (generally nonpathogenic, but can cause bacteremia/liver abscess).
- Fecal enemas or colonoscopic stool transfer from healthy donor (eg, spouse): effective reconstitution of colonic flora.

Operative Treatment

Indications
- Fulminant disease.
- Toxic megacolon.
- Colonic perforation.
- Failure of medical therapy with refractory or worsening disease: warning signs among others include secondary organ dysfunction (respiratory, renal, neurologic, hemodynamic), vasopressor use, steroid use, WBC > 20,000.

Operative approach
Total abdominal colectomy with end-ileostomy for all patients (no exceptions).

Outcome

Symptomatic improvement in > 95% of patients after 10 days of combined conservative efforts. Persistent *C difficile* in stool: 3.5% of "cured" patients, 20% of patients whose colitis recurs. Risk of first relapse: 20–35%, risk of subsequent relapse 45–65% → repeat antibiotics, no single effective treatment.

Overall 30-day attributable mortality: 6–7%.

Emergency colectomy: mortality 10–40% (mostly related to delayed decision to intervene).

Follow-up

Emergency surgery: planning of subsequent surgery, ie, elective restoration of intestinal continuity, after complete physical/nutritional recovery.

Cross-reference

Topic	*Chapter*
Diarrhea	1 (p 12)
Megacolon	1 (p 31)
Colonoscopy	2 (p 71)
CT scan	2 (p 117)
Ischemic colitis	4 (p 303)
Infectious enterocolitis	4 (p 315)
IBD—ulcerative colitis	4 (p 320)
Colonic pseudoobstruction	4 (p 360)
Total abdominal colectomy	5 (p 557)

INFECTIOUS ENTEROCOLITIS *(002-009.X)*

Overview

Infectious colitis is a group of acute and chronic inflammatory diseases of the colon that have an identifiable cause and represent an important differential diagnosis to idiopathic IBD. The clinical picture shows variations and may range from acute self-limiting diarrhea to fulminant toxic and potentially fatal presentation.

Pathogenesis: enterotoxic organisms preserve mucosal integrity but cause secretory diarrhea; enteroinvasive organisms cause mucosal injury with combined secretory, ulcerative symptoms. Immunosuppression (eg, HIV infection) may predispose to specific pathogens (Table 4–6).

Epidemiology

Exact incidence unknown as patients with many minor forms do not seek medical care. Sporadic local epidemics achieving attention in news media.

Symptoms

Universal enterocolitis symptoms (acute/chronic: see Table 4–6): diarrhea, passage of mucus, urgency, tenesmus, incontinence; bleeding per rectum associated with certain pathogens.

Possible systemic effects: anorexia, dehydration, mental status change, abdominal pain, fever.

Complications: abdominal distention, toxic megacolon, perforation.

Differential Diagnosis

Idiopathic IBD (ulcerative colitis, Crohn colitis), microscopic colitis, collagenous colitis, IBS, radiation enterocolitis/proctitis, ischemic colitis, diversion colitis, eosinophilic colitis, diverticulitis, STD proctitis (eg, lymphogranuloma venereum, gonorrhea), noninfectious causes (drugs, food allergies, celiac disease).

Pathology

Inflammatory process with or without microscopically identifiable organisms.

Pathogens (see Table 4–6):

- Acute: Salmonella, *Campylobacter, Shigella, Cryptosporidium, E coli* O157:H7, *Campylobacter jejuni, C difficile,* norovirus, *Staphylococcus aureus, Yersinia enterocolitica, Listeria, Vibrio cholerae,* etc.

TABLE 4-6. Pathogens of Infectious Enterocolitis.

Type	Pathogen	Diarrhea	Colitis	Acute	Chronic	Immuno-suppression
Bacterial	*Bacillus cereus*	+		+		
	Bacteroides fragilis	+		+		
	Campylobacter	+	+	+		+
	Clostridium difficile	+	+	+		+
	Clostridium perfringens	+		+		
	Enterohemorrhagic E coli		+	+		+
	Salmonella enteritidis	+	+	+		+
	Salmonella typhimurium	+	+	+		+
	Shigella		+	+		
	Staphylococcus aureus	+		+		+
	Vibrio cholerae	+		+		
	Yersinia enterocolitica	+	+	+		
	Yersinia paratuberculosis	+		+		
Mycobacterial	*Mycobacterium avium complex* (MAC)	+	+		+	+
	M tuberculosis	+	+		+	+

Parasitic					
Cryptosporidium	+			+	+
Cyclospora cayetanensis	+		+	+	+
Entamoeba histolytica	+	+		+	+
Giardia	+			+	+
Isospora	+		+	+	+
Microsporidium	+			+	+
Viral					
Adenovirus	+			+	+
Astrovirus	+			+	+
Cytomegalovirus	+		+	+	
Norovirus	+				+
Rotavirus	+				+

+, positive.

317

- Chronic: *Entamoeba histolytica, Cryptosporidium, Microsporidium, MAC*/tuberculosis, CMV, *Cyclospora, Giardia, Isospora.*
- Bloody diarrhea: *E coli* O157:H7, *Shigella, Campylobacter, Salmonella* species, *C difficile,* amebic colitis.

Evaluation

Required minimal standard

History: symptom characterization, endemic area, risk factors, recent travel, underlying HIV infection or immunosuppression, simultaneously affected family members, bowel function prior to onset, etc.

Clinical examination: general appearance, vital signs, dehydration, abdominal distention, focal tenderness, peritoneal signs, bowel sounds.

Rigid/flexible sigmoidoscopy or colonoscopy: evaluation of extent/severity of morphologic changes → biopsy.

Stool cultures, O&P, *C difficile* toxins: rule out specific, infectious etiology: → 20% positive.

Emergency presentation: plain abdominal x-rays—rule out perforation or colonic dilation > 6 cm ($1^1/_2$ vertebrae) in transverse colon or > 12 cm for cecum.

Additional tests (optional)

Stool WBCs: positive if epithelial injury.

Classification

- Acute vs chronic presentation.
- Specific vs idiopathic colitis.
- Segmental colitis vs pancolitis.
- Enteroinvasive vs enterotoxic colitis.
- Nontoxic colitis vs toxic colitis.

Nonoperative Treatment

Unspecific/symptomatic treatment: rehydration, antidiarrheals, empirical antibiotics (quinolone, metronidazole).

Pathogen-specific treatment: targeted antibiotic treatment.

Identification of source of infection?

Operative Treatment

Indications

- Life-threatening complications: fulminant colitis, toxic megacolon, colonic perforation, massive bleeding.

• Lack of response or deterioration within 3–5 days of conservative treatment.

Operative approach
Total abdominal colectomy with end-ileostomy (ie, sparing rectum and pelvic dissection).

Outcome

Fulminant/toxic colitis rare → significant morbidity/mortality. Nontoxic colitis → complete recovery expected.

Follow-up

Upon resolution of infection: no specific follow-up needed.

Carrier status (eg, *Salmonella*), eg, in gallbladder → need for cholecystectomy?

Cross-reference

Topic	*Chapter*
Diarrhea	1 (p 12)
Megacolon	1 (p 33)
Radiation proctitis/enteritis	4 (p 299)
Ischemic colitis	4 (p 303)
IBD—ulcerative colitis	4 (p 320)
Colonic pseudoobstruction	4 (p 360)
Diversion colitis	4 (p 399)
Total abdominal colectomy	5 (p 557)

IBD—ULCERATIVE COLITIS *(556.9)*

Overview

Ulcerative colitis (UC), a subentity of idiopathic inflammatory bowel diseases, is a complex chronic autoimmune disease of unknown etiology characterized by relapsing and remitting course of an acute ulcerating inflammation of the colorectal mucosa. Lacking a specific cause, treatment remains unspecific. Surgery is largely curative, but does not completely normalize the functional aspects. Approximately 30–40% of UC patients will at some point require an operative treatment.

Epidemiology

Annual incidence in Western countries: 5–16 new cases per 100,000. Age at onset most commonly but not exclusively between 15 and 45 years. Prevalence: 50–220 cases per 100,000 with familial, geographic, ethnic, and cultural variations. Nicotine use may exert favorable effect in UC (in contrast to Crohn disease). At any time, 50% of patients are relatively asymptomatic, 30% with mild symptoms, 20% with moderate to severe symptoms. Despite periods of complete remission, cumulative probability of remaining relapse-free only around 20% after 2 years, < 5% after 10 years.

Cancer risk: 5% after 10 years, increase of 1–2% per year, about 15–25% after 20 years. Average risk of established cancer in presence of dysplasia 20%, in presence of severe dysplasia or DALM 40–50%.

Cancer screening: 2% of patients with regular colonoscopies end up with cancer; 25% of UC patients with colorectal carcinoma show no dysplasia except in immediate proximity to the cancer; 18% of patients with colorectal cancer in UC are less than 8 years post onset of the disease.

Symptoms

Variations in severity of the disease, alternating exacerbations and remissions: diarrhea, passage of mucus and blood per rectum, urgency/incontinence, tenesmus. Systemic effects associated with longstanding or fulminant course of the disease: anemia, anorexia, malnutrition/weight loss, retardation of growth, general debility, abdominal pain, fever.

Extraintestinal manifestations (15–25% of patients): paralleling colonic disease activity: peripheral arthritis (15–20%), skin lesions (pyoderma gangrenosum, erythema nodosum), ocular (episcleritis), hypercoagulability. Independent of colonic disease activity: ankylosing spondylitis and sacroiliitis (1–6%), hepatobiliary disease (pericholangitis, primary sclerosing cholangitis; 3–5%), ocular (anterior uveitis, iritis), cardiac complications (pericarditis), hypercoagulability.

Complications: massive bleeding, toxic megacolon (5%), perforation (may be masked by steroids), malignant transformation.

Differential Diagnosis

Crohn disease, indeterminate colitis (7–15%), ischemic colitis, diverticulitis, infectious colitis (including pseudomembranous *C difficile* colitis), STD proctitis (eg, lymphogranuloma venereum, gonorrhea), radiation proctitis, IBS.

Pathology

Macroscopic

- Confluent inflammation starting at dentate line and extending proximally, sharp demarcation between distal involved colon and more proximal uninvolved colon (Figure 4–13A), or pancolitis (Figure 4–13B).
- Ulcerations in distal ileum in 10% of patients with pancolitis (backwash ileitis).
- Edematous, hyperemic and very friable mucosa, large mucosal erosions and ulcerations, margins may protrude into the lumen and form pseudopolyps.
- Chronically involved colon segments lose haustral folds, become foreshortened, flat, and rigid pipelike ("burned-out colitis").
- Cancer developing in UC often does not form a mass!

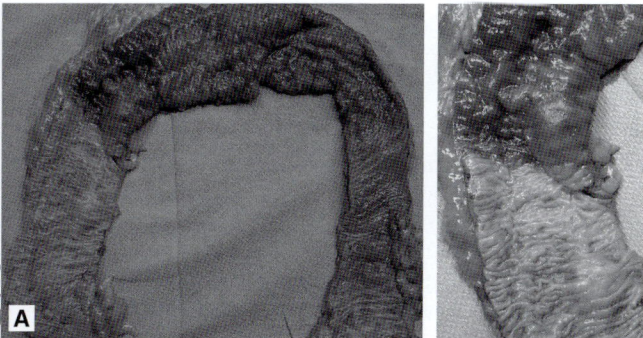

Figure 4–13A. Ulcerative colitis: extended colitis with sharp demarcation.

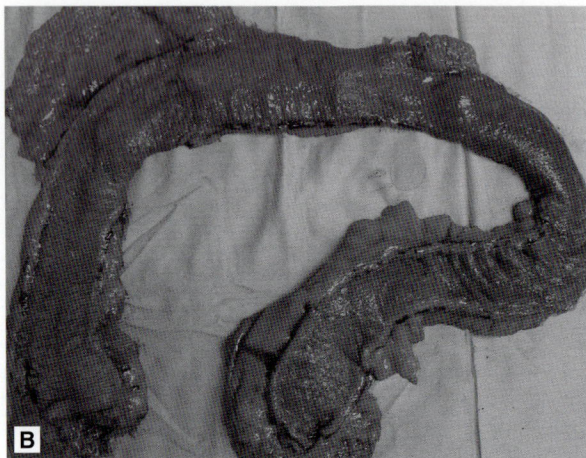

Figure 4–13B. Ulcerative colitis: pancolitis.

Microscopic
- Superficial acute (neutrophils) and chronic (lymphocytes) inflammation limited to mucosa and submucosa (except in toxic megacolon).
- Crypt abscesses, vascular congestion, hemorrhage (acute episodes), distortion of the crypt architecture (gland branching, shortening, loss of parallel arrangement), Paneth cell metaplasia, infiltration of lamina propria with mononuclear cells (chronic disease).

Caveats: overlap of morphologic picture with Crohn disease in 7–15% of patients (indeterminate colitis). Relative rectal sparing: "burned-out proctitis," treatment effect (steroid enemas).

Evaluation

Required minimal standard
Rigid or flexible sigmoidoscopy: sufficient to establish diagnosis, always needed prior to elective surgery to rule out cancer in rectum (as that would change the management).

Colonoscopy: gold standard to evaluate the extent and activity of the disease, but increased risk of perforation in acute disease. (Bi-)annual surveillance starting no later than 7 years post onset.

Stool cultures, O&P, *C difficile* toxins: → rule out specific, infectious etiology.

Emergency presentation: plain abdominal x-rays → rule out perforation or colonic dilation > 6 cm ($1^1/_2$ vertebrae) in transverse colon or > 12 cm for cecum.

Caveat: extent of the colonic diameter does not accurately predict risk of perforation.

Additional tests (optional)

Contrast studies (barium or Gastrografin enema): mucosal pattern as well as foreshortening and stricturing of the colon; procedures are contraindicated in patients with acute disease (may precipitate deterioration with toxic dilation).

Virtual colonoscopy: role not defined, risk of perforation.

MRI, PET, PET-CT: role not yet defined, may be useful for detection of fistulae or skip lesions, for assessment of the disease activity, and for differentiation between Crohn disease and UC.

Capsule endoscopy: not indicated.

Markers: pANCA-positive (60–80% positive in UC), ASCA-negative (60% positive in Crohn disease): definitive role remains controversial.

Classification

- Proctitis or proctosigmoiditis (45–60%), left-sided colitis (distal to the splenic flexure), extensive colitis (involving the transverse colon), pancolitis (20%).
- Minor forms of UC (?): microscopic colitis, collagenous colitis.

Nonoperative Treatment

Principle: control symptoms, suppress disease activity, maintain remission.

- Antidiarrheals/antispasmodics (contraindicated in acute exacerbation: may precipitate toxic dilation).
- Enemas containing corticosteroids or 5-ASA (mesalamine, olsalazine, sulfasalazine) for limited disease (proctitis, left-sided colitis) or chronic pouchitis.
- Oral 5-ASA, prednisone for mild to moderate UC and to maintain remission in 75–80% of patients.
- Hospitalization, intravenous steroids (or ACTH), intravenous nutritional support, transfusions for severe forms of the disease with systemic signs and symptoms
- Cyclosporine A, azathioprine, or 6-mercaptopurin induce and maintain remission (3–6 months delay to establish an effect).
- Newer developments: nicotine, thalidomide, or infliximab.

• Antibiotics not indicated except for medical management of fulminant/toxic colitis.

Operative Treatment

Indications

• Life-threatening complications: fulminant colitis, toxic megacolon, colonic perforation, massive bleeding. Lack of response or deterioration within 3–5 days of conservative treatment.

• Malignancy: established cancer, any level of dysplasia (low grade, high grade), stricture, cancerophobia. Caveat: rectal cancer should always be treated with neoadjuvant chemoradiation first to avoid radiating the pouch!

• Treatment-refractoriness of the disease: failure of or side effects from conservative treatment, steroid dependency, unacceptable quality of life.

Operative approach

Goal: cure from the disease and/or from toxic effects of medications, reconstruction with low morbidity but high quality of life, minimization of morbidity/mortality.

Surgical principle: combination of surgical modules (Figure 4–13C): (1) elimination of disease → (2) reconstruction → (3) protection → (4) completion.

Urgent/Emergency

Total abdominal colectomy with end-ileostomy (ie, sparing rectum and pelvic dissection) for all high-risk patients. Complete excision (ie, proctocolectomy with reconstruction and diversion) acceptable in selected cases. Turnball blowholes: more of historical than practical interest.

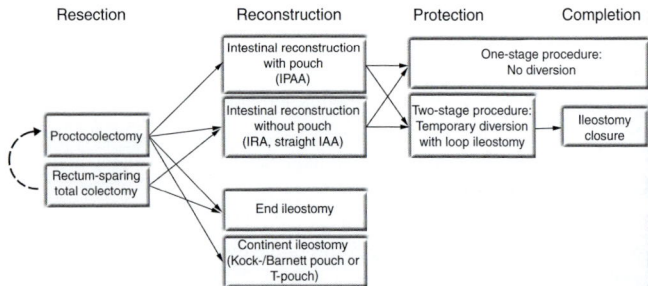

C

Figure 4–13C. Ulcerative colitis: surgical treatment algorithm.

Elective

Most common approach: proctocolectomy, ileal J-pouch anal anastomosis (with/without temporary ileostomy). Mandatory criteria to consider one-stage operation: perfect tension-free anastomosis, normal nutritional status, no immunosuppressive medication (steroid, infliximab, etc). Caveat: For patient, the adjustment period is more difficult (bowel frequency, urgency, control) after one-stage than after two-stage operation.

Less frequent approach: proctocolectomy with end ileostomy or continent ileostomy.

Rarely performed: total abdominal colectomy/ileorectal anastomosis in selected patients (relative rectal sparing, maintained rectal compliance).

Outcome

Emergency colectomy: mortality dropped from 30% to 1%. Massive hemorrhage: leaving rectum in → continued bleeding in 10–12% of the patients.

Elective: Mortality 1%, satisfaction 90–95%, 4–8 bowel movements per day.

Complications: SBO 15–35%, wound infections 5–6%, bleeding 4%, leak with/without pelvic sepsis 4–10%, abscess formation, fistula (perirectal, vaginal pouch), ileostomy-related complications: ≥ 1 episode of pouchitis 20–50%, ATZ cuffitis (UC pathology in rectal remnant), ATZ dysplasia. Pouch loss 3–10%. Sexual dysfunction in males 1–3%, dyspareunia 5–25%, decreased fertility 25–40%.

Follow-up

Emergency surgery: planning of subsequent surgeries after complete physical/nutritional recovery.

Elective surgery: ileostomy takedown > 6 weeks if clinically and radiologically (pouchogram) no evidence of leak and steroids tapered off.

Long-term: antidiarrheals and fibers may be needed. (Bi-)Annual routine follow-up with pouchoscopy and biopsy of ATZ, or as needed. Education about pouchitis symptoms and management.

Cross-reference

IBD—CROHN DISEASE *(555.X)*

Overview

Crohn disease ("terminal ileitis"), a subentity of idiopathic inflammatory bowel diseases, is a complex chronic autoimmune disease of unknown etiology characterized by relapsing and remitting inflammation anywhere in the GI tract between mouth and perianal area.

Pathogenesis reflects complex interaction between genetic susceptibility, environmental triggers (diet, infections, etc), and the immune system: initiating factors result in a leaky mucosa, which allows for antigen presentation and sensitization. Perpetuation and amplification of immune response subsequently cause the autodestructive action.

Lacking a specific cause, treatment remains unspecific. In contrast to ulcerative colitis (UC), surgery is generally not curative in Crohn disease and is therefore only indicated for complications of the disease. Nonetheless and paradoxically, > 50% probability that patients will need surgery in first decade, > 70–90% lifetime risk. Repeated interventions result in significant risk of secondary morbidity (ostomy, short bowel syndrome).

Epidemiology

Annual incidence in Western countries: 6–8 new cases per 100,000, prevalence 50–100 per 100,000. Bimodal age peak: 15–30 and 60–80 years. North-south gradient: higher incidence in industrialized countries, urban areas > rural areas. No severity differences among ethnicities.

Positive family history in 15–25%. Disease concordance among twins: 30–67% monozygotic vs 4% dizygotic. Smoking results in increased primary risk, increased risk for disease relapse (contrast: nicotine beneficial in UC). Higher mortality of Crohn patients compared with non-Crohn population. Crohn disease is associated with increased risk of colorectal and small bowel cancer in areas of chronic inflammation.

Symptoms

Variations of the disease in severity and duration with alternating exacerbations and remissions:

- General symptoms (particularly in childhood onset): anorexia, weight loss, malnutrition, anemia (blood loss, vitamin B_{12} deficiency), growth retardation.
- Abdominal symptoms: diarrhea (from epithelial damage combined with decreased bile acid absorption, causing cathartic effect in colon), bleeding, abdominal pain and cramping, inflammatory mass, fever, sepsis, obstructive symptoms (stricture).

- Perianal manifestations: edematous skin tags, suppurations/abscess, fistula, nonhealing fissures/ulcers, anal stenosis.
- Extraintestinal manifestations: cholelithiasis (decreased bile acid absorption in ileum), urolithiasis (bile acids binding calcium → increased absorption of oxalate → increased urinary oxalate concentration), sclerosing cholangitis, skin pathology (erythema nodosum, pyoderma gangrenosum), ophthalmopathy (uveitis, conjunctivitis, iritis), rheumatologic pathology (polyarteritis nodosa, arthralgias, rheumatoid spondylitis), bronchopulmonary disease.

Complications: massive bleeding, sepsis, retroperitoneal abscess, toxic megacolon, malignant transformation.

Differential Diagnosis

UC, indeterminate colitis (7–15%), ischemic colitis, appendicitis, diverticulitis (sigmoid, right-sided), drug-induced colitis (eg, NSAIDs), infectious colitis (including pseudomembranous *C difficile* colitis), STD proctitis (eg, lymphogranuloma venereum, gonorrhea), radiation proctitis, IBS, celiac disease, Whipple disease, Behçet disease.

Pathology

Distribution pattern: anywhere in the GI tract: 40–50% small and large bowel, 30% small bowel, 20% colon (Figure 4–14A), 15–40% perianal involvement (3–5% of patients have only perianal disease).

Macroscopic

- Patchy discontinuous inflammation (skip lesions, Figure 4–14A), longitudinal ulcers (bear claw, rake), cobblestoning, aphthoid ulcers, deep ulcers and fissures that may form into fistulae, mesenteric fat wrapping or creeping, mesenteric thickening and lymphadenopathy.
- Perianal lesions: skin tags, hemorrhoids, fissures, anal ulcers, fistulas, rectovaginal fistulas, perianal abscesses, anorectal strictures, anal cancer.
- Caveat: cancer developing in Crohn disease does not often form a mass!

Microscopic

Transmural acute and chronic inflammation (neutrophils, lymphocytes), ulcerations, formation of noncaseating granulomas (overall present in 50–60%, but only rarely in superficial biopsy!), penetrating fissures → fistulae, abscesses; chronic inflammation → fibrosis, stricturing.

Caveat: morphologic overlap with UC in 7–15% of patients (indeterminate colitis).

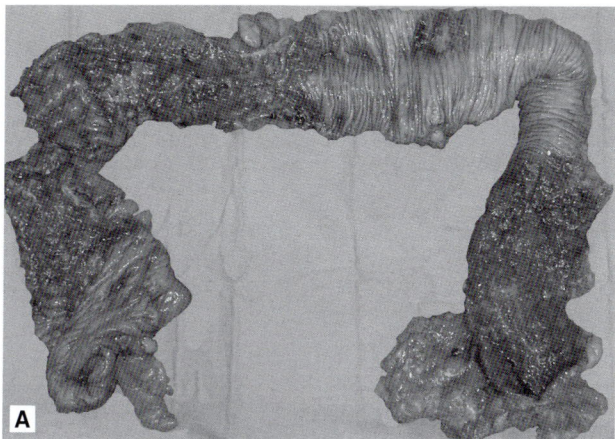

Figure 4–14A. Crohn colitis: acute inflammation with skip areas.

Evaluation

Required minimal standard

History: family history of IBD? Bowel function, perianal manifestations (current, past), course of symptoms, extraintestinal manifestations, preexisting fecal incontinence, smoking? Risk factors for other differential diagnoses?

Clinical examination: stigmata of Crohn disease (perianal disconfiguration, fistulae, etc), strictures?

Endoscopy:
  – Rigid or flexible sigmoidoscopy: rectal involvement, biopsy?
  – Colonoscopy: gold standard to evaluate extent and activity of large bowel disease.

Stool cultures, O&P, *C difficile* toxins: → rule out specific, infectious etiology.

Blood work: C-reactive protein (CRP), CBC, liver parameters, nutritional parameters.

Small bowel evaluation: small bowel follow-through, CT-enterography, or capsule endoscopy (caveat: presence of strictures!).

Emergency presentation: plain abdominal x-rays → rule out perforation or colonic dilation.

Additional tests (optional)

Markers: ASCA-positive (60% positive in Crohn disease), pANCA-negative (60–80% positive in UC): → combination ASCA-positive/pANCA-negative 80% predictive of Crohn disease, definitive role remains controversial.

CT: > 70% sensitivity and > 90% accuracy for Crohn-specific changes.

MRI: evaluation of complex pelvic and perirectal fistulae.

Contrast studies (barium or Gastrografin enema): mucosal pattern, intestinal macroconfiguration, strictures, fissures, and fistulae (Figure 4–14B); procedures are contraindicated in patients with acute disease (may precipitate deterioration with toxic dilation).

Virtual colonoscopy: role not defined, risk of perforation.

PET, PET-CT: role not yet defined, may be useful for detection of fistulae or skip lesions, for assessment of disease activity, and for differentiation between Crohn disease and UC.

Classification

- Disease behavior: stricturing, nonstricturing, penetrating, nonpenetrating (inflammatory).
- Anatomic location: terminal ileum (distal one-third of small bowel), colonic (no small bowel involvement), ileocolonic (both small and large bowel), upper GI tract (proximal to distal one-third of small bowel), perianal.
- Severity (reflected in Crohn activity index): mild, moderate, severe, fulminant, in remission.

Nonoperative Treatment

Conservative management = treatment of choice; defining goals: induction of remission (symptom control, disease activity suppression), maintenance of remission, prevention of relapse after surgery; in severe cases: need for bowel rest and TPN.

Drug categories:

- Salicylates: mild to moderate disease.
- Corticosteroids: moderate to severe disease, rapid suppression of activity in 70–80%.
- Antibiotics: moderate to severe disease, active suppurations and abscesses.
- Conventional immunosuppressants (azathioprine, 6-mercaptopurine (6-MP), methotrexate, cyclosporine, tacrolimus, mycophenolate mofetil): maintenance for long-term activity suppression, avoidance of chronic steroid dependency; may take 3–6 months until visible effect.

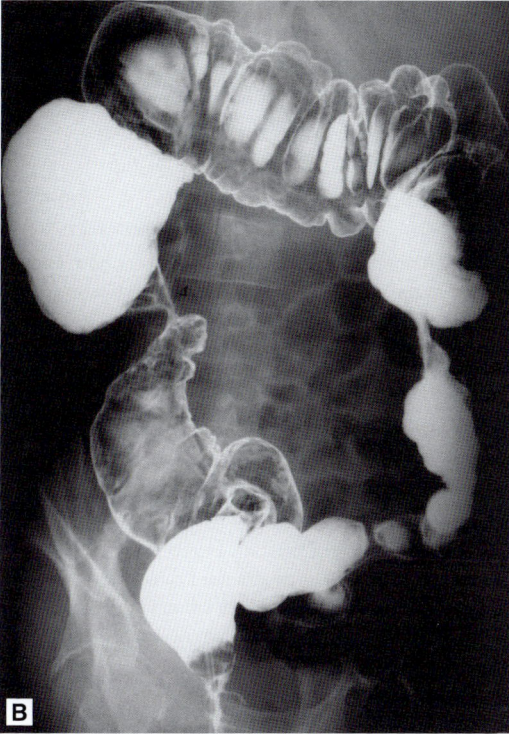

Figure 4–14B. Crohn colitis: chronic strictures and perirectal fistulae.

- Biologic immunosuppressants (infliximab, natalizumab, adalimumab): rapid suppression of activity, steroid-resistant disease (20–30%).

Operative Treatment

Indications

- Symptomatic subacute/chronic disease complications: recurrent/persistent abscess (not manageable with percutaneous drainage), fistulae, stricture.
- Acute life-threatening complications: fulminant colitis, toxic megacolon, perforation, sepsis, massive bleeding → lack of response or deterioration within 3–5 days of conservative treatment.

- Malignancy: established cancer, any level of dysplasia (low grade, high grade), nonsurveillable colonic strictures (5–10% risk of malignancy).
- Treatment-refractoriness of limited-extent disease: failure of or side effects from conservative treatment, (risk of) steroid-dependency.

Operative approach
Principles
- Goal: optimized symptom control vs reconstruction with low morbidity/mortality and high quality of life (eg, avoidance of ostomy).
- Small intestine nonrenewable resource → need for bowel conservation: no benefit from radical surgery → no difference in terms of recurrence between limited and wide resection margins.
- Laparoscopic approach (if appropriate) → decreased long-term risk of adhesive SBOs.

Elective/Semi-elective
- Limited resection with/without primary anastomosis, possible Hartmann-type resection, possible proximal diversion.
- Single/multiple stricturoplasty/-ies (different techniques).
- Isolated Crohn colitis: total colectomy or proctocolectomy. In that situation, IPAA may be offered at experienced centers as an option (even if 5–10 times higher risk of failure) if both criteria fulfilled: (1) small bowel disease absent; (2) perianal manifestations absent.

Urgent/Emergency
Fulminant/toxic colitis: total abdominal colectomy with end-ileostomy (ie, sparing rectum and pelvic dissection) for all high-risk patients; alternative: complete excision (ie, proctocolectomy with permanent ileostomy).

Outcome
Relapse after discontinuation of steroids: 40–50%.

Risk of enterocutaneous fistula: open abscess drainage > percutaneous abscess drainage.

Postsurgical recurrence rate at 2 years for small bowel disease: 70–80% without medical treatment, 55–60% with 5-ASA, 50% with 6-MP.

Recurrence rate for colitis only: ~25% after proctocolectomy.

Follow-up
Careful guidance of patients, monitoring of disease activity, surveillance, teamwork with gastroenterologist.

Cross-reference

"POUCHOLOGY"—THE SCIENCE OF POUCHES

Overview

Pouches reflect an important concept in continence-preserving procedures: creation of an internal reservoir from the intestines, to serve as a low-pressure/high-volume storage area for feces or urine and/or to slow or interrupt propulsive waves and hence decrease urgency.

Effects

Pouch physics

Goal: low-pressure reservoir, increased volume, reversed peristalsis: $\rightarrow$ higher compliance, reduced urgency/frequency.

Pouch bacteriology

• Colonic pouch: normal colonic flora unchanged.

• Small bowel pouch: adaptation of microenvironment $\rightarrow$ adaptation of bacterial density and composition such that it lies in between normal small bowel or end-ileostomy and normal colonic flora.

Histology

• Colonic pouch: unchanged.

• Ileal pouch: adaptation of mucosa to more colon-like architecture; varying degrees of inflammatory changes.

Classification

Different aspects to be considered when classifying pouches:

• Organ of origin: colon, small bowel.

• Specific location of anastomosis: ileoanal, coloanal, urinary, ileocutaneous.

• Type of construction: J-pouch (ileal, colonic), transverse coloplasty, S-/W-/H-pouches, continent ileostomy pouch (T-pouch, Kock pouch, BCIR [Barnett continent intestinal reservoir]). Urinary pouches (T-pouch, Kock/Studer/Indiana pouches, ileal conduit).

• Connection: internal anastomosis (anus, urethra), skin-level ostomy.

Common Problems (for All Types of Pouches)

Early

• Patient anxiety/frustration, mismatch between expectations and true function: need for continued patient education and support (ideally to start before surgery: patient support group, Internet chat rooms; caveat: clustering of negative outcomes!).

- Leak: correlation with overall length of anastomotic suturing, tension, blood supply (ischemic edges), nutritional status, concomitant immunosuppression/steroid medication, malnutrition.

After healing

- Pouchitis: unclear etiology, bacteriologic imbalance, increase in sulfide concentration. Defined by either (1) clinical criteria: increased frequency, diarrhea, gas formation, flulike symptoms; or (2) morphologic criteria: mucosal inflammation, ulcerations.
- Pouch prolapse: ileal J-pouch anal anastomosis, continent ileostomy → pouchopexy, local trimming of redundancy, complete pouch revision.
- Stricture: result of chronic leak, ischemic segment, or postradiation → treatment with serial dilations, stricturoplasty, salvage pouch.
- Fistula: result of anastomotic leak, underlying Crohn disease, cryptoglandular origin → proximal diversion, drainage procedure, pouch revision with axial rotation and reinsertion, collagen plug, advancement flap, muscle interposition.
- Sinus: confined anastomotic leak → marsupialization/incorporation into pouch vs pouch revision.
- Pouch polyp → risk for pouch cancer: definitive risk in FAP, low but not negligible risk in IBD. Prophylaxis: adequate pouch surveillance; once cancer present → oncologic resection and management.
- Pouch outlet obstruction: low-pressure reservoir anastomosed to high-pressure segment, ie, S-pouch with long efferent limb, J-pouch to high rectum: → functional outlet obstruction (as opposed to morphologic stricture) → surgical revision vs supportive measures (tube insertion, stool management).

Assessment Tools

Clinical assessment: inspection, digitalization, etc.

Endoscopy: rigid or flexible, often narrow instruments needed.

Contrast studies (pouchogram): road map, leak, sinus, fistula, size, configuration, distance to the sacral curvature (on lateral view).

Defecation proctogram/pouchogram.

CT/MRI → possible 3D reconstruction.

Specific Pouch Characteristics

Colonic pouch

- Example: LAR/TME.
- Purpose: creation of larger storage area, reversal of peristaltic wave, reduction of urgency. Functional benefit mainly in the first 6–12 months

postoperatively; thereafter advantage compared with straight coloanal anastomosis is less obvious.

- Technical aspects:
  - J-pouch: length 5–6 cm. Risk of outlet obstruction if too long limb or too long rectal stump. Rule of thumb: creation of J-pouch is indicated if (1) possible and (2) proximal colon is too narrow to accept 33-mm stapler.
  - Transverse coloplasty: ~3–4 cm vertical colotomy with transverse closure about 4 cm proximal to distal end of colon to be anastomosed. Possible alternative to J-pouch if colon would otherwise not reach. Increased leak rate. Less effective than J-pouch.
- Output: generally formed, depending on length and condition of residual colon.
- Advantage: decreased frequency, urgency, improved continence. Potentially lower anastomotic leak rate with J-pouch (initial claim unproven).
- Disadvantage: need for additional colon mobilization, depending on patient's anatomy insufficient space for loop (eg, narrow pelvis after radiation or in obese male patient). Increased leak rate with transverse coloplasty.

Specific problems
- Incomplete separation of pouch septum from inadequately stapled J-pouch creation → endoscopic linear stapler division of the septum or pouch revision.
- Functional outlet obstruction.

Ileal J-pouch
- Example: ileoanal pull-through procedure (ileal J-pouch anal anastomosis [IPAA]): J-pouch most common form of ileoanal anastomosis: simple, easy, predictable.
- Purpose: after proctocolectomy → creation of new storage area, reversal of peristaltic wave, reduction of urgency.
- Technical aspects: J-pouch: length ~12 cm (2–2$^1/_2$ firings of 75-mm linear stapling device). Risk of outlet obstruction if too long limb or too long residual rectal stump.
- Output: semiliquid (oatmeal-like consistency), rarely almost formed, more liquid stool not uncommon (baseline or during episodes of pouchitis).
- Advantage: decreased frequency, urgency, improved continence. Definitively preferable to straight ileoanal anastomosis!
- Disadvantage: occasionally difficult to achieve adequate small bowel mobilization; in very obese patients potentially insufficient space for loop

or difficulty to get sufficient length: → alternatives: S-pouch (risk of outlet obstruction, see below) or straight ileoanal anastomosis (poor functional result).

Specific problems
- Pouch leak: order of frequency for J-pouch: (1) pouch–anal anastomosis; (2) staple line of most distal bowel segment; (3) any of the anastomotic lines in between.
- Incomplete separation of pouch septum: inadequately stapled J-pouch → endoscopic linear stapler division or pouch revision.
- Functional outlet obstruction.
- ATZ cuffitis: frequently inflammatory changes on pathology, but clinically not relevant. If patient symptomatic → mesalamine suppositories. If no success and unclear whether frequency caused by cuffitis or pouchitis → transanal mucosectomy and pouch advancement to dentate line.
- ATZ dysplasia: Prophylaxis: adequate ATZ surveillance with visualization and biopsies every 1–3 years → transanal mucosectomy and pouch advancement to dentate line.

Continent ileostomy pouch (T-pouch, Kock pouch, BCIR/Barnett pouch)
- Example: alternative to IPAA or end-ileostomy after proctocolectomy, fallback option after failed IPAA.
- Purpose: skin-level stoma (in lower location than regular ileostomy), consisting of low-pressure, high-volume internal storage area, equipped with a continence mechanism (valve) to prevent inadvertent discharge of stool. Evacuation of stool through insertion of ileostomy tube 3–5 times per day. Obviates the need for an external appliance.
- Technical variations (in historical order):
  - Kock pouch (1969): valve mechanism consisting of intussuscepted efferent bowel segment, reservoir commonly as folded U. Functional pouches result in high patient satisfaction. But increased perioperative morbidity (leak rate) and high probability of reoperation: valve slippage (desintussusception), most commonly either within the first 6 months or after 15–20 years → kinking of efferent segment with increasing leakage and difficulty to intubate the pouch, or valve prolapse with leakage.
  - Comment: despite high reoperation rate, these patients are generally so convinced of the continent ileostomy concept that they would rather undergo one or several reoperation(s) than consider an end-ileostomy.
  - BCIR (Barnett continent intestinal reservoir; 1984): Expanded but more complex Kock pouch concept: Valve mechanism consisting of

intussuscepted efferent bowel segment in combination with additional bowel wrap at the pouch outlet/neck to form collar with additional pressure on valve as pouch fills; reservoir like in Kock pouch but front suture anastomosed to bowel wrap. Concept developed in response to problems with intussuscepted valve; construction more complex and using more small bowel. Results comparable.

– T-pouch (Kaiser, 2002): Completely different valve concept using an interposed separate bowel segment with preserved vascular arcades → concept of intussusception abandoned and risk of valve disintegration and slippage decreased. Design of pouch reservoir of no importance and therefore variable according to individual needs: folded U, S-pouch, long U-pouch configuration. Pouch may be constructed completely new from scratch, or incorporate parts of preexisting pouches, or augment just a new T-pouch valve on an existing reservoir.

- Output: like ileostomy—oatmeal-like, opaque, 600–1000 mL/24 hours.
- Advantage: no need for external appliance with improved quality of life, permitting active physical lifestyle, improved body image, fewer social and workplace restrictions, fewer sexual restrictions (patient and partner).
- Disadvantage: need for patient selection, increased perioperative morbidity, long-term dysfunction, pouchitis. Rarity of this type of stoma → other physicians (eg, in emergency department) are not familiar with concept. Food restrictions: size of holes in tube limited → raw vegetables, seeds, etc, may be a problem.

Specific problems
- Pouch leak: regardless of type of continent ileostomy, there is a 10–15% leak rate (correlation with overall length of anastomotic suturing).
- Skin-level stoma → need for minor "maintenance" operations: (1) tendency to form stricture → widening in local anesthesia; (2) mucosal redundancy → trimming with infrared coagulation or surgical shortening.
- Stone formation: particularly in inadequately drainable pouch area.
- Inability to intubate → emergency because of risk that pouch ruptures → use of narrow rigid sigmoidoscope to intubate under visual control and decompress pouch, followed by sliding in small guiding tube over which larger tube can be inserted.

Other pouches (S-/W-/H-pouches)
- Example: design alternatives to J-pouch for ileoanal pull-through procedure.
- Purpose: S-pouch improves ability to reach pelvic floor, W-/H-pouches increase reservoir (usually not necessary!).

• Disadvantage: S-pouch—too-long efferent limb → low-pressure reservoir situated proximal to high-pressure segment → fecal outlet obstruction. S-/W-/H-pouches—technically much more complex and challenging construction than J-pouch.

Urinary pouches (T-pouch, Kock/Studer/Indiana pouches, ileal conduit)

• Purpose: neobladder or conduit formation after complete cystectomy, eg, during pelvic exenteration.

• Details: see urology literature.

Cross-reference

POUCHITIS—ILEOANAL DYSFUNCTION *(569.60)*

Overview

Restorative proctocolectomy (IPAA) is the surgical treatment option of choice for patients with treatment refractoriness or (pre-)malignant transformation in ulcerative colitis and FAP. Overall outcome and satisfaction are excellent with expected benchmarks of 4–8 bowel movements per day, good fecal control, ability to defer defecation until socially convenient, ability to work, and improved quality of life.

Ileoanal dysfunction is defined as failure to meet these goals. Acute vs recurrent episodes or chronic ileoanal dysfunction. Pouchitis is the most frequent long-term complication after IPAA or continent ileostomy for ulcerative colitis, represents the most common cause of ileoanal dysfunction of an intact pouch. Pathogenesis remains unclear (bacterial overgrowth or imbalance, sulfide concentration, IBD autoimmunity, nutritional etiology, etc).

Poor correlation between morphologic (endoscopic) and functional parameters → use of clinical criteria for diagnosis of pouchitis:

- Intact pouch, not defunctionalized by diverting ileostomy.
- Sudden change in the clinical course (onset of diarrhea, fever, malaise, urgency, incontinence).
- No evidence of pouch stricture or pelvic symptoms from Crohn disease, pelvic abscess, pouch fistula.
- Negative bacteriology.
- Rapid response to antibiotics (eg, metronidazole, ciprofloxacin, rifaximin).

Pouchitis disease activity index (PDAI): scoring system based on clinical, endoscopic, and histologic parameters.

Epidemiology

Ulcerative colitis: 40–50% of patients develop at least one episode of pouchitis, 60% of patients with one pouchitis episode will experience recurrent episodes; 5–10% of patients per decade develop treatment-refractory ileoanal dysfunction → risk of pouch loss. FAP: risk of pouchitis is lower (10–15%).

Symptoms

Primary symptoms: diarrhea, increased/unacceptable frequency/urgency above expected normal range of 4–8 bowel movements per day, fecal incontinence or soilage, gas formation, passage of mucous and blood.

Secondary symptoms: perianal dermatitis with/without excoriations → perianal/perirectal pain, itching/burning.

Systemic symptoms: fever, flulike symptoms may occur, particularly in acute-onset pouchitis; flare-up of extraintestinal manifestations.

Differential Diagnosis

Pouchitis: most common long-term adverse event after technically successful IPAA, nonspecific pouch inflammation of unknown etiology. Defined by (1) clinical criteria: increased frequency, diarrhea, gas formation, flulike symptoms; (2) morphologic criteria: mucosal inflammation, ulcerations.

Irritable pouch syndrome (IPS): same symptoms as pouchitis but complete absence of inflammatory changes.

Anal transitional zone (ATZ) cuffitis: morphologically normal-appearing pouch (pouchogram, pouchoscopy) but significant acute and chronic ATZ cuff inflammation with/without ulcerations → topical mesalamine or steroid suppositories, mucosectomy with pouch-anal advancement if treatment-refractory cuffitis.

Specific pouch infection: *C difficile*, candidiasis, CMV → specific treatment.

Insufficient pouch volume: technical problem (too-short limbs, incomplete division) or result of extrinsic or intrinsic process (abscess, desmoids, pouch tumor, etc) → pouch augmentation or revision, completion of septum division (transanal endoscopic linear stapler division or pouch revision), pelvic "clean-out" depending on etiology.

Pouch prolapse (IPAA, continent ileostomy) → pouchopexy, local trimming of redundancy, complete pouch revision.

Stricture: result of chronic leak, ischemic segment, postradiation, desmoid formation → treatment with serial dilations, stricturoplasty, salvage pouch.

Fistula: result of anastomotic leak, underlying Crohn disease, cryptoglandular origin → rediversion, drainage procedure, pouch revision with axial rotation and reinsertion, collagen plug, advancement flap, muscle interposition.

Sinus: resulting from confined anastomotic leak → marsupialization/incorporation into pouch vs pouch revision.

Pouch polyp → pouch cancer. Prophylaxis: adequate pouch surveillance; once cancer present → oncologic resection and management.

Pouch outlet obstruction: low-pressure reservoir anastomosed to high-pressure segment, ie, S-pouch with long efferent limb, J-pouch to high rectum: → functional outlet obstruction (as opposed to morphologic stricture) → surgical revision vs supportive measures (tube insertion, stool management).

Crohn disease: incidence 2–7%. Diagnosis difficult: mucosal inflammation/ulcerations in afferent small bowel mucosa proximal to the pouch, pouch fistula or other perianal complication more than 3 months after closure of temporary ileostomy.

Pathology

Macroscopic

Diffuse or focal erythema and granularity, loss of vascular pattern, friability of the mucosa with bleeding tendency, exudates, focal ulcerations, aphthoid lesions; while changes are generally diffuse, the posterior pouch portions are more exposed to the stool stasis and may show more extensive inflammation; afferent limb to pouch unaffected, otherwise suspicious for secondary Crohn disease.

Microscopic

Depending on the course and acuity of pouchitis: varying degrees of inflammatory infiltrates (chronic: lympho-/plasmocytes; acute/subacute: neutrophils and eosinophils), focal epithelial ulceration with fibrinoid exudates, superficial acute (neutrophils) and chronic (lymphocytes).

Evaluation

Required minimal standard

Clinical assessment: inspection: perianal skin irritation with/without excoriations. Digital rectal exam: stricture, evidence for fistula, etc.

Pouchoscopy (rigid or flexible): assessment of mucosa in ATZ cuff and the pouch (suspicion of Crohn disease only if ulcerations in afferent small bowel).

Contrast studies (pouchogram) → road map, leak, sinus, fistula, stricture, pouch configuration, volume and size, distance to the sacral curvature.

Additional tests (optional)

Defecation proctogram/pouchogram: configuration, prolapse.

CT/MRI with possible 3D reconstruction: extrinsic problem (compression, abscess, etc).

Pouch cultures (in treatment-refractory or recurrent episodes): *C difficile* toxin, Candida, CMV, stool cultures (*Salmonella, Shigella, E coli, Campylobacter*, etc).

Classification

- Idiopathic pouchitis: acute, recurrent, chronic.
- Specific pouchitis: identifiable/treatable pathogen.
- Morphologic ileoanal dysfunction.

Nonoperative Treatment

General measures

- Improvement of perianal skin care: barrier creams; avoidance of moisture; petroleum jelly–based creams (eg, Vaseline) are generally counterproductive. Severe skin excoriations/ulcerations → application of topical Maalox mixed with nystatin powder until area improved.
- Adjustment or change of antidiarrheal medication, addition of fibers.
- Adjustment of diet and meal schedule.

Specific measures

1. Pouchitis:

    a. Empirical initial treatment of suspected pouchitis:

    (1) Antibiotic treatment (eg, metronidazole, ciprofloxacin, rifaximin): 10–14 days.

    (2) Optimization of diet, antidiarrheal medication (diphenoxylate/atropine, loperamide, glycopyrrolate), protection of perianal skin.

    b. Treatment options for recurrent pouchitis episodes:

    (1) Same as above, but tapering of medication, prolonged low-dose antibiotic maintenance therapy (caveat: metronidazole-induced polyneuropathy), alternating antibiotic schedules.

    (2) Specific pouchitis → adjustment of antibiotic regimen according to culture result.

    (3) Oral bismuth medication.

    (4) Antibiotic course, followed by probiotics prophylaxis.

    (5) Mesalamine enemas.

2. Stricture: dilation → digital, or with dilator (eg, Hegar), Foley catheter balloon (office), or self-dilation by patient using dilators (expensive) or candle (cheap).

3. Cuffitis: mesalamine suppositories.

4. Functional outlet obstruction: insertion of tube for evacuation, possible combination with enemas.

Operative Treatment

Indications

- Failure of nonoperative management with unacceptable quality of life.
- Morphologic ileoanal dysfunction.

Operative approach
Transanal approach
- Examination under anesthesia.
- Dilation of stricture.
- ATZ mucosectomy.
- Local fistula repair.
- Septum division with stapler.
- Marsupialization of sinus.

Abdominal approach
- Pouch revision, redo pouch.
- Pouchopexy.
- Pouch excision → end-ileostomy or continent ileostomy.

Outcome

Depending on underlying cause of ileoanal dysfunction: 5–10% pouch loss per decade. Risk of peripheral neuropathy with long-term metronidazole use.

Follow-up

Careful patient guidance and reassurance.

Pouch surveillance (bi-)annually.

Cross-reference

KOCK POUCH DYSFUNCTION

Overview

Continent ileostomy remains one of the options (rarely used since IPAA) for patients who are either not candidates for an IPAA, have failed an IPAA, or for other reasons ended up with a permanent ileostomy. A continent ileostomy consists of an internal reservoir equipped with a valve that prevents stool leaking through a skin-level ostomy. The pouch is emptied several times per day by inserting a tube through the stoma.

Invented in 1969 by Dr Nils Kock, subsequently several different modifications/alternatives:

- 1969 Kock pouch.
- 1984 Barnett pouch (BCIR [Barnett continent intestinal reservoir]).
- 2002 T-pouch (Kaiser).

The valve mechanism in the first 2 techniques relies on an intussuscepted bowel segment. Paradox: naturally occurring intussusception usually is not considered a good thing, but it is intentionally created for these pouches. This construction triggers the problem that natural force tends to disintussuscept the valve over time (Figure 4–15A): common either early (within the 1 year) or long term (after 15–20 years):

- Axial transfascial desintussusception: → leakage and stoma prolapse.
- Subfascial desintussusception: unfolding and kinking of valve segment → leakage and difficulty intubating the pouch.

Epidemiology

Rare.

Symptoms

Chronic: leakage of gas or feces, increasing difficulty to intubate the pouch, stoma prolapse. Secondary symptoms: peristomal skin irritation.

Acute: sudden inability to intubate a pouch that is still continent → closed loop, SBO → risk of pouch rupture.

Differential Diagnosis

Pouchitis in the continent reservoir.

Pouch-valve fistula.

Pathology

As described above: shortened effective valve segment.

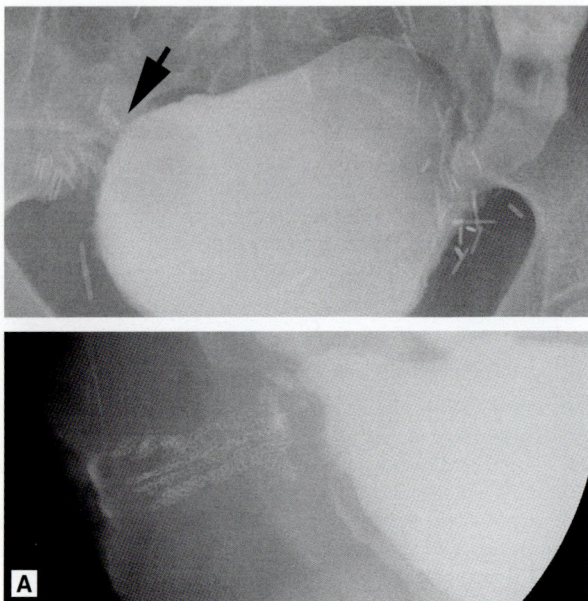

Figure 4–15A. Kock pouch dysfunction from valve desintussusception.

Evaluation

Required minimal standard

History: suggestive circumstances and symptoms.

Clinical examination: pouchoscopy: difficult course of the valve? Pouchitis? Traumatized valve segment? Visible fistula opening?

X-rays: pouchogram or CT-pouchogram (3D reconstruction).

Additional tests (optional)

Stool analysis: *C difficile* toxin, cultures (including fungi).

Small bowel follow-through: assessment of residual small bowel length.

Classification:

• Transient vs progressive Kock pouch dysfunction.
• Valve dysfunction vs reservoir dysfunction.

- Functional pouch dysfunction: clogged system from lack of dietary compliance, inadequate intubation, kinking of intubation tube.
- Morphologic pouch dysfunction: secondary Crohn disease, leak, fistula, chronic pouchitis.

Nonoperative Treatment

Optimization of drainage schedule.

Antibiotic trial → suppress element/variable of pouchitis.

Operative Treatment

Indication

- Chronic Kock pouch dysfunction.
- Acute inability to intubate.
- Need for minor service operations.

Operative approach
Inability to intubate

- Emergency pouch decompression: insert narrow rigid sigmoidoscope and advance to reservoir to decompress the pouch → slide in an adequate guidance tube that fits through the scope, followed by a larger tube with cut-off tip that is slipped over guidance tube.
- Common mistake: placement of NGT only because of assumption that lack of output results from "garden-variety" SBO rather than from the valve → insertion of tube is mandatory!

Options for chronic Kock pouch dysfunction

- Minor revision.
- Detachment of existing valve → pouch rotation and creation of new intussuscepted valve.
- Conversion of Kock pouch into T-pouch (Figure 4–15B).
- Shortening of competent but kinked valve segment.
- Pouch removal with creation of end-ileostomy.

Minor service operations

- Stenosis of skin-level stoma → stricturoplasty.
- Mucosal redundancy of stoma → infrared coagulation, formalin ablation, surgical trimming of redundancy.
- Dilatation of valve segment stricture.

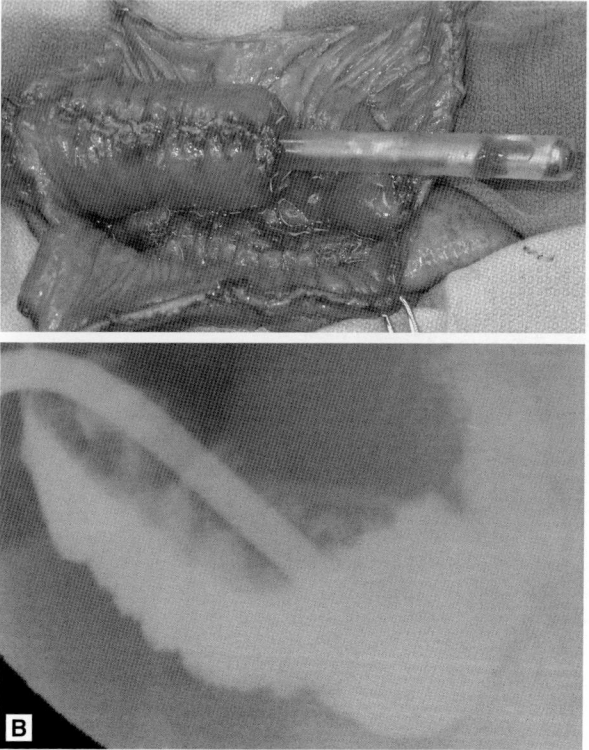

Figure 4–15B. T-pouch valve intraoperatively and on a pouchogram.

Outcome

Continent ileostomy business time-consuming but rewarding: most patients are convinced of the continence concept → they would rather undergo several operations than abandon bag-free life. Increased perioperative morbidities (eg, 10–15% leak, abscess or enterocutaneous fistula formation) → need to carefully select patients and document information to minimize risk of litigation.

Follow-up

Functional reassessment in regular intervals. FAP → pouch surveillance.

Cross-reference

TOXIC MEGACOLON *(556.9)*

Overview

Toxic megacolon is the common final pathway of numerous unrelated pathologies of the colon and carries a high risk of fatal outcome. Definition: combination of segmental or total colonic distention (superimposed on acute colitis) and signs of systemic toxicity (Jalan criteria: fever, tachycardia, elevated WBCs). Proactive aggressive treatment is the only chance for survival. Very high probability that patient will require colectomy—emergency, urgent, or in future.

Variety of underlying diseases: IBD (ulcerative colitis, Crohn colitis), infectious colitis (*C difficile, Salmonella, Shigella, Campylobacter, Yersinia, Entamoeba,* CMV, etc), ischemic colitis, etc.

Pathogenesis: inflammation with complex mediator interaction with cytokine and nitric oxide release → colonic dysmotility → impaired smooth muscle contractility → reduction of luminal pressure via dilation. Toxic decompensation may be triggered in an acute episode of colitis by instrumentation or contrast enemas.

Complications: perforation, sepsis, coagulopathy, abdominal compartment syndrome, multiorgan failure, death.

Epidemiology

Incidence: depends on cause; eg, up to 5–10% risk in admissions for ulcerative colitis, up to 3% of *C difficile* colitis.

Symptoms

Signs of severe/fulminant exacerbation of colitis: diarrhea, bleeding, passage of mucus per rectum, abdominal pain.

Later development of systemic effects: fever, anemia, anorexia, malnutrition/weight loss, dehydration, transition of diarrhea to ileus with increasing abdominal distention.

Differential Diagnosis

Other causes of colonic distention (without signs of toxicity, without inflammatory trigger):

• LBO.
• Colonic pseudoobstruction (Ogilvie syndrome).
• Hirschsprung disease, Chagas disease.

Severe/fulminant colitis without toxic dilation.

Pathology

Macroscopic
Massive colonic distention, colonic wall either paper-thin or thickened/edematous (edema extension to retroperitoneum), focal areas of hemorrhagic and ischemic necrosis, covered or free perforation, mucosal pathology according to underlying disease.

Microscopic
Combination of mostly acute and some chronic inflammation involving all layers of colonic wall, with muscle necrosis, vascular congestion, hemorrhage.

Evaluation

Required minimal standard
History: Known underlying colitis vs toxic megacolon as primary presentation, abdominal pain, diarrhea or constipation, nausea, vomiting, fever? Triggering events: instrumentation, contrast studies, opiates, antidiarrheals? Previous medications: steroids ($\rightarrow$ masking of clinical signs), other immunosuppressives?

Clinical examination: vital signs: high fever, tachycardia, hemodynamic instability, mental status change, signs of systemic toxicity? Abdominal tenderness and distention, decreased bowel sounds, peritoneal signs (may often be absent)?

Blood work: CBC (WBC?, anemia?, thrombocytopenia?), electrolyte imbalances, renal failure, coagulopathy, increased lactate?

Imaging:
- Plain abdominal x-rays: colonic dilation > 6 cm ($1^1/_2$ vertebrae) in transverse colon or > 12 cm for cecum, abnormal haustration, rule out perforation (Figure 4–16). Caveat: extent of colonic diameter does not accurately predict risk of perforation!
- CT abdomen/pelvis: colonic dilation, wall thickening, mucosal edema/hyperemia, pericolonic stranding, ascites, free extraluminal air, pneumatosis intestinalis, portal vein gas?

Additional tests (optional)
Colonoscopy (for diagnosis and decompression) in selected patients.

Contrast studies (barium or Gastrografin) contraindicated in acute colitis: may precipitate toxic deterioration.

Classification
- Toxic megacolon without associated organ dysfunction.
- Toxic megacolon with associated organ dysfunction (kidney, liver, cardiopulmonary, etc), perforation, or peritonitis.

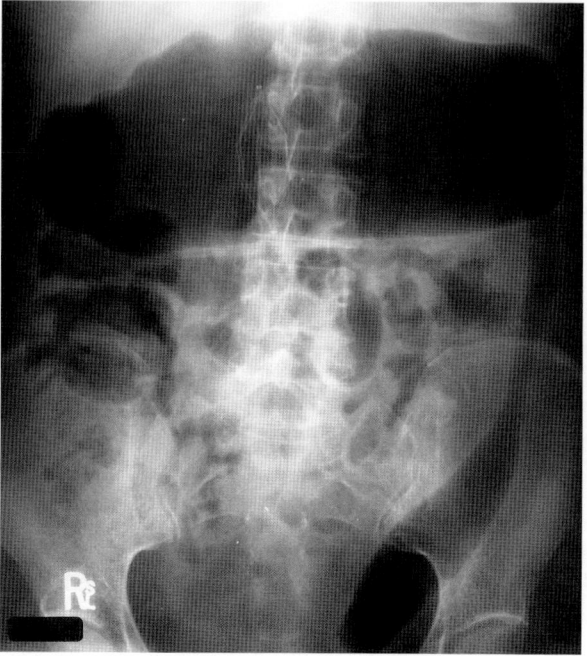

Figure 4–16. Toxic megacolon and rigid pipe in ulcerative colitis.

Nonoperative Treatment

Initial conservative management acceptable only if no evidence of perforation, compartment syndrome, or multiorgan dysfunction → serial examinations: no deterioration but marked improvement should be noted in all parameters within maximal 3–5 days, otherwise surgical management.

• Supportive care with ICU monitoring, hemodynamic resuscitation.

• Antibiotics → appropriate adjustment (and possible addition of antiviral medication) if specific infectious cause or *C difficile* colitis found.

• Immunosuppressives (for IBD-related toxic megacolon only): steroids (and/or steroid stress dose if on steroids < 6 months), cyclosporine A, etc.

Operative Treatment

Indications
Surgery generally is indicated unless favorable circumstances allow for conservative treatment trial:

- Definitive indications: colonic perforation, progressive dilation, abdominal compartment syndrome, beginning multiorgan dysfunction.
- Lack of response or deterioration within 3–5 days of conservative treatment.

Operative approach
- Total abdominal colectomy with end-ileostomy (ie, sparing rectum and pelvic dissection).
- Turnbull blowholes: more of historical than practical interest as it leaves the disease burden on the patient.

Outcome

True toxic megacolon still carries high mortality:

- Any resection less than total colectomy is associated with poor outcome.
- Decision to operate comes too late!
- Poor prognostic parameters: secondary organ dysfunction, perforation, peritonitis, coagulopathy, delayed intervention.

If patient is still hemodynamically stable and not coagulopathic → mortality has dropped from 30% to 1%.

Probability that patient will require colectomy: 50–90% (depending on series).

Follow-up

Emergency surgery: planning of subsequent surgeries after complete physical/nutritional recovery.

Recovery with conservative management: close monitoring of clinical course, elective surgery?

Cross-reference

LARGE BOWEL OBSTRUCTION *(LBO, 560.9)*

Overview

LBO is a partial or complete mechanical obstruction distal to the ileocecal valve. Complete LBO: no passage of stool and gas. Partial LBO: abdominal distention, cramping, but still occasional passage of gas or stool.

Numerous causes: neoplasm (intrinsic, extrinsic), benign stricture (chronic diverticulitis, ischemic, radiation, Crohn disease), adhesions (more often resulting in SBO than LBO), colonic volvulus, intussusception, hernia, endometriosis.

Obliteration of large bowel lumen results in prestenotic stalling of stool. The initial compensatory hypermotility (increased and tympanitic bowel sounds) weakens and shifts into paralytic ileus (late phase, absence of bowel sounds). Increased intraluminal pressure results in bowel dilation with subsequent impairment of microcirculation, followed by increased mucosal permeability and bacterial translocation. Third-spacing of fluids into bowel wall and into the bowel lumen + decreased oral intake + loss from nausea/vomiting, transudation result in hypotension that perpetuates vicious circle with downward spiral.

Complications: electrolyte and metabolic imbalance, malnutrition, colonic perforation (at site of obstruction, eg, perforating cancer, or in dilated prestenotic colon, particularly if ileocecal valve competent), colon gangrene, feculent peritonitis, septic shock.

Epidemiology

Causes: 60–80% malignancies, 10–20% diverticular stricture, 5% colonic volvulus.

Synchronous tumor: in nonobstructing tumors 2–5%; in obstructing cancer 10–25% incidence of synchronous polyps and 5–10% of synchronous cancers in proximal colon.

Symptoms

Depending on cause: gradual or sudden onset of crampy abdominal pain, distention, constipation followed by lack of passage of stool and gas, decreased appetite, dehydration, weight loss. Late symptoms: nausea and vomiting (miserere = fecal vomiting).

Change of stool consistency over course of the colon (right side: soft/liquid, left side: more compact and formed) → earlier development of clinical symptoms in left-sided colon obstruction.

Differential Diagnosis

SBO, paralytic ileus (eg, pancreatitis).

Constipation (LLQ pain, no fever, no WBC elevation, improvement on Fleet enema, colon full of stool).

Colonic pseudoobstruction (Ogilvie syndrome).

Megacolon (toxic, Hirschsprung, Chagas diseases).

Pathology

Underlying pathology causing the obstruction.

Evaluation

Required minimal standard

History: time frame of symptoms, previous similar episodes, change in bowel habits, bleeding per rectum, anemia, last passage of stool/gas. Previous surgeries (eg, bowel resection, appendectomy, hysterectomy, etc)? Previous colonic evaluations (flexible sigmoidoscopy, colonoscopy, contrast enema)? Comorbidities (coronary artery disease, COPD, diabetes, liver/kidney disease, etc).

Clinical examination: vital signs → signs of toxicity, fever? distended/meteoric abdomen, diffuse vs localized tenderness, guarding and peritoneal signs? Increased and tympanitic bowel sounds? Rectal mass? Inguinal hernia!! Fluid status/dehydration?

X-rays: supportive but not sufficient to make diagnosis of LBO:

– Upright chest x-ray: free intraperitoneal air?
– Abdominal x-ray: colonic distention; ie, diameter of cecum > 12 cm, transverse colon > 6 cm ($1^1/_2$ vertebrae)? Small bowel distention? Transition point? Evidence of volvulus?

Rigid (or flexible) sigmoidoscopy: always indicated unless perforation.

Lab work: increased WBC? Anemia? Renal failure (prerenal: dehydration; postrenal: obstruction involving urinary system).

Urinalysis: urinary tract infection → sign of fistulizing process?

Limited water-soluble contrast enema (up to obstruction point but not beyond)!: → road map, but risk of perforation if hyperosmolar contrast trapped proximal to stenosis.

Colonoscopy (with possible stenting): assessment of obstruction site, biopsy, possible stenting (see operative treatment) → full colonic evaluation prior to surgery.

Additional tests (optional)

CT abdomen/pelvis (Figure 4–17A) with dual (oral + IV) or triple (oral + IV + rectal) contrast: site and nature of obstruction, colonic diameter,

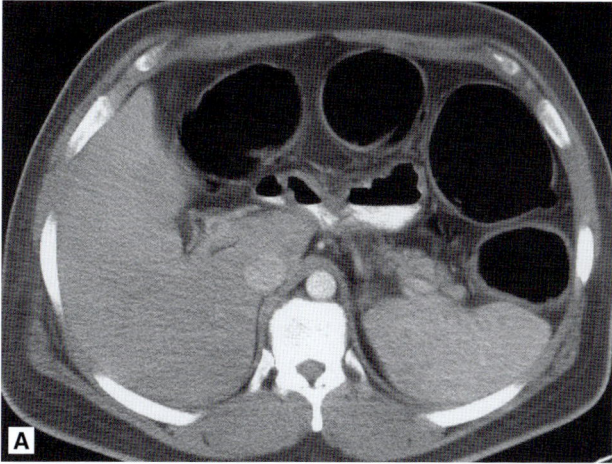

Figure 4–17A. CT scan of LBO.

pneumatosis coli, extraluminal and free intraperitoneal air? Evidence of tumor spreading (carcinomatosis, liver metastases), ascites? Assessment of kidneys, NGT, abdominal aorta, visceral arterial blood supply (celiac, SMA, IMA), portal vein, pleural effusion, etc.

Spiking temperatures: blood cultures.

Fecal occult blood test: only if no macroscopic bleeding per rectum.

Classification

- Partial vs complete LBO.
- LBO with perforation: at site of obstruction vs distant from obstruction (most commonly in the cecum).
- Right-sided LBO vs left-sided LBO.

Nonoperative Treatment

General measures: adequate monitoring, fluid resuscitation, nothing by mouth, NGT placement, IV antibiotics only with defined target.

Local measures if partial LBO:

- Enemas, mild orthograde bowel cleansing.
- Volvulus: endoscopic decompression, possible tube placement.
- Hernia: attempt to reduction unless incarcerated.

Operative Treatment

Indication

Every true LBO is an indication for surgery, unless special circumstances ask for less aggressive approach (eg, end-stage carcinomatosis):

- Complete obstruction → emergency.
- Partial obstruction → semi-urgent, workup possible (eg, full colonic clearance).

Operative Approach

Disobstruction without resection (eg, incarcerated hernia)
Need to check colonic viability, resection if in doubt.

Colonic decompression
- Prestenotic colostomy (Figure 4–17B): eg, loop transverse or sigmoid colostomy is simplest (temporary) operation to allow effective decompression (potentially even in local anesthesia) → stabilization and further investigation of fragile patients. (Caveat: tube cecostomy is not indicated/sufficient because it does not allow for proper decompression/elimination of stool).
- Stenting of left-sided colonic obstruction: definitive palliation or bridging to (semi-)elective resection 1–2 weeks post stenting after stabilization, bowel preparation, and colon clearance.

Resection
- Right-sided obstruction: direct resection with ileocolostomy (regardless of bowel preparation).

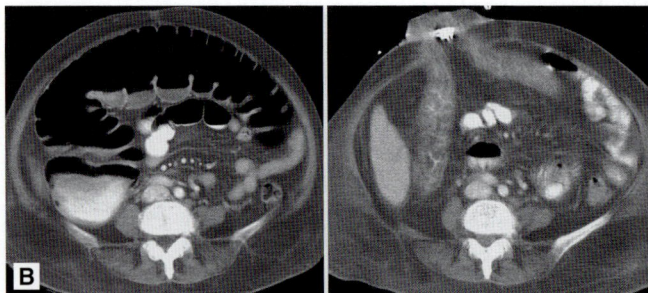

Figure 4–17B. CT scan of LBO before and after transverse loop colostomy.

• Left-sided obstruction:
  – Hartmann resection with end-colostomy and blind distal stump.
  – Resection with primary anastomosis and proximal diversion.
  – (Sub-)total colectomy with ileosigmoidostomy or ileorectostomy.
  – Resection with on-table lavage and primary anastomosis.

Outcome

Surgical mortality historically very high (up to 30–40%), more recently 3–14%.

Stenting: successful in ~90%, risk of perforation, migration.

Follow-up

Confirmation of diagnosis, full colonic evaluation.

Assess effectiveness of resuscitation (vital signs, urine output).

Planning of subsequent surgeries: after temporary decompression without resection, stoma reversal after discontinuous resection.

Cross-reference

COLONIC PSEUDOOBSTRUCTION
(OGILVIE SYNDROME, 560.89)

Overview

Colonic distention without a mechanical obstruction resulting from acquired diffuse colonic dysmotility disorder, usually secondary to general illness or surgery. Numerous extrinsic triggering factors in 95% of cases, which typically occur in the setting of hospitalization or nursing facility: cardiac disease (congestive heart failure, post–cardiopulmonary bypass), retroperitoneal or mediastinal pathology (hematoma, neoplasia), trauma (eg, spinal fractures), pulmonary disease (pneumonia, embolus), metabolic disturbances, drug adverse effects (narcotics, anticholinergics, calcium-channel blockers, antidepressants), extra-abdominal surgeries (eg, orthopedic), prolonged immobility; 5% of cases idiopathic.

Most commonly, pseudoobstruction not associated with any intrinsic colonic pathology, but it can occasionally be a first manifestation of *C difficile* or ischemic colitis.

Rupture of cecum is the most frequent complication (La Place law: pressure inversely proportional to diameter). Treatment is initially conservative including pharmacologic intervention, colonoscopic decompression, rarely surgical.

Epidemiology

Incidence essentially unknown: 0.3–1.5% of major orthopedic procedures. Age generally increasing, average 5th–6th decade. Male predominance.

Symptoms

Abdominal distention → increasing abdominal discomfort, labored breathing, risk of perforation (mainly in cecum) → peritoneal signs.

Variable symptoms: constipation, diarrhea, nausea/vomiting, tachycardia, progressive weight loss.

Differential Diagnosis

Mechanical LBO: identifiable site of obstruction (transition point).

Toxic megacolon (IBD, *C difficile*, other colitis): fever, tachycardia, abdominal tenderness, etc.

Nontoxic megacolon (Hirschsprung, Chagas).

Volvulus.

Postoperative ileus.

Pathology

No intrinsic pathology in majority of cases.

Evaluation

Required minimal standard

History: presence of triggering factors? Past colonic evaluations? Bleeding?

Clinical examination: distended, tympanitic abdomen, presence/absence of bowel sounds, peritoneal signs ($\rightarrow$ suggestive of impending perforation) $\rightarrow$ serial abdominal exams.

Abdominal and chest x-ray: colonic distention, free air? If no immediate surgery $\rightarrow$ serial abdominal x-rays.

At least limited colonic evaluation (water-soluble contrast enema, colonoscopy $\rightarrow$ also decompression) to rule out distal obstruction.

Additional tests (optional)

CT scan: if other pathology or complication suspected (eg, abscess, mass, aortic rupture, etc).

C difficile toxin.

Classification

- Pseudoobstruction without or with intrinsic colonic pathology.
- Compensated vs decompensated colonic contractility.

Nonoperative Treatment

Absence of severe pain or critical colonic distention (> 12 cm cecum, > 6 cm transverse colon):

- Optimization of conservative management: treatment of underlying disease, correction of electrolyte imbalances, bowel rest, IV fluid, nasogastric suction, removal of precipitants (narcotics, anticholinergics, etc).
- Drugs or enemas to stimulate colonic motility.
- Alternating body positioning.

Colonic stimulation:

- Neostigmine 2 mg IV over 2–4 hours (alternative: IV within 10 minutes).
- Side effects (more frequent if shorter administration period): bradycardia, abdominal pain, diaphoresis, salivation, vomiting.
- Precautions: supine position, telemetry monitoring, atropine available as antidote.
- Contraindications: mechanical obstruction, perforation, heart rate < 60, bronchospasm.

Colonoscopic decompression (ideally followed by neostigmine):

• Diagnostic clarification (rule out obstruction, inflammation, ischemia), rapid decompression (particularly if critical colonic diameter), potential guidewire-assisted placement of decompression tube.

Operative Treatment

Indication
• Failed medical and endoscopic management.
• Signs of peritonitis.
• Perforation: ischemia, serosal splitting, mucosal herniation.

Operative approach
Not perforated
• Open (vs percutaneous) cecostomy tube placement for venting of the colon (caveat: does not divert stool!).
• Creation of loop ileostomy (with decompressive catheter through efferent limb → through ileocecal valve into ascending colon).
• Creation of loop colostomy.

Perforated
• Total abdominal colectomy with ileostomy.
• Hartmann-type procedure.

Outcome

Depending on underlying condition:

• Conservative management (including neostigmine): 85–90% success, 20% recurrent distention → require repeated decompression; 3–20% morbidity, 1% (–14%) mortality.
• Need for surgical intervention: 5–15% due to intestinal ischemia or perforation → higher mortality rate (up to 50%, comorbidities!).

Follow-up

Resolution under conservative management: no specific follow-up needed, colonic evaluation per guidelines.

Postsurgical intervention: planning of subsequent surgeries once triggering circumstances eliminated.

Cross-reference

COLONIC VOLVULUS *(560.2)*

Overview

Volvulus is a rotation of the colon segment around its pedicle, which may result in obstruction, strangulation, closed loop, necrosis, and perforation. It is the third most common cause of LBO (3–10%). Subvolvulus with single or recurrent episodes of incomplete rotation and/or quick spontaneous detorsion: very difficult to verify, may precede manifest volvulus (in up to 50%).

Predisposing factors: anatomic hypermobility due to inadequate retroperitoneal attachments, narrow mesenteric base and redundant bowel loop, fiber-rich diet (geographic high-incidence zone around equator: "volvulus-belt"). Multiple other conditions associated with volvulus: age, pregnancy, psychotropic medications, constipation, diarrhea, Parkinson disease, pregnancy, Chagas disease, peptic ulcer, ischemic colitis, diabetes.

Location: sigmoid volvulus (60–75%) > cecal volvulus (20–35%) > transverse colon (3–5%). Two different mechanisms: axial rotation (90%, all sites), volvulus en bascule (10%, cecum) = horizontal and upward folding of cecal pole.

Epidemiology

Geographic variation of incidence: 2–5% of all LBO in US, 15–30% (up to 80%) in geographic belt (South America, Africa, Middle East, India, Pakistan, Eastern Europe). Age in US: 60–70 years, rare in children. Gender: males > females.

Symptoms

Clinical triad:

- Acute abdominal pain, often initially crampy in nature.
- Abdominal distention.
- Cessation of bowel activity.

Late signs: fever, chills, nausea, vomiting, hypotension and shock, peritoneal signs.

Differential Diagnosis

Other causes of LBO:

- Neoplasm (intrinsic, extrinsic).
- Stricture (diverticulitis, ischemia, anastomotic, Crohn disease).
- Hernia.

• Colonic pseudoobstruction.

• Fecal impaction.

Other causes of SBO, ileus.

Acute ischemic colitis or mesenteric ischemia.

Pathology

Nonspecific: ischemic changes with vascular congestion, hemorrhage, necrosis.

Evaluation

Required minimal standard

History: underlying bowel function, time of onset, preceding history of subvolvulus?

Clinical examination: assessment of general hemodynamic condition and fluid status, fever, abdominal distention, presence/absence of peritoneal signs, bowel sounds hyperperistaltic (early), absent (late). Digital rectal exam: empty rectal vault.

Imaging:

• Abdominal x-ray: diagnostic in 70–90% when dilated colon with "bent inner tube" or "coffee-bean sign" with axis from LLQ to RUQ (sigmoid volvulus) or RLQ to LUQ (cecal volvulus).

• Contrast studies (typically not necessary): "bird's beak" or "ace of spades."

Endoscopy (rigid or flexible): "whirl sign"—spiraling narrow segment → therapeutic attempt to overcome obstruction by untwisting (particularly for sigmoid volvulus).

Additional tests (optional)

CT: only if diagnosis in doubt (eg, suspected ischemia): "whirl sign," evidence of necrosis (eg, pneumatosis)?

Classification

• Based on location: sigmoid vs cecal vs transverse colon.

• Based on mechanism: torsion (classical form), cecal volvulus en bascule.

• Based on severity: nongangrenous, gangrenous.

Nonoperative Treatment

Sigmoid volvulus

• Rigid proctosigmoidoscopy (or flexible sigmoidoscopy) with rectal tube insertion (eg, chest drain).

- Contrast enema.
- Colonoscopy.
- → 70–90% successful detorsion (showing as explosive passage of liquid stool and gas), but high risk for recurrence (> 50%)

Cecal/transverse volvulus
- Contrast enema.
- Colonoscopy.
- → high chance of immediate failure, high recurrence rate (75%).

Operative Treatment

Indication
Any volvulus in operable patient:
- Peritoneal signs, inability to detorse: emergency surgery.
- Successful detorsion: semi-elective surgery during same admission: resect or correct hypermobility.

Operative approach
General
Determine bowel viability; resection mandatory if irreversible damage.

Sigmoid volvulus
- Viable: (1) resection with primary anastomosis; (2) mesosigmoidoplasty—incision/widening of mesenteric base.
- Nonviable: Hartmann procedure vs primary anastomosis with/without ileostomy.
- Not proven to be efficacious: percutaneous endoscopic catheter sigmoidopexy (analogous technique of percutaneous endoscopic gastrostomy tube placement).

Cecal volvulus
- Viable: (1) resection with anastomosis, (2) cecopexy and tube cecostomy.
- Nonviable: (1) resection with ileocolonic anastomosis, (2) resection with ileostomy and long Hartmann pouch or mucous fistula.

Volvulus of transverse colon
- Viable: segmental resection vs extended right hemicolectomy.
- Nonviable: (1) extended right hemicolectomy with ileocolonic anastomosis, (2) resection with ileostomy and long Hartmann pouch or mucous fistula.

Outcome

Mortality: 3–12% if viable bowel, 10–20% (up to 50% in some series) if nonviable bowel.

Follow-up

Functional reassessment (constipation, incontinence) after 3 and 6 months.
Full colonic evaluation under elective conditions.

Cross-reference

Topic	*Chapter*
LBO	1 (p 27), 4 (p 355)
Megacolon	1 (p 33)
Conventional x-ray	2 (p 94)
CT scan	2 (p 117)
Sigmoid resection	5 (p 544)
Right hemicolectomy	5 (p 550)
Creation of colostomy	5 (p 596)

DIVERTICULAR DISEASE *(DIVERTICULOSIS, DIVERTICULITIS, 562.1X)*

Overview

Most frequent noncancerous pathology of the colon, related to constipation and age. Clinical presentation ranges from mild disease to life-threatening condition. Diverticulosis: colonic muscular hypertrophy with mucosal prolapse through gaps at entry site of arterial blood supply; complications of diverticulosis: diverticulitis, acute (massive) bleeding per rectum. Diverticulitis: inflammation of colonic wall due to stasis within diverticulum; microperforation/microabscess results in either confined or expanding inflammation with potential complications. Complications of diverticulitis: abscess, microperforation or macroperforation: free perforation with feculent peritonitis, development of fistulae (colovaginal fistula (particularly after previous hysterectomy!), colovesical fistula, etc, chronic inflammation with formation of diverticulotic stricture (caveat: suspicious for cancer until proven otherwise!!).

Diverticular disease is not a risk factor for colon cancer, but it has the same age distribution as colon cancer. But: cancer may present like diverticulitis: 5% of "diverticulitis" episodes are caused by a colon cancer!!

Epidemiology

Western cultures: diverticula increase with age: ie, after age of 50 almost as frequent as the patient's age (rule of thumb); true incidence/prevalence unknown. Caveat: young age does not rule out diverticulosis/-itis. Estimated 10–20% of patients with diverticulosis will have an episode of diverticulitis within a period of 20 years. Risk of second attack of diverticulitis is ~10–20%, of a third attack 40–60%.

Symptoms

Diverticulosis: most frequently asymptomatic, chronic constipation, acute bleeding.

Acute diverticulitis: increasing abdominal pain, fever, peritoneal signs (may be masked in immunosuppressed patients!), small or large bowel obstruction, initially less frequently nausea/vomiting. Caveat: sepsis, dehydration.

Chronic diverticulitis: obstructive symptoms, fistular symptoms.

Differential Diagnosis

Colon cancer (masking with typical symptoms of diverticulitis).

Constipation (LLQ pain, no fever, no WBC elevation, improvement on enemas).

Ischemic colitis.

IBD, particularly Crohn disease.

Postactinic colitis (history of radiation treatment).

IBS.

Noncolonic pathology (tubo-ovarian abscess, endometriosis, appendicitis, pyelonephritis, etc).

Perforation of other hollow viscus (peptic ulcer, small bowel, etc).

Pathology

Muscular hypertrophy, diverticula with acute/subacute/chronic inflammation (polymorphonuclear leucocytes, lymphocytes), abscess formation.

Evaluation

Required minimal standard

History: time frame of symptoms, previous similar episodes, change in bowel habits, bleeding per rectum, anemia, passage of stool/gas through vagina or urethra? Previous surgeries (eg, appendectomy, hysterectomy, etc)? Previous colonic evaluations (flexible sigmoidoscopy, colonoscopy, barium enema)? Comorbidities (coronary artery disease, COPD, diabetes, liver/kidney disease, immunosuppression, etc).

Clinical examination: localized tenderness/guarding vs diffuse peritoneal signs? Rectal mass? Fever? Fluid status/dehydration?

Lab work: increased WBC? Anemia? Prerenal kidney dysfunction (dehydration!). Spiking temperatures: blood cultures. Urinalysis: rule out obvious urinary tract infection, some WBCs and RBCs in urine are still consistent with diverticulitis. Guaiac test in acute setting (diverticulitis, macroscopic bleeding) is of little value.

X-rays: upright chest x-ray/abdominal x-ray in left decubitus: → free intraperitoneal air?

Unless diffuse peritonitis: CT abdomen/pelvis with dual (PO + IV) or triple (PO + IV + rectal) contrast: most sensitive/specific investigation! Look for: pericolonic phlegmon (Figure 4–18A), (drainable) abscess (Figure 4–18B and 4–18C), extraluminal air, free intraperitoneal air, ascites, bladder thickening, air in bladder, other pathologies.

Additional tests (optional)
Acute

Water-soluble contrast enema (barium contraindicated in acute setting): amputated diverticula as sign of diverticulitis, localized perforation, evidence of extravasation, stenosis; visualization of the whole colon is not

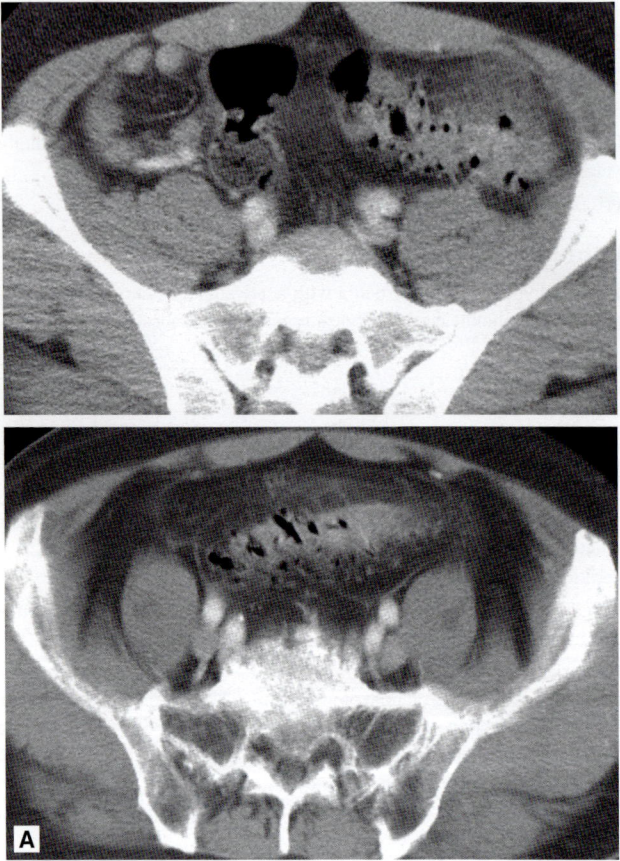

Figure 4–18A. Diverticular disease: acute phlegmon.

necessary at this (!) time, but later. Second best primary investigation if CT not available, however, a limited enema with water-soluble contrast should be considered during the initial hospitalization to rule out cancer-suspicious morphology!

Chronic/elective situation

Barium/air double contrast study (Figure 4–18D) to obtain a "road map": distribution pattern of diverticula, stricture, fistula?

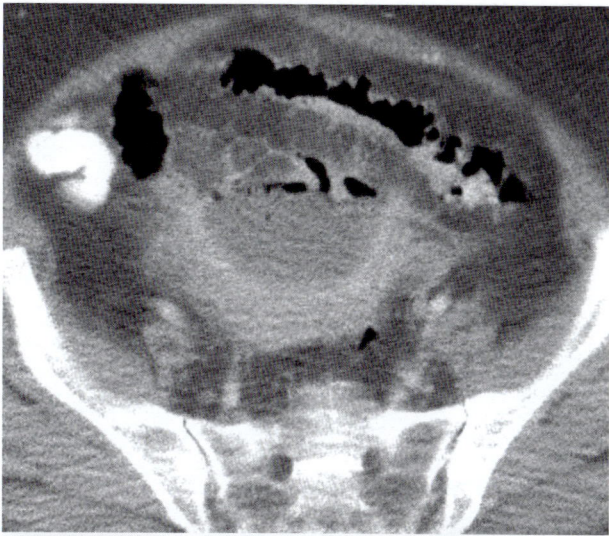

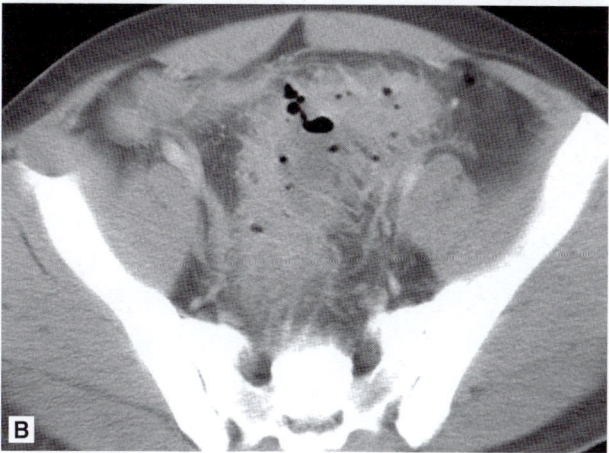

Figure 4–18B. Diverticular disease: pericolonic abscess.

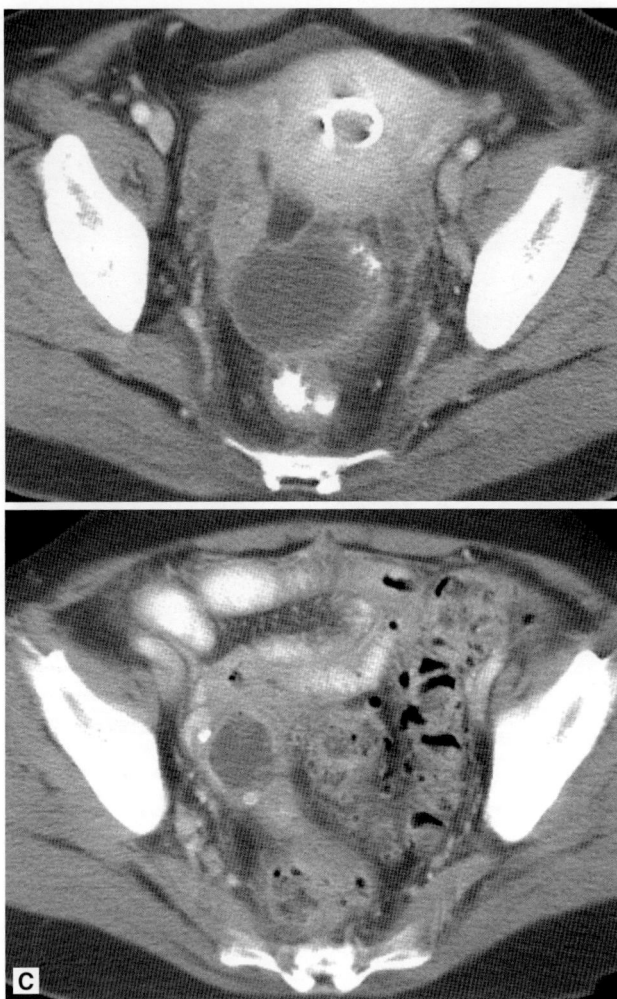

Figure 4–18C. Diverticular disease: pelvic abscess.

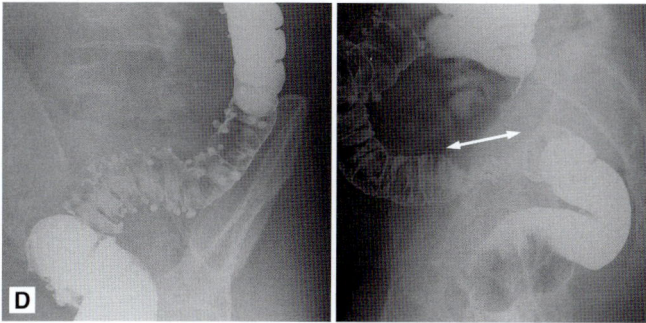

Figure 4–18D. Diverticular disease: chronic stricture.

Classification

Hinchey or modified Hinchey classification: Table 4–7.

Nonoperative Treatment

Conservative: antibiotics for 1–3 weeks, temporary bowel rest vs active bowel stimulation with small aliquots of bowel cleansing, stool regulation with fibers, stool softener, dietary changes, limited water-soluble contrast enema during initial hospitalization to rule out obvious cancer, formal barium enema, or colonoscopy 6 weeks after episode.

CT-guided drainage of abscess.

Operative Treatment

Indication

Emergency or urgent/nonelective resection: diffuse peritonitis, free perforation, nonresponsive to conservative management within 72 hours or worsening under conservative treatment, suspicion of cancer on limited water-soluble contrast enema.

Elective colon resection:

- Two or more episodes of diverticulitis (any age, increasingly debated indication), one episode of diverticulitis in young patient (< 40 years old, increasingly debated indication), one(?) episode in immunosuppression (transplant patient, diabetes, chemotherapy, leukemia, etc), but taking overall prognosis (eg, tumor) into consideration!
- Colonic fistula (colovaginal, colovesical, colocutaneous, etc), colonic stenosis (Figure 4–18D).

TABLE 4–7. Modified Hinchey Classification for Diverticulitis.

Hinchey Classification		Modified Hinchey Classification (Imaging- or Surgery-Defined)		Comment
		0	Mild clinical diverticulitis	LLQ pain, elevated WBC, fever, no confirmation by imaging or surgery
I	Pericolic abscess or phlegmon	Ia	Confined pericolic inflammation: phlegmon	
		Ib	Confined pericolic abscess	
II	Pelvic, intra-abdominal, or retroperitoneal abscess	II	Pelvic, distant intra-abdominal, or retroperitoneal abscess	
III	Generalized purulent peritonitis	III	Generalized purulent peritonitis	No open communication with bowel lumen (ruptured abscess)
IV	Generalized fecal peritonitis	IV	Fecal peritonitis	Free perforation, open communication with bowel lumen
		FIST	Colovesical/-vaginal/-enteric/-cutaneous fistula	
		OBST	Large and/or small bowel obstruction	Acute or chronic

LLQ, left lower quadrant; WBC, white blood count.

374

• Controversial: one episode of complicated diverticulitis (eg, post–CT-guided abscess drainage), which responded to conservative treatment.

Operative approach
• Commonly two-stage vs one-stage colon resection, ie, resection of inflamed segment and creation of stoma. Three-stage almost always obsolete as patient's recovery is faster if diseased segment can be primarily removed, yet in so-called "malignant" diverticulitis, inflammation is too extensive to allow safe mobilization of sigmoid without injury to other structures (ureters, etc), and proximal diversion is the only first option.

• As cancer can never be ruled out, resection should always follow oncologic principles. Extent of resection starts distally at rectosigmoid junction (confluens of teniae) and extends proximally until normal bowel wall consistency is found; removal of all diverticula-bearing colon is not indicated.

Emergency
Typically two-stage resection: (1) Hartmann resection, ie, removal of diseased colon segment, blind distal end, proximal end as end-colostomy; (2) after recovery (± 3 months) Hartmann reversal, ie, descendo-rectostomy (after previous colonic evaluation!!), possibly laparoscopically.

Alternatively: resection and primary anastomosis with or without proximal diversion in appropriate patients and healthy appearing bowels.

Elective
Typically 1-stage resection with primary anastomosis, possible temporary ileostomy. Ideally laparoscopically assisted! Consider preoperative ureteral stents (recurrent severe attack).

Outcomes

Acute: > 70% recover with conservative treatment.

Surgery: complete recovery, recovery with stoma (20–40% of which are never closed), sepsis/death (13th most frequent cause of death).

Recurrent attacks, long-term sequelae (fistula, stricture).

Follow-up

Appropriate duration of antibiotics: 1–3 weeks, depending on severity and normalization of WBCs and clinical parameters.

Stool management with fibers, stool softener, dietary changes (popcorn/peanuts allowed).

Limited water-soluble contrast enema during initial hospitalization: rule out obvious cancer with barium enema or colonoscopy ~6 weeks after acute episode.

Evaluate for prophylactic surgery.

Cross-reference

COLOVAGINAL AND COLOVESICAL FISTULA
(619.1, 596.1)

Overview

Direct communication between abdominal or pelvic intestines and either vagina (uterus) or bladder. Depending on the pressure gradient, pathologic flow most commonly occurs from the intestines to the secondary organ, ie, passage of fecal material and gas with urine; occasionally reverse direction (leaking of urine with stool). Amount of material passing depends on the diameter and length of the fistula track, its exact location, the stool consistency, and the absolute intestinal pressure build-up.

Symptoms alone are not specific for high or low location: abnormal passage (stool/gas in vagina, pneumaturia/fecaluria) and mandates distinction between distal rectal/anal origin and abdominal origin: necessary because of different treatment approach (abdominal vs perineal).

Most common causes: diverticulitis, cancer, Crohn disease, postsurgical complications (enterotomy, leak, etc). Erosion into the vagina or the bladder is more frequent after previous hysterectomy.

Treatment (type of repair, timing) depends on the severity of symptoms, the underlying etiology, the tissue quality (eg, after recent surgery, postradiation, etc), and the level of the fistula (in reach from perineum or not?): need to distinguish rectovaginal fistula from colovaginal or enterovaginal fistula (high).

Epidemiology

Incidence: overall unknown because of various different etiologies. Up to 50% of patients do not recall acute abdominal episode prior to onset of symptoms.

Symptoms

Vaginal fistula: vaginal passage of stool or gas, frequent urinary tract infections, incontinence, perianal skin irritation.

Urinary fistula: urinary passage of stool (fecaluria) or gas (pneumaturia), urinary tract infection, urosepsis, drainage of urine per rectum.

Differential Diagnosis

Diverticulitis.

Cancer.

Crohn disease.

Postsurgical (eg, anastomotic leak, enterotomy).

Radiation enteropathy.

Pathology

Depending on underlying disease: most important to differentiate between malignant and benign.

Evaluation

Required minimal standard

History: onset and characterization of symptoms, altered bowel habits, underlying abdominal pathology, previous surgeries, previous colonic evaluations, systemic disease.

Clinical examination: rectovaginal exam including anoscopy/rigid sigmoidoscopy to rule out distal origin (rectovaginal or rectourinary fistula), abdominal exam (mass, tenderness).

Complete colonic evaluation.

Visualization:

- CT scan: air in bladder, thickened bladder wall, adjacency of colon (Figure 4–19)?
- Cystoscopy/colposcopy: visible stool, visible defect, inflammatory changes?
- Contrast enema: direct contrast translocation from colon into bladder/vagina?

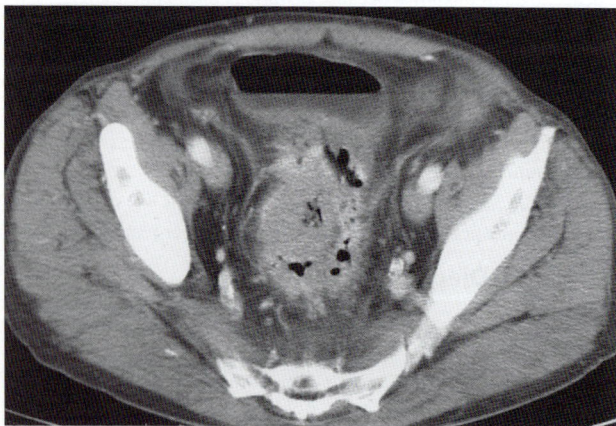

Figure 4–19. Colovesical fistula on CT scan.

Additional tests (optional)

Imaging studies: cystogram, vaginogram (colpogram).

Small bowel study: small bowel follow-through, CT enterography, capsule endoscopy.

Classification

- Colovaginal/-vesical.
- High rectovaginal/-vesical.
- Enterovaginal/vesical.

Nonoperative Treatment

Bulking of stool.

Operative Treatment

Indication

Any symptomatic colovaginal/-vesical fistula.

Operative approach

- Benign disease: resection with primary anastomosis of the intestines, most commonly without major surgery on bladder/vagina side (possibly simple oversewing).
- Malignant disease: en-bloc resection with appropriate reconstruction.
- Acute symptoms, hostile pelvis: proximal fecal diversion to gain time → later appropriate repair.
- Inability to reconstruct: palliative measure → fecal (and urinary) diversion only, no plan for repair.

Outcome

Depending on underlying etiology: benign nature → complete recovery, malignant → tumor-related prognosis.

Follow-up

Colovesical fistula: Foley catheter for 10 days, possible cystogram prior to removal.

Benign cause: clinical follow-up after 2–4 weeks, once fistula problem resolved, no specific follow-up needed; routine cancer screening (per guidelines).

Malignant cause: oncologic treatment and follow-up.

Cross-reference

RECTOURINARY FISTULA *(596.1)*

Overview

Rectourinary fistula is a direct communication of the rectum or anal canal with the bladder or urethra. This is a problem of male patients (in women, vagina/uterus are interposed).

Common causes: congenital anomaly (anorectal malformations); acquired—postsurgical (iatrogenic: prostatectomy, low anterior resection, etc), pelvic malignancy, radiation injury, inflammatory bowel disease, trauma (perineal, rectal, urethral). The communication may result in bidirectional flow of feces/bacteria into the urine or leakage of urine through the rectum.

Treatment (type of repair, timing) depends on the severity of symptoms, underlying etiology, tissue quality (eg, after recent surgery, postradiation, etc), and level of the fistula (in reach from perineum or not?): need to distinguish rectourinary fistula (low) from colovesical or enterovesical fistula (high).

Epidemiology

Rare, but significant number in tertiary referral centers. Overall incidence unknown because of various different etiologies.

Symptoms

Symptomatic: pneumaturia, fecaluria, urinary tract infection/sepsis, hematuria, rectal bleeding and leakage of urine, pelvic pain.

Asymptomatic.

Differential Diagnosis

Colovesical fistula (see separate discussion earlier).

Rectourinary fistula:

- Local abscess (perirectal abscess, etc).
- Posttraumatic: Foley catheter insertion, foreign body, etc.
- Postsurgical: prostatectomy, hemorrhoidectomy, LAR, IPAA, etc.
- Malignancy.
- Crohn disease.
- Radiation-induced (particularly brachytherapy, eg, prostatic seeds, etc).
- Lymphogranuloma venereum.
- Congenital rectourinary fistulae (eg, in conjunction with imperforate anus).

Pathology

Depending on underlying etiology.

Evaluation

Required minimal standard

History: exact description and sequence of symptoms? Previous diseases, previous surgeries, timing, previous radiation therapy → educated guess: abdominal or pelvic origin? Previously attempted repair? Comorbidities?

Clinical examination: rectal exam, anoscopy/rigid sigmoidoscopy → visible opening? Cystoscopy → identification and location of defect? Abdominal exam → distinction between low- or mid-level rectourinary fistula (trigonum or below) from high rectourinary/colovesical fistula (bladder dome).

Setting priority for further tests.

Additional tests (optional)

Imaging studies: cystogram/urethrogram, contrast enema (Figure 4–20), CT/MRI.

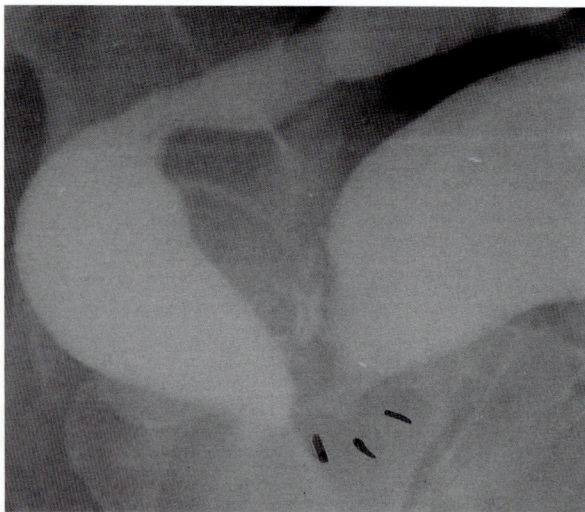

Figure 4–20. Rectourinary fistula.

Endoscopy (colonoscopy, flexible sigmoidoscopy): (1) for evaluation, (2) for screening purposes according to guidelines.

Classification

• High: colovesical, enterovesical, high rectovesical fistula.
• Mid-level: rectourinary fistula.
• Low: rectourinary fistula, anourinary fistula.

Nonoperative Treatment

No/minimal symptoms → conservative management: bulking of stool, antibiotics, Foley or suprapubic catheter, possibly percutaneous nephrostomy tubes.

If patient already diverted → waiting 3–6 months and reassessment.

Operative Treatment

Indication
Any symptomatic rectourinary fistula.

Operative approach
Temporizing approach: proximal fecal diversion to gain time (eg, highly symptomatic, shortly after previous surgery) → appropriate repair electively 3–6 months later.

Primary/secondary repair (depending on etiology, timing): perineal vs transabdominal approach:

• Transanal/transrectal approach (through York-Mason approach) → layered closure and rectal advancement flap.
• Transperineal approach with tissue interposition: eg, gracilis muscle, Dartos flap, urethral grafting (eg, buccal mucosal graft).
• Transabdominal approach:
  – LAR/coloanal, omentum interposition.
  – Cystectomy/urinary conduit, abdominal repair of rectal defect.

Definite palliative measure with no plan for repair/reconstruction: fecal diversion, APR/pelvic exenteration.

Outcome

Dependent on underlying etiology, tissue quality, number of previous attempts, nutrition, type of reconstruction.

Follow-up

Recheck patient after 2–4 weeks of initiated or performed treatment. Once fistula problem resolved → planning of ostomy takedown; otherwise no fistula-specific, but potentially disease-specific follow-up needed.

Cross-reference

RECTOVAGINAL FISTULA *(619.1)*

Overview

Rectovaginal fistula is a direct communication of the rectum or anal canal with the vagina. Following a high-to-low pressure gradient, both stool and gas may pass through the vagina. The amount of material passing depends on the diameter and length of the fistula track, its exact location, the stool consistency, and the absolute endorectal pressure build-up.

Most rectovaginal fistulae are acquired, eg, postobstetric injury or anorectal surgery (rectocele repair, hemorrhoidectomy, LAR), radiation injury, perirectal/-neal abscesses (cryptoglandular, Crohn disease).

Treatment (type of repair, timing) depends on the severity of symptoms, underlying etiology, tissue quality (eg, after recent surgery, postradiation, etc), and level of the fistula (in reach from perineum or not?): need to distinguish rectovaginal fistula from colovaginal or enterovaginal fistula (high).

Epidemiology

Incidence: overall unknown because of various different etiologies. Obstetric injuries in 0.1–1% associated with rectovaginal fistula, radiation in 1–6%, Crohn disease in 5–10%.

Symptoms

Passage of gas or stool through vagina.

Associated symptoms: pain, bleeding, altered bowel habits, diarrhea, fever/sepsis, urinary tract infections, perianal/-vulvar skin irritation.

Very small fistulae may be asymptomatic.

Differential Diagnosis

Colovaginal fistula (see separate discussion in this chapter).

Rectovaginal fistula:

• Local abscess (perirectal abscess, Bartholin abscess, etc).
• Posttraumatic: obstetric injury, foreign body, etc.
• Postsurgical: hemorrhoidectomy, rectocele repair, LAR, IPAA, etc.
• Malignancy.
• Crohn disease.
• Radiation-induced (particularly brachytherapy, eg, cervical cap, etc).
• Lymphogranuloma venereum.
• Congenital rectovaginal fistulae (eg, in conjunction with imperforate anus).

Pathology

Dependent on underlying etiology.

Evaluation

Required minimal standard

History: exact description and sequence of symptoms? Previous diseases, previous surgeries, timing → educated guess: abdominal or pelvic origin? Previously attempted repair?

Clinical examination: rectovaginal exam, anoscopy/rigid sigmoidoscopy, abdominal exam → distinction between low- or mid-level rectovaginal fistula from high rectovaginal or colovaginal fistula.

Setting priority for further tests.

Additional tests (optional)

Air bubbling test: colposcopy (in Trendelenburg position, saline in vagina), rectal air insufflation via rigid sigmoidoscope → air bubbling on vaginal side?

Tampon test: insertion of vaginal tampon, rectal instillation of $1/2$ ampulla of methylene blue in ~200 mL saline, check tampon 30 minutes later → positive if blue at tip of tampon, but base clear), vs false positive (distal overflow), negative, false negative.

Imaging studies: contrast enema, vaginogram (colpogram), CT/MRI.

Endoscopy (colonoscopy, flexible sigmoidoscopy): (1) for evaluation, (2) for screening purposes according to guidelines.

Classification

- High: colovaginal, enterovaginal, high rectovaginal fistula.
- Mid-level: rectovaginal fistula.
- Low: rectovaginal fistula, anovaginal fistula.

Nonoperative Treatment

Bulking of stool.

If patient already diverted → wait 3–6 months and reassess.

Operative Treatment

Indication

Any symptomatic rectovaginal fistula.

Operative approach

Temporizing approach: proximal fecal diversion to gain time (eg, highly symptomatic, shortly after previous surgery) → appropriate repair electively 3–6 months later.

Definite palliative measure with no plan for repair/reconstruction: fecal diversion, APR.

Primary/secondary repair (depending on etiology, timing): perineal vs transabdominal approach:

- Endorectal advancement flap.
- Transfistular rectoperineovaginotomy with layered reconstruction of rectovaginal septum/perineum.
- Insertion of collagen plug.
- Seton management.
- Transperineal interposition: eg, collagen, muscle—gracilis muscle, rectus abdominis, bulbocavernosus muscle (= Martius flap).
- Transabdominal approach: LAR/coloanal anastomosis, omentum interposition.
- Not indicated: fistulotomy, vaginal flap.

Outcome

Dependent on underlying etiology, tissue quality, number of previous attempts, nutrition, type of reconstruction.

Follow-up

Recheck patient after 2–4 weeks of initiated or performed treatment. Once fistula problem resolved → planning of ostomy takedown; otherwise no fistula-specific, but potentially disease-specific follow-up is needed.

Cross-reference

ENDOMETRIOSIS *(617.X)*

Overview

Endometriosis is the presence of functional endometrium outside the uterus. As pathogenesis remains unclear, different theories have evolved: endometriosis foci stemming from retrograde menstruation vs celomic metaplasia vs direct dissemination during GYN surgery.

Epidemiology

Typical age: 20–40 years. Endometriosis involving intestines in 10–30%, majority of which show at least some symptoms.

Symptoms

Depending on the location:

- GYN symptoms: infertility, dysmenorrhea, dyspareunia, etc.
- Bowel symptoms: cyclic bleeding, obstruction with constipation/diarrhea, cyclic pain/tenesmus; if near surface (perineum, rectovaginal septum) → cyclic swelling and pain; perforation rare.
- Bladder symptoms: bleeding, dysuria, urgency.
- Incidental finding of pelvic mass (CT scan, MRI, ultrasound).

Differential Diagnosis

Bowel symptoms or mass related to other causes: cancer, diverticulitis, Crohn disease, etc.

Pathology

Functional endometrium (no neoplastic activity) in ectopic sites, either extrinsic or involving mucosa, desmoplastic reaction, formation of adhesions. Locations: cul-de-sac, sigmoid colon, ovary, appendix, small bowel, other colon.

Evaluation

Required minimal standard

History: careful evaluation of symptoms and relationship to menstrual cycle → clinical suspicion. Further hint from responsiveness to hormonal therapy (eg, gonadotropin-releasing hormone agonists, danazol, etc).

Clinical examination (ideally around menstrual bleeding), including bidigital exam of rectovaginal septum (→ visible/palpable lesions?)

Rigid/flexible sigmoidoscopy: extrinsic fixation and angulation, tethering of mucosa.

Full colonic evaluation: colonoscopy vs contrast enema, biopsies rarely con-clusive if mucosa not involved (but rules out colorectal cancer).

GYN evaluation.

Additional tests (optional)
CT/MRI abdomen/pelvis.

Endorectal/transvaginal ultrasound.

Classification

Based on:
- Number and distribution pattern of endometriosis implants.
- Depth of implants penetration: deeply penetrating vs superficial.
- Severity of perifocal scar tissue (adhesions).

Nonoperative Treatment

Asymptomatic or little symptomatic intestinal endometriosis: oral contra-ceptives, danazol, gonadotropin-releasing hormone agonists (eg, leuprolide, goserelin, etc).

Operative Treatment

Indications
- Symptomatic treatment-refractory endometriosis.
- Intestinal endometriosis: obstruction, or if diagnosis in doubt (eg, pelvic mass).
- Incidental finding during surgery for other cause.

Operative approach
- Laparoscopic/open removal of endometriosis foci, complete whenever possible.
- Segmental bowel resection vs focal bowel wall excision.
- Preservation of fertility → no oophorectomy/hysterectomy without consent!

Outcome

Postoperatively, symptomatic pain relief > 80%, nearly complete relief of cyclic bleeding and obstructive symptoms, satisfaction in 50–80% of patients (depending on whether oophorectomy performed or not).

Follow-up

Functional reevaluation at regular intervals. Role for postoperative prophy-lactic medical management not corroborated.

Cross-reference

ACUTE LOWER GI BLEEDING *(578.9)*

Overview

Acute lower GI bleeding may be brisk and life-threatening unless decisive management prevents a patient's fatal deterioration. Immediate resuscitation and transfusions are key to maintaining hemodynamic stability. Active intervention is desirable but requires identification of a target. However, there is no universally applicable sequence of investigations, and positive identification of the bleeding source often remains elusive for several reasons:

- Bleeding is a common symptom of a wide spectrum of different causes and locations.
- Bleeding may originate from any segment of the GI tract and unselectively accumulate in others.
- Severity may vary with time: severe bleeding may often occur intermittently with often long and equally unpredictable interval periods in between.

Emergency surgery with educated guess of likely bleeding source may be the only option but carries associated morbidity and mortality and may not prevent recurrent bleeding.

Epidemiology

Incidence: unknown, 0.5–1% of hospital admissions; 75–85% of bleeding episodes spontaneously stop. Recurrent bleeding in 25–40% (depending on etiology).

Symptoms

Bleeding per rectum: bright red, dark red, melena—rectal evacuation potentially significantly delayed to actual bleeding episode.

Depending on magnitude of bleeding: associated hemodynamic impact.

Differential Diagnosis

Colonic origin
- AV malformation (angiodysplasia): right colon > left colon.
- Diverticulosis: left colon > right colon.
- Neoplasm: epithelial, nonepithelial.
- Colitis: ischemic, infectious, idiopathic, postradiation.
- Stercoral ulcers.
- Endometriosis → cyclic bleeding.
- Iatrogenic: post-polypectomy/-biopsy.

Anorectal origin
- Radiation proctitis.
- Hemorrhoids.
- SRUS.
- Rectal varices.
- Dieulafoy ulcer.
- Fissure.
- Traumatic/posttraumatic.

Origin proximal to colon
- Upper GI bleeding: esophageal varices, peptic ulcer disease, Mallory-Weiss, aortoduodenal fistula, tumor.
- Small intestine: tumor (epithelial, nonepithelial), Crohn disease.
- Meckel diverticulum.

Pathology

Dependent on underlying cause of bleeding.

Evaluation

Required minimal standard

Overall clinical and hemodynamic assessment, ICU monitoring if unstable.

Lab work: evidence of coagulopathy/thrombocytopenia?, type and cross, transfusion if critical.

Anoscopy/rigid sigmoidoscopy: rule out anorectal bleeding source (even if colonoscopy planned).

Further tests depending on acuity of presentation:

- Acute:
  - NGT placement: discrimination of upper GI bleeding vs lower GI bleeding.
  - Colonoscopy/EGD: acute setting—limited by poor visibility (unprepped colon, strong light absorption of blood → darkness); distribution of blood in the colon has only limited value in localization of bleeding source; after acute bleeding stopped: evaluation after bowel prep.
  - Tagged red blood cell scan: sensitive if > 0.5 mL bleeding, particularly the first 15–30 minutes are meaningful for localization.
  - Angiography with possible embolization: sensitive if > 1 mL/min bleeding.

- Not acute or outpatient:
  - Colonoscopy, EGD.
  - Further tests depending on findings.

Additional tests (optional)

Capsule endoscopy: indicated for GI bleeding not amenable to EGD or colonoscopy.

Meckel scan.

Classification

- Origin: upper GI bleeding, lower GI bleeding, anorectal bleeding, GI bleeding of unknown origin.
- Severity: transfusion-requiring bleeding, mild/sporadic bleeding, occult bleeding, anemia.

Nonoperative Treatment

Patient stable and no evidence of localized morphologic problem → watchful waiting, correction of coagulopathy, possible platelet transfusion, periodical reassessment.

Super-selective embolization.

Operative Treatment

Indication

Localizable bleeding source.

Bleeding not localizable, but ongoing, massive bleeding, unstable patient:

- Acute life-threatening hemorrhage with persistent hypotension.
- Transfusion requirements:
  - > 1500 mL of blood (> 6 units of blood) transfused and continuation of bleeding.
  - > 2000 mL (> 6–8 units of blood) of blood needed to maintain vital signs within 24-hour period.
  - Perform surgery prior to 10 units of transfusion.
- Continued bleeding after 72 hours.
- Significant rebleeding within 1 week after initial cessation.

Operative approach

- Localization successful: appropriate segmental resection/treatment.
- Efforts to localize lower GI bleeding unsuccessful: laparotomy with intraoperative assessment of small bowel, including enteroscopy: if bleeding

still most likely from colon → empirical total abdominal colectomy with ileorectal anastomosis.

Outcome

Majority of bleeding stops spontaneously without surgical or endovascular intervention. Recurrent bleeding episodes in 25–40%.

Risk of intestinal necrosis after embolization: 5–10%.

Emergency surgery: historical mortality 30–40% down to 10–20%.

Risk of recurrent bleeding:

• Minimal after surgery for identifiable bleeding source.

• 3–10% after total colectomy for unidentifiable bleeding source.

• 50–75% after "blind" segmental colectomy.

Mortality commonly related to shock-induced organ failures: myocardial infarction, shock liver, kidney failure, brain injury, ARDS.

Follow-up

Dependent on nature and severity of the bleeding.

Repeat colonoscopy under elective conditions once patient stabilized.

Potential capsule endoscopy to rule out bleeding from small bowel.

Cross-reference

Topic	*Chapter*
Bleeding per rectum	1 (p 4)
Capsule endoscopy	2 (p 76)
Angiography	2 (p 128)
Nuclear scintigraphy	2 (p 131)
Colorectal cancer	4 (pp 252–265)
IBD—Crohn disease	4 (p 327)
Diverticular disease	4 (p 368)
Total abdominal colectomy	5 (p 553)

ENTEROCUTANEOUS FISTULAE *(569.81)*

Overview

Enterocutaneous fistulae (in contrast to ostomies) are unintended abnormal communications between the intestines and the skin. The loss of intestinal integrity with leakage of intestinal content results in intra-abdominal abscesses, sepsis, and decompression through wound or other skin areas.

Most common scenarios: intraoperative enterotomies (eg, after adhesiolysis: primarily not recognized vs leak after repair), anastomotic leak, eroding foreign bodies (eg, mesh), neoplastic bowel erosion (eg, carcinomatosis), IBD, diverticulitis.

Enterocutaneous fistulae are associated with significant long-term morbidity and a mortality of 5–20%. The individual degree of symptoms and output depends on the number of fistulae, the primary site(s) in the intestine (proximal > distal), and the overall size/diameter, ie, high output vs low-output fistula.

Some enterocutaneous fistulae will spontaneously close; others remain open → FRIEND (Foreign body, Radiation, Infection, Epithelialization, Neoplasm, Distal obstruction).

Epidemiology

Incidence unknown; 85–90% related to previous intervention, 10–15% spontaneous (IBD, diverticulitis).

Symptoms

Primary symptoms:

- Prodromal stage: bowel dysfunction, ileus, erythematous wound, wound dehiscence, sepsis.
- Established fistula: various degrees of constant or intermittent leakage of fecal content, gas, pus, resolving vs persistent sepsis.

Secondary symptoms: skin irritation with significant pain, fluid loss, dehydration, malnutrition, weight loss, decubitus, etc; need for parenteral nutrition with TPN-induced problems (hepatopathy, line sepsis); depression.

Differential Diagnosis

Draining abscess/hematoma/fascial dehiscence without communication to the intestines.

Delayed wound healing.

Ulcerating cancer implant.

Urachus fistula.

Wet umbilicus.

Pancreatic fistula.

Pathology

Dependent on the nature of the cause.

Evaluation

Required minimal standard

History: previous interventions → collection of all reports: operative notes, pathology, previous imaging studies → understanding time frame of events, problems, underlying tissue condition, mesh implants, etc.

Clinical examination: general appearance, vital signs, nutritional status, abdominal distention, focal tenderness, underlying induration, skin condition → photographic documentation.

Assessment of nutritional status: weight loss, albumin, prealbumin, lymphocyte count, transferrin.

Imaging: CT abdomen with oral and IV: persistent active abscesses, visible contrast extravasation, anatomy.

Additional tests (optional)

Confirmation of enterocutaneous fistula: measuring amylase in output, oral ingestion of charcoal → positive if black particles show up in fistula output.

Contrast studies: small bowel follow-through, contrast enema (to rule distal obstruction), fistulogram; timing of these investigations: no impact on management at time of acute fistula occurrence, only in planning phase prior to corrective surgery.

Classification

- Output per 24 hours: low (< 200 mL), moderate (200–500 mL), high (> 500 mL).
- Manageable vs unmanageable.
- With/without secondary pathology.
- FRIEND-positive vs FRIEND-negative.

Nonoperative Treatment

Fistula management → gaining time for tissue and nutritional recovery:

- Nutrition: optimization of nutritional parameters—oral diet/enteral feeding preferable if tolerated (ie, not resulting in unmanageable increase of output), potentially fistuloclysis (feeding through fistula), parenteral nutrition (total or complementary in addition to oral/enteral feeding).

- Wound management: need for creativity and individual adjustments; wound-VAC (vacuum-assisted closure), suction drains, skin protection, catheter for collection of enteric content.

- Antibiotic and antifungal treatment: to continue as long as active internal infection, not for fistula as such.

- Output control: no benefit from long-term NGT; no proven benefit from somatostatin or other drugs, except for Crohn disease: infliximab improves fistula symptoms even though it rarely results in lasting closure; role for fibrin glue injection?

Operative Treatment

Indications

- Acute unmanageable enterocutaneous fistula.
- Chronic/persistent symptomatic enterocutaneous fistula after minimum of 6–12 weeks (up to 6 months) of conservative optimization.

Operative approach

- Acute: proximal fecal diversion.
- Chronic: abdominal exploration with most careful adhesiolysis → isolation of defective bowel segment and removal of all foreign material (eg, mesh).
- Segmental resection of involved bowel with primary anastomosis.
- Complete exclusion of segment → continued minimal mucus drainage but no enteric content.
- Not recommended: simple fistula closure (> 40% recurrence).
- Abdominal wall closure without mesh → direct closure; if needed component separation or flaps.

Outcome

Even under best circumstances: 10% failure rate (depending on the nature of the problem). Once healed → complete recovery.

Follow-up

Functional and nutritional follow-up until complete normalization. Additional follow-up if underlying disease (cancer, Crohn disease).

Cross-reference

DIVERSION COLITIS *(V44.2)*

Overview

Reversible morphologic (and symptomatic) changes in the large intestine that develop from a lack of nutrients as a result of proximal fecal diversion (ostomy). Common scenarios: status diverting ileostomy/colostomy, status post Hartmann resection.

Pathogenesis:

• 70% of colonic mucosal nutrition comes from lumen.

• Short-chain fatty acids (SCFAs: acetate/propionate/n-butyrate) are of particular importance for the colon.

(Contrast: for small intestine, glutamine is the most relevant component for nutrition.)

Epidemiology

To some degree present every time diversion is performed (100% prevalence) but only fraction of these patients are symptomatic.

Symptoms

Rectal bleeding, mucus or mucopurulent discharge, occasionally cramps.

Differential Diagnosis

IBD: ulcerative colitis, Crohn colitis (caveat: assessment of IBD activity impossible after diversion → has to be described at the time of diversion).

Radiation proctitis.

Pathology

Mild: friability of colonic mucosa → difference between colonoscopy on way in (normal appearance) and out (diffuse injuries from contact with instrument).

Moderate to severe; diffuse and increasingly confluent ulcerations.

Microscopic: crypt atrophy and distortion with acute (polymorphonuclear) and chronic (lymphoplasmocellular) infiltrates.

Evaluation

Required minimal standard
History: suggestive circumstances.

Clinical examination: endoscopic evaluation.

Additional tests (optional)
Evaluation for options to reverse ostomy.

Classification
- Symptomatic vs asymptomatic diversion colitis.
- Diversion colitis with/without prospect of ostomy reversal.

Nonoperative Treatment
Asymptomatic patients.

Symptomatic patients: SCFA enemas (good but pharmacologically unstable) → more practical to use milk or tube feed enemas (daily to weekly).

Operative Treatment
Indication
Treatment-refractory symptomatic diversion colitis.

Operative approach
- Reversal of ostomy possible → ostomy takedown.
- Reversal of ostomy not possible → resection of diverted colon segment.

Outcome
Generally relatively benign course.

Follow-up
Functional reassessment at regular intervals.

Cancer surveillance of diverted segments is still indicated.

Cross-reference

"STOMATOLOGY"—THE SCIENCE OF OSTOMIES (V44.2)

Overview

Stoma/ostomy is an intentionally created intestinal opening to the skin in order to allow controlled decompression and elimination of waste, to provide access for nutrition, or to divert stool from a more distal area of concern (anastomosis, inflammation, rectovaginal fistula, incompetent sphincter muscle, etc). Ostomies are overall less frequently needed than in the past, but remain one of the "necessary evils" of colorectal surgery. Much worse than having an ostomy is having a bad ostomy.

Classification

Different aspects to be considered when classifying ostomies:

- Organ of origin: → colostomy, ileostomy, jejunostomy, gastrostomy; urostomy.
- Specific colonic location: cecostomy, transverse colostomy, descending/sigmoid colostomy, perineal colostomy.
- Type of construction: end- vs loop ostomy, blowhole, continent ostomy, tube/catheter ostomy
- Intended appearance: nipple, skin-level, rose, catheter.
- Planned duration: temporary ostomy vs permanent ostomy.
- Purpose of ostomy: waste management, diversion of stool from more distal area of concern, decompression/venting of stomach or intestines, nutrition.

Common Problems (All Types of Stomas)

- Patient anxiety/frustration: need for continued patient education and support (ideally to start before surgery), enterostomal nurse, ostomy support group, Internet chat rooms.
- Inadequate stoma location: preoperative marking—ideally through rectus muscle, avoidance of folds, belt line, uneven/concave surface, bony prominences. Skinny patients → below umbilical transverse line. Obese patients → generally much higher location (upper abdomen) needed because of down-shift of abdominal pannus in upright position.
- Inadequate configuration and maturation (Figure 4–21A): mainly a problem in obese patients or if bowels significantly distended.
- Peristomal skin irritation: insufficient management vs insufficient ostomy (→ enterostomal nurse), allergic reactions (→ change of products),

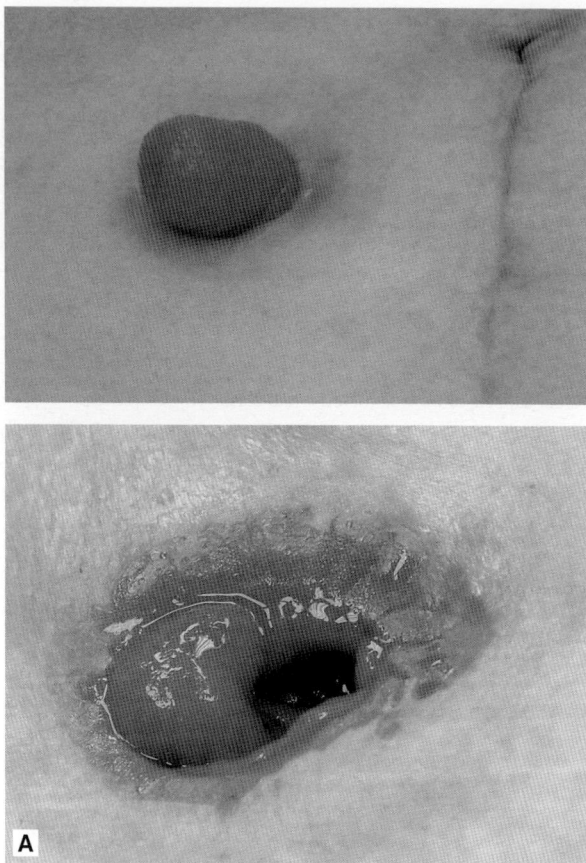

Figure 4–21A. Ileostomy: correct (top) and incorrect configuration (bottom).

peristomal candidiasis (→ topical antifungal medications), peristomal pyoderma gangrenosum (→ topical or systemic immunosuppressives).

- Inflammatory polyps: on exposed mucosa or mucocutaneous junction → ablation with topical silver nitrate or with cautery.
- Stoma prolapse (Figure 4–21B): increasing protrusion with discomfort, bleeding, and aesthetic problem → resection, relocation, possible extraperitoneal tunnel, button-fixation.

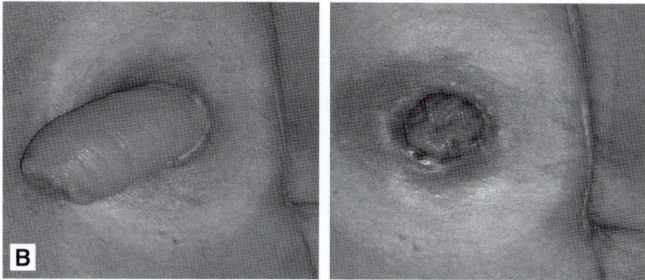

Figure 4–21B. Colostomy prolapse: before and after correction.

- Peristomal herniation: increasing bulging and management difficulties → fascial narrowing and reinforcement with implant (Gore-Tex or collagen: keyhole technique vs Sugarbaker onlay technique), stoma relocation. Mesh not recommended as sharp edges risk erosion into bowel.

Stoma necrosis/retraction (acute): (1) epifascial → conservative management possible, acceptance of stricture/retraction → later complete stoma revision or final takedown; (2) subfascial → risk of free bowel perforation → urgent stoma revision.

- Stoma retraction, stricturing (chronic): → takedown if possible, otherwise complete stoma revision, possible relocation.
- Internal hernia/wrapping of small bowel around ostomy-bearing bowel with resulting bowel obstruction. Prevented at least in permanent stomas by closing lateral aspect.
- Peristomal abscess: drainage either close (into the bag) or far (not to be located right underneath the appliance wafer).
- Peristomal fistula: depending on output → doing nothing, fibrin glue/collagen plug, complete revision/relocation (if related to mesh implant → mesh removal necessary), placement of coated stent (?).
- High ostomy output: possible causes include idiopathic/incomplete adjustment (→ regular food, fibers, antidiarrheals), partial SBO (→ avoid antidiarrheals), excessive oral fluid consumption (→ reduce excessive oral fluids), "serositis" (→ trial with antibiotics).
- Peristomal varices (portal hypertension): (1) prevention: avoid long-term ostomy wherever possible in patients with liver cirrhosis; (2) treatment: reseparation of mucocutaneous junction and reimplantation of stoma.
- Leakage of ascites (eg, liver cirrhosis): → avoid stoma, routine placement of peritoneal overflow drain until healed (even in low severity cirrhotics).

Stoma Takedown

Generally simpler for loop ostomies, often complex for discontinuous resection/stoma (Hartmann type). Takedown facilitated by application of anti-adhesion products (Seprafilm, SprayGel, etc). Laparoscopic vs open approach. Timing preferably not before 6–12 weeks after previous surgery.

Preoperative evaluation of current anatomy (water-soluble contrast studies).

In case of stoma complication: evaluate whether ostomy still needed ($\rightarrow$ revision) or not needed anymore, eg, healed distal anastomosis $\rightarrow$ ostomy takedown.

Assessment Tools

Clinical assessment: inspection, digitalization, flash light/test tube to determine the level of viability above or below the fascia, positional changes ($\rightarrow$ hernia?), etc.

Endoscopy.

Contrast studies: road map.

CT/MRI: herniation, abscess, etc?

Specific Ostomies

End colostomy

- Example: Hartmann resection $\rightarrow$ anus/rectal stump maintained. APR $\rightarrow$ closed perineum. (Special situation: perineal colostomy—see below.)
- Purpose: result of resection where (immediate) restoration of intestinal continuity not possible or not desired. If distal anatomy still preserved $\rightarrow$ elective takedown possible.
- Target location (unless adjusted): LLQ, through rectus muscle.
- Appearance: relatively flat rose, < 2–4 mm elevation, 3–4 cm diameter (Figure 4–21B).
- Output: formed; while most patients carry an external appliance, this stoma may be trained with scheduled enemas, etc, to obtain planned/controlled evacuation once per day only $\rightarrow$ no need for external appliance in-between.
- Advantage: fluid balance unaffected, avoidance of anastomosis under suboptimal conditions.
- Disadvantage: potentially challenging operation for reversal. Odor.

Loop colostomy

- Example: sigmoid loop colostomy, transverse loop colostomy.
- Technical variations: (1) true loop with afferent and efferent limb $\rightarrow$ both afferent and efferent limb decompressed but potentially incomplete

diversion; (2) Prasad-type loop: open afferent limb, efferent limb closed off/attached to afferent limb or fascia or matured into ostomy as mucous fistula → complete diversion, to be avoided in case of (pending) distal obstruction. Temporary bridge for 10–14 days.

- Purpose: colonic decompression, fecal diversion (complete, incomplete). Ostomy of choice in emergency case of acute distal problem (anastomotic leak, obstructing tumor, pelvic sepsis, etc).
- Target location (unless adjusted): (1) LLQ, through rectus muscle; (2) RUQ/LUQ, not too close to costal margin. Caveat: double-check actual colonic vascularization post previous resection and plan ostomy proximal to feeding vascular pedicle to avoid creation of avascular segment!
- Appearance: relatively flat (2–4 mm) rose; efferent limb clearly visible (true loop), or mucous fistula only (Prasad type).
- Output: left side of colon → formed stool; right side → liquid stool.
- Advantage: allows access to colon; both afferent and efferent limb may be decompressed/washed out, no risk of closed loop. Reduced risk of electrolyte imbalances (compared with ileostomy). If needed, surgery can even be performed in local anesthesia. In morbidly obese patients, colostomy may better reach than ileostomy.
- Disadvantage: incomplete diversion for true loop, prolapse, peristomal hernia formation, odor (compared with ileostomy).

Double-barrel colostomy
- Same as loop but two separate exits.
- Advantage: efferent end can be removed during subsequent surgery without disturbing otherwise healed afferent ostomy.

End-ileostomy (Brooke ileostomy)
- Example: total abdominal colectomy (anus/rectal stump maintained), total proctocolectomy (closed perineum).
- Purpose: result of resection where (immediate) restoration of intestinal continuity not possible or not desired. If distal anatomy still preserved → elective takedown vs possible further resection/restoration (eg, ileoanal pull-through procedure) possible.
- Target location (unless adjusted): RLQ, through rectus muscle.
- Appearance: symmetric nipple (2.5–3.5 cm, Figure 4–21A).
- Output: oatmeal-like, opaque, 600–1000 mL/24 hours.
- Advantage: predictability, avoid anastomosis, allow for physical and nutritional recuperation. Less odor.
- Disadvantage: high output, risk of electrolyte imbalances, difficulty in obese patients.

Loop ileostomy
- Example: elective proximal diversion, eg, after LAR or PC/IPAA.
- Technical variations: (1) true loop with afferent and efferent limb; (2) Prasad-type loop: open afferent limb, efferent limb closed off/attached to afferent limb or fascia or matured into ostomy as mucous fistula. Occasionally temporary bridge for 10–14 days.
- Purpose: fecal diversion (complete, incomplete). Ostomy of choice in elective cases with risk of distal problem (anastomotic leak, pelvic sepsis, etc).
- Target location (unless adjusted): RLQ, through rectus muscle.
- Appearance: symmetric nipple (2.5–3.5 cm).
- Output: oatmeal-like, opaque, 600–1000 mL/24 hours.
- Advantage: easier takedown (compared with colostomy or Hartmann), less odor, does not tether the colon or compromise its blood supply → permits full colonic mobilization if needed.
- Disadvantage: incomplete diversion for true loop, high output, risk of electrolyte imbalances, does not decompress colon if competent ileocecal valve, difficulty in obese patients.

Double-barrel ileostomy
- Same as loop but two separate exits.

Continent ileostomy (Kock pouch, Barnett pouch/BCIR, T-pouch)
- Example: post–proctocolectomy (IBD, FAP), inability to reconstruct, failure of J-pouch.
- Purpose: ileostomy continent for feces and gas (valve mechanism), storage area, no need for external appliance.
- Target location (unless adjusted): as low as possible, ideally hiding in underwear.
- Appearance: skin-level, symmetric, 1 cm diameter (Figure 4–21C).
- Output: Only upon intubation (3–5× per day): oatmeal-like, opaque, 600–1000 mL/24 hours.
- Advantage: avoidance of appliance (covered with bandaid only), elimination of ileoanal dysfunction, permitting active physical lifestyle, improved body image.
- Disadvantage: need for patient selection, increased perioperative morbidity, long-term dysfunction, pouchitis, concept and management familiar to only limited number of physicians.

Perineal colostomy
- Example: status post colonic pull-through procedure for imperforate anus or secondary abdominoperineal reconstruction post APR.

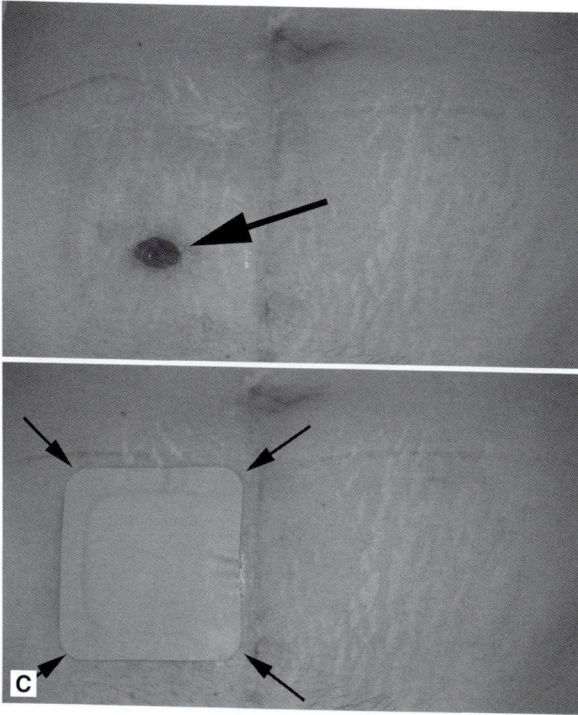

Figure 4–21C. Skin-level stoma of continent ileostomy, covered with bandaid.

- Purpose: restoration of anatomy, for functionality may need implantation of artificial bowel sphincter.
- Target location: center of perineum (sufficient tissue coverage toward coccyx and vagina).
- Appearance: flat, no anal verge, no anal canal.
- Output: stool.
- Advantage: body image. Up to 60–70% acceptable control despite lack of sphincter muscle.
- Disadvantage: lack of or insufficient spontaneous control, lack of blood supply from distance, development of mucosal ectropion.

Tube cecostomy
- Example: cecal volvulus, colonic pseudoobstruction (Ogilvie syndrome).
- Purpose: venting of colon, colopexy. Caveat: tube cecostomy is not a fecal diversion!
- Target location: RLQ.
- Appearance: large-diameter Foley catheter.
- Output: air, some stool (needs daily irrigation with fluid).
- Advantage: spontaneous closure once catheter removed.
- Disadvantage: does not allow fecal diversion, need for irrigation.

Tube gastrostomy
- Example: carcinomatosis or massive adhesions with expected recurrent/progressive SBO.
- Purpose: decompression of stomach, ability to insert tube feeding.
- Target location: LUQ.
- Appearance: large-diameter Foley catheter or percutaneous endoscopic gastrostomy (PEG).
- Output: stomach retention.
- Advantage: avoidance of NGT. Spontaneous closure once catheter removed.
- Disadvantage: leakage, need for irrigation.

Tube jejunostomy
- Same as tube gastrostomy, but tube placed more distally (jejunum), used for enteral feeding.

Appendicostomy for MACE (Malone antegrade colonic enema)
- Example: fecal incontinence, cases of severe constipation (eg, in cystic fibrosis).
- Purpose: maturation of appendix into umbilicus to allow insertion of tube → irrigation of colon with > 2 L of fluid every day.
- Target location: umbilicus.
- Appearance: as little visible as possible.
- Output: None.
- Advantage: lavaging and/or liquefaction of stool in colon.
- Disadvantage: time-consuming: after completion → continuation of liquid discharge for up to 2 hours.

Urostomy
- Urinary conduit.

Blowholes (Turnbull)

- Example: historically used in fulminant colitis; today mostly obsolete except under very unusual circumstances.
- Technical variations: flat suturing of (friable) bowel to the fascia.
- Purpose: venting/decompression of toxic intestines while avoiding emergency resection.
- Target location (unless adjusted): loop ileostomy, 3–5 colonic locations.
- Appearance: skin-level, no maturation.
- Advantage: avoidance of risky emergency resection (rarely a true advantage).
- Disadvantage: diseased colon left in place (→ continued sepsis), need for secondary resection.

Cross-reference

TRAUMA *(863.X)*

Overview

Colorectal trauma is a major cause of morbidity and often involves patients of younger age. Number of injury patterns is unlimited, but four main mechanisms include:

1. Penetrating trauma, ie, focal impact through body surface:
   a. Direct internal injury limited to path: eg, stab wound, impalement.
   b. Combined injury from trajectory as such and the much more serious cavitation effect: gunshot wounds, particularly if high-velocity projectiles.

2. Blunt abdominal and/or pelvic trauma, ie, broad impact to body surface which causes indirect internal injury.

3. Internal trauma, ie, direct impact onto anorectum or intestines:
   a. Inside-out: eg, endoscopic perforation, enema perforation, foreign body insertion/ingestion, sexual assault, internal overpressure (eg, air or water jet), fall straddling, jumping, bouncing, suction.
   b. Outside-in: eg, intraoperative laceration, obstetric injury.

4. Devascularization: mesenteric avulsion, aortic dissection, retroperitoneal hemorrhage, compartment syndrome.

Management depends on the severity and location of colorectal and associated injuries. Circumstances (war vs civilian) are major factor affecting outcome for major injuries of comparable severity: delay to therapy, recognition and treatment of associated injuries, overall condition (shock, blood loss, contamination).

Surgical options include diversion, local debridement, and/or primary repair—by suturing or resection/anastomosis. Exteriorization of repaired bowel segments largely abandoned (obstruction).

Classical contraindications for primary colon repair (as opposed to fecal diversion):

- > 1000 mL of blood in peritoneum (or transfusion of > 6 units of blood).
- More than just minimal fecal contamination.
- Delay in surgical intervention > 6–8 hours.
- Hemodynamic instability (or preoperative blood pressure < 80/60).
- > 2 other organs injured (or penetrating abdominal trauma index > 25).
- Peritonitis.

Current contraindications for primary repair: delayed presentation (> 24 hours), gross fecal contamination, need for damage control.

Epidemiology

Colon injury (frequently not isolated): 30% of all penetrating injuries, 5% of all blunt abdominal traumas. Vice versa: 90% of colorectal injuries caused by gunshot or stab wounds, 5% by motor vehicle crashes.

Rectal injury: 95% due to penetrating trauma, blunt rectal trauma and pelvic fractures, endorectal trauma. Penetrating rectal injuries: gunshot 80–90%, impalement (rare); blunt rectal trauma (eg, deceleration: crashes, falls).

Symptoms

All traumata: possibly more serious symptoms in other organ systems (eg, cardiovascular, pulmonary, cerebral, etc).

Anorectal trauma: visible wound(s) or marks, rectal bleeding (→ at least mucosal injury), "rectal pain," abdominal pain (ominous sign → peritonitis), symptoms of associated injury.

Abdominal trauma: visible wound(s) or marks, bleeding (external/internal), hemodynamic instability, abdominal wall pain vs peritoneal pain, nausea, vomiting, fever, abdominal distention, compartment syndrome.

Differential Diagnosis

Based on the history of trauma, the diagnosis is not typically in question, more the extent of damage.

Pathology

Depending on trauma mechanism, location, secondary underperfusion (shock, hemorrhage, etc).

Evaluation

Required minimal standard
All traumas

History: trauma mechanism? Coherence of the story (involvement of others, possible crime?), current symptoms (hematuria, bleeding per rectum, pain etc)? Injury causing object still in patient? Pregnancy?

Inspection of whole body: locations of primary and secondary wounds/marks (consistent with reported trauma type?), suspected wound extent and path (entry and exit sites → possible photographic documentation)!

Whole body examination.

Anorectal trauma

Clinical examination: careful palpation of the perineum (urethral injury? sphincter avulsion or lacerations?), digital rectal exam (rectal wall integrity/defect? sphincter tone? position of prostate? Sacrum/coccyx not palpable → presacral hematoma?), vaginal exam (vaginal/uterine injury, extent of the anorectal injury). Associated neurologic deficits from spine/pelvic injuries?

Anoscopy/rigid sigmoidoscopy evaluation: careful to avoid aggravation of injury.

Urinalysis: micro-/macrohematuria.

Abdominopelvic and chest x-rays: evidence for free peritoneal air? Retained foreign body? Associated skeletal injuries?

CT scan (if possible with triple water-soluble contrast, ie, oral, IV, rectal): extent of injury, perforation, etc.

Abdominal trauma

Clinical examination: hemodynamic, respiratory, and neurologic assessment, careful abdominal evaluation (wounds, marks, evisceration, peritoneal signs, tension), digital rectal exam (rectal wall integrity? sphincter tone? sacrum/coccyx not palpable → presacral hematoma?).

X-rays: evidence for free peritoneal air? Involvement of other organ system (eg, traumatic diaphragmatic hernia, chest, mediastinum, retroperitoneum), retained foreign body? Associated skeletal injuries?

Urinalysis: micro-/macrohematuria.

CT scan (if possible with triple water-soluble contrast, ie, oral, IV, rectal): extent of injury, evidence for colon perforation, associated injuries (abdominopelvic/retroperitoneal organs, vascular and osseous structures, etc).

Additional tests (optional)

Contrast studies with water-soluble contrast:

– Urethrography/cystography vs IV urography.

– Contrast enema.

Diagnostic peritoneal lavage (DPL) vs abdominal ultrasound: intra-abdominal fluid?

CT/MRI with 3D reconstruction of skeletal and soft tissue injuries.

Cystoscopy.

Angiography with possible embolization: diagnostic and therapeutic.

Measurement of bladder pressure: abdominal compartment syndrome?

TABLE 4–8. AAST Score for Colorectal Injury.

Grade[a]	Description of Colon/Rectal Injury
I	Hematoma (contusion without devascularization)
	Laceration (partial thickness, no perforation)
II	Laceration < 50% circumference
III	Laceration > 50% circumference without transection
IV	Laceration transection of colon
V	Laceration transection with segmental tissue loss

[a]Grade for single injury; for multiple injuries → upgraded by one to grade III.

Classification

- Nondestructive vs destructive intestinal trauma: colon/rectal injury score (by American Association for Surgery for Trauma): Table 4–8.
- Anorectal and sphincter trauma.

Nonoperative Treatment

All traumata: adequate resuscitation (fluid and electrolytes, blood products as needed), broad-spectrum antibiotics, tetanus prophylaxis, close observation with serial assessments, Foley catheter (unless high index of suspicion for urethral disruption!).

Blunt and penetrating abdominal trauma:

- Nonoperative management in selected patients → serial examinations → physical examination reliable in detecting significant injuries: minimizing rate of unnecessary laparotomies.
- Patient selection: hemodynamically stable, local abdominal tenderness only, no peritoneal signs, absence of factors making clinical examination unreliable (ie, severe head or spinal cord injury, intoxication, need for sedation/intubation).

Operative Treatment

Indication

- Any trauma with proven, suspected, or pending intestinal disruption/perforation, unless very favorable individual circumstances permit a conservative approach.
- Patients with (initially or in the course of serial exams):
  – Hemodynamic instability.

– Diffuse abdominal tenderness after penetrating abdominal trauma.
– Unreliable clinical examination (ie, severe head injury, spinal cord injury, severe intoxication, or need for sedation or intubation).

Operative approach
Intraperitoneal colon/rectal injuries
• Nondestructive colon/rectal injuries: primary repair.
• Destructive colon/rectal injuries:
– Resection with primary anastomosis if possible.
– Resection with ostomy if: shock, hemorrhage, comorbidities, blast wounds, crush injuries, radiated tissue, distal obstruction, mesenteric vascular damage or otherwise impaired blood supply, massive infection.

Extraperitoneal rectal injuries
• Nondestructive injuries: distal rectal washout, antibiotics, possible ostomy.
• Destructive injuries:
– Repair with/without proximal fecal diversion.
– Presacral drainage, colostomy for fecal diversion, distal rectal washout.
– Low anterior resection with primary anastomosis (unless diffuse pelvic trauma) with or without protective ileostomy/colostomy.

Infralevator injuries (minor to moderate)
• Examination under anesthesia, debridement, suture repair of essential structures (sphincter), drainage, possible fecal diversion.
• Perineal wounds left open → post-primary wound closure or healing by secondary intention.

Outcome
Survival determined by extracolonic injuries, mortality of isolated colorectal injury low (if managed timely).

Morbidity: anastomotic leak, colostomy-related complications, presacral abscess, pelvic or abdominal abscess, fistula formation (enterocutaneous, enterovesical, enterovaginal, perianal, pelvic plexus damage, fecal/urinary incontinence).

Follow-up
Functional reassessment (constipation, incontinence) after convalescence.
Planning of secondary surgeries (ostomy takedown, etc).

Cross-reference

SPINAL CORD INJURY–ASSOCIATED COLORECTAL PATHOLOGY

Overview

Severe spinal cord injury (SCI) causes multiple irreversible physical changes that require lengthy adjustments. Acute abdominal and intestinal problems are relatively rare (eg, acute GI dilation) unless related to direct traumatic impact. However, irreversible neurologic damage after spinal cord injury is associated with significant long-term GI and pelvic organ management issues and morbidity. Acute management centered around damage control, chronic management on rehabilitation and maintenance of functionality.

Extent of neurologic dysfunction primarily depending on level of trauma (cervical injury → tetraplegia; thoracic/lumbar injury → paraplegia) and completeness of motor-sensory damage.

Epidemiology

Annual incidence of SCI in the US: each year ~ 40 cases per million population or 11,000 new cases. Prevalence: estimated 225,000–300,000 persons in the US. Age at time of injury: most frequently between 16–30 years. Gender: 75% male.

Symptoms

Acute symptoms (immediately/early after the injury):

- Acute colonic dilation with risk of perforation.
- Acute gastric dilation with risk of necrosis/perforation.
- Direct trauma to abdominal organs.

Chronic symptoms (most common problems):

- Overall patient mobility, transfers, ability to sit (eg, on toilet).
- Baseline bowel function: bowel control, constipation, manual stimulation of evacuation.
- Baseline urinary function: bladder emptying, need for suprapubic or Foley catheter vs intermittent catheterization, bladder reservoir, bladder stone formation, urinary tract infections, sepsis.
- Spasticity of paralyzed extremities.
- Relaxation of pelvic floor with perineal descent, rectal prolapse, hemorrhoids.
- Lack of protective sensory input → decubitus, abscess/fistula formation.

Issues not directly related to spinal injury:

- Unchanged need for colon cancer screening per guidelines.
- Constipation → increased risk for diverticulosis/it is (caveat: lack of abdominal pain!).

Differential Diagnosis

Depending on presenting symptomatology.

Pathology

Neurogenic colon (lack of nervous control): may lead to fecal impaction (80% of patients with spinal cord injury), bowel distention, incontinence, discoordination of defecation.

Autonomic dysreflexia: chronic constipation with resulting risk of developing autonomic dysreflexia in spinal cord injury above T6: potentially life-threatening condition: sudden increase in blood pressure, severe, pounding headache, profuse sweating, goose pimples of the skin, bradycardia, cardiac arrhythmias. Dysreflexia resolves when triggering cause removed, ie, evacuation of fecal impaction. Prophylaxis prior to manual evacuation: calcium antagonists or topical local anesthesia.

Impaired rectal sensation and sphincter function: periodic mass movements in the colon lead to rectal fullness → reflex relaxation with incontinence.

Diverticulosis: chronic constipation with increased intraluminal pressures → overdistention of the bowel resulting in diverticula formation.

Rectal prolapse: passage of large hard stools in combination with weakened pelvic and anorectal tonus.

Hemorrhoids: frequent problem (70–80%), result from combination of constipation, lack of pelvic floor muscle tone, chronically high pressures in the anorectal marginal veins.

Bladder dysfunction:

- Spastic (reflex) bladder: automatic triggering of bladder voiding.
- Flaccid (nonreflex) bladder: decreased/absent bladder reflexes lead to urinary retention with urinary tract infections.
- Bladder dyssynergia: lack of sphincter relaxation on bladder contraction → retention, incomplete emptying, reflux.

GERD: autonomic dysfunction → colonic and gastric overdistention → incompetence of gastroesophageal sphincter.

Evaluation

Required minimal standard

History: exact time and level of injury, residual sensory or motor function? Specific current complaints (abdominal, anorectal)? Change in baseline bowel function and management?

Clinical examination:

- Abdominal exam: distention, fecal impaction, mass?

- Anorectal exam: perineal descent, prolapse, ulcerations, tone?
- Anoscopy/rigid sigmoidoscopy: polyps, mass, hemorrhoids, proctitis?

Except in emergency: full/partial colonic evaluation as per general screening guidelines and prior to any planned intervention.

Additional tests (optional)

Depending on likely diagnoses.

Urinalysis: rule out urinary tract infection or hematuria.

Decubitus: imaging to rule out osteomyelitis.

Classification

Grading of spinal cord injury according American Spinal Injury Association (ASIA) scale:

A. Complete: no sensory or motor function in sacral segments S4–S5.

B. Incomplete: sensory, but not motor, function below the neurologic level and extends to sacral segments S4–S5.

C. Incomplete: preserved motor function below neurologic level, strength of most key muscles below the neurologic level < grade 3.

D. Incomplete: preserved motor function below neurologic level, strength of most key muscles below the neurologic level ≥ grade 3.

E. Normal: normal sensory and motor functions.

Bowel function in relation to level of SCI:

- Lower motor neuron (LMN) colon (SCI below T12).
- Upper motor neuron (UMN) colon (SCI above conus medullaris).

Nonoperative Treatment

Bowel management:

- Bowel emptying programs: evacuation of rectum on fixed schedule (eg, daily or every other day) to minimize fecal impaction and avoid reflex relaxation of internal sphincter with incontinence. Triggering of defecation reflex: digital stimulation, manual evacuation, rectal stimulant suppository, enemas.
- Between scheduled emptyings: stool softeners (eg, docusate sodium), colonic stimulants (eg, bisacodyl), supplemental dietary fiber to induce better defecatory response.

Bladder management: intermittent catheterization, indwelling Foley catheter, external condom catheter for males.

Local problems → primary conservative approach:

- Hemorrhoids: dietary changes, mild laxatives.
- Decubitus: primarily conservative management with optimized wound care, sitting aids.

Operative Treatment

Indication

Specific local symptoms/problems:

- Extensive external hemorrhoids (interfering with hygiene).
- Treatment-refractory hemorrhoids with bleeding/prolapse.
- Rectal prolapse.
- Abscess/fistula.
- Anorectal stricture.
- Acute treatment-refractory, complicated, or recurrent diverticulitis.
- Treatment-refractory functional outlet obstruction.

Operative approach

- Office interventions for internal/external hemorrhoids, abscess, superficial fistula (premedicate with topical lidocaine gel).
- Appropriate local procedures: excisional vs stapled hemorrhoidectomy, drainage of abscess, fistulotomy vs seton placement, stricturoplasty (with/without flap), perineal prolapse repair.
- Abdominal procedures: segmental colectomy, rectopexy, creation of diverting colostomy.

Outcome

Leading causes of death after SCI: renal failure in the past; nowadays pneumonia, pulmonary embolism, septicemia. Colorectal issues: matter of quality of life.

Follow-up

Dependent on primary presenting symptom.

Cross-reference

Topic	*Chapter*
Hemorrhoids	4 (p 167)
Fecal incontinence	4 (p 189)
Trauma	4 (p 410)
Chronic constipation	4 (p 427)
Hemorrhoid treatment	5 (pp 506–512)

PELVIC FLOOR DYSFUNCTION *(618.X)*

Overview

Pelvic floor dysfunction is a complex combination of problems related to the relaxation of the pelvic floor and suspension structures for the pelvic organs. Associated with parity, increasing age, and obesity, pelvic floor dysfunction causes significant morbidity and has a negative impact on the quality of life in aging women: dysfunction of urinary and/or fecal control or evacuation, pelvic pain syndromes, pelvic organ prolapse syndrome (cystocele, rectocele, enterocele, vaginal prolapse).

Epidemiology

Among women > 55 years of age, 50% have some symptoms of pelvic relaxation; ~75% by age of 75. Bladder-related complaints increase threefold between ages 45 and 75 years. Pelvic organ prolapse: > 10% of women seek operative repair by age 80.

Symptoms

Various combinations of urinary and/or fecal incontinence, urinary obstruction, obstructed defecation, perineal descent, and pelvic organ prolapse, which is either visible or sensed as pelvic/perineal pressure or vaginal bulging of cystocele, rectocele, enterocele, or uterine/vaginal prolapse, rectal prolapse, solitary rectal ulcer syndrome, sexual dysfunction.

Differential Diagnosis

Other causes of urinary and anorectal dysfunction.

Other causes of pelvic pain.

Pathology

Absence of primary pathology. Secondary pathology from prolapse, eg, solitary rectal ulcer syndrome.

Evaluation

Required minimal standard

History: careful evaluation of symptoms, questionnaires on primary and secondary problems.

Clinical examination: general appearance, habitus/nutritional status; anorectal exam—perineal descent, flattening of anal "verge," visible rectal or vaginal prolapse (at rest, upon straining); rigid sigmoidoscopy, colposcopy.

Colonic evaluation as per guidelines.

Anophysiology testing, including balloon expulsion test.

Imaging:

   – Dynamic MRI (Figure 4–22).

   – Defecating proctogram (see Figure 2–6).

Urodynamics and GYN evaluation.

Additional tests (optional)

Sitzmark study?

CT abdomen/pelvis?

Classification

• Anterior pelvic compartment: bladder, urethra.

• Middle pelvic compartment: vagina, uterus.

• Posterior pelvic compartment: rectum, anus.

Nonoperative Treatment

Lifestyle alteration, dietary modification, supplemental fibers.

Behavioral therapy, physical therapy, biofeedback training.

Pessary placement.

Electrogalvanic stimulation.

Pharmacologic treatment: eg, detrusor or levator hyperactivity, muscle-relaxing drugs, hormone-replacement therapy?

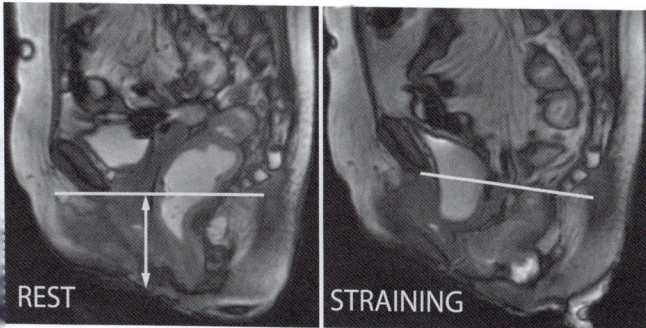

Figure 4–22. Pelvic floor dysfunction on dynamic MRI.

Operative Treatment

Indications

Isolated or combined pelvic organ prolapse, not responding to conservative management.

Operative approach

- Pelvic organ resuspension: rectopexy, sacrocolpopexy, and cystopexy (multidisciplinary approach).
- Resection: sigmoid resection with/without rectopexy, hysterectomy.
- Transanal/-perineal/-vaginal rectocele repair.
- Sacral nerve stimulation.

Outcome

Persistent/recurrent symptoms (20–30%), discrepancy between imaging results and functional performance.

Follow-up

Functional reevaluation at regular intervals. Even after surgical approach → role for physical therapy and biofeedback training to further strengthen and recoordinate muscle function.

Cross-reference

RECTAL PROLAPSE *(569.1)*

Overview

Protrusion of the rectum below the anal verge: full-thickness prolapse *(Figure 4–23)* or mucosal prolapse. Associated with a primary or secondary lack of pelvic suspension structures. Characteristic low peritoneal reflection, underdeveloped mesorectum, and lack of lateral attachments. May occur alone or in conjunction with pelvic floor dysfunction and prolapse of other pelvic organs. Etiology essentially unclear, reports on role of parity are controversial. Predisposing factors: age, chronic constipation, malnutrition, consuming diseases (eg, cancer, tuberculosis), neuroleptic medications, neurologic diseases (spinal cord, multiple sclerosis); in children: malnutrition,

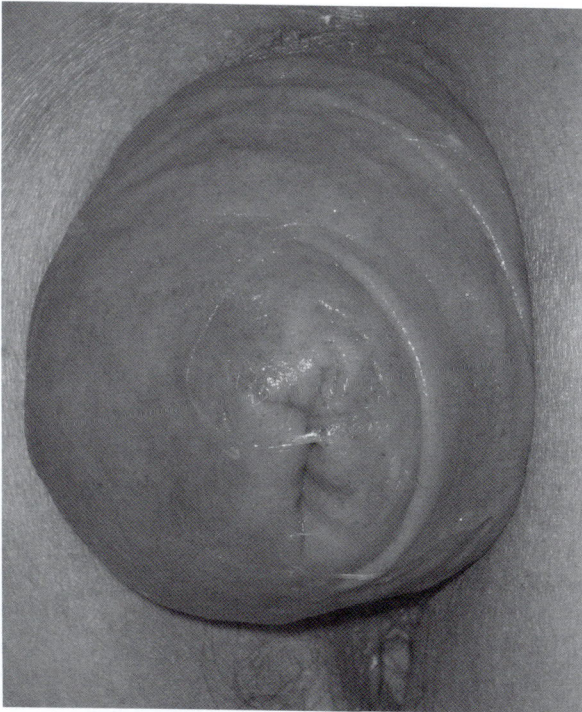

Figure 4–23. Rectal prolapse.

cystic fibrosis, diarrhea. Rectal tumor may be a "lead point" and needs to be ruled out (rigid sigmoidoscopy). Chronic/recurrent prolapse may result in secondary pathologies: sphincter distention with reduced contractility and fecal incontinence (partially reversible); solitary rectal ulcer syndrome; myoinflammatory polyps.

Epidemiology

Most common in elderly females (impact of nulliparity vs multiparity controversial) or males < 50 years of age.

Symptoms

Occult/internal prolapse (rectal intussusception): pelvic pressure, fullness, constipation, pencil-like stools, mucous discharge.

External prolapse: bleeding, moisture, discomfort/pain, itching, fecal incontinence.

Nonreducible prolapse: pain, spasm; fever = alarming late sign.

Differential Diagnosis

Hemorrhoidal prolapse: radial pattern.

Protrusion of polyp, mass, hypertrophic anal papillae, condylomata.

Urogynecologic prolapse, rectocele.

Pathology

Chronic/recurring prolapse: solitary rectal ulcer syndrome with myofibrosis of lamina propria.

Acute prolapse: elements of acute inflammation (neutrophils), ischemia.

Evaluation

Required minimal standard

History: extent of prolapse (length)? Site of prolapse (rectum, vagina)? Constipation/diarrhea? Change in bowel habits? Incontinence (fecal/urinary)? Previous surgeries (eg, prolapse, hysterectomy, etc)? Previous colonic evaluations (flex sigmoidoscopy, colonoscopy, barium enema)? Comorbidities (coronary artery disease, COPD, diabetes, liver/kidney disease, weight loss, etc).

Clinical examination:

- Elective: best to let patient take sitting position on toilet and trigger the prolapse by Valsalva maneuver: concentric pattern vs radial pattern?
- Acute setting: viability of prolapsed tissue? Local tenderness? Rectal mass? Fever? Fluid status/dehydration?

Rigid sigmoidoscopy: lead point?

Colonic evaluation prior to elective surgery.

Additional tests (optional)
Defecating proctogram (if unable to provoke prolapse during clinical exam).

Dynamic MRI.

Urogynecologic evaluation.

Classification
- Occult/internal prolapse (intussusception) vs external prolapse.
- Full-thickness prolapse vs mucosal prolapse.
- Circumferential vs asymmetric prolapse.
- Reversible prolapse vs irreducible/incarcerated prolapse.

Nonoperative Treatment

Elective situation, minimal prolapse, or inoperable patient: banding, stool regulation, injection of sclerosing agent.

Reduction of incarcerated prolapse with circumferential and axial pressure: perianal/pudendal nerve block (local anesthesia) for sphincter relaxation and/or application of granular table sugar to reduce edema may facilitate maneuver.

Operative Treatment

Indication
Any rectal prolapse if patient operable, potential need to combine with urogynecologic procedure.

Operative approach
Numerous procedures for rectal prolapse, but two major categories: abdominal approach vs perineal approach. Choice of specific procedure dependent on patient fitness, history and type of previous prolapse operation, risk of recurrent prolapse, patient preference for large vs small operation and willingness to accept recurrence, underlying constipation/diarrhea and/or fecal incontinence.

Abdominal approach
- Laparoscopic vs open sigmoid resection with complete posterior rectal mobilization, with/without rectopexy: lowest recurrence rate, preferred approach for operable patients with significant constipation and patients in whom lifting the rectum out of the pelvis would result in significant redundancy.

- Laparoscopic vs open rectopexy after complete posterior rectal mobilization: preferred approach for operable patients with element of incontinence → preservation of colonic length or for patients with previous Altemeier operation (vascular supply). Variations: suture rectopexy, posterior implant rectopexy (Wells rectopexy, using mesh/collagen/Ivalon sponge), anterior implant rectopexy (Ripstein rectopexy, using mesh/collagen sling: risk of constipation due to kinking and narrowed passage).

Perineal approach
- Delorme procedure: complete mucosal stripping of prolapsed segment with muscular plication: possible benefit for incontinence?
- Altemeier procedure: perineal proctectomy, with/without levatorplasty: primary approach for emergency, better perineal approach for every prolapse (compared with Delorme procedure); contraindicated after previous sigmoid resection (blood supply!).
- Thiersch repair: insertion mesh/wire/collagen cerclage to narrow anal canal and prevent exteriorization of hypermobile rectum.

Outcome

Recurrence of rectal prolapse: 5–30% (depending on type of surgery).

Fecal incontinence: 60–70% improvement within 6 months, possibility of worsening control.

Constipation: worsening in up to 50% of patients with nonresective procedures.

Implant complication: overall low risk of implant erosion or migration, but synthetic implants can potentially cause major problems that might require ostomy and complete removal of material.

Follow-up

Functional reassessment (constipation, incontinence) after 3 and 6 months.

Cross-reference

FUNCTIONAL DISORDERS—CHRONIC CONSTIPATION *(564.0X)*

Overview

Constipation is one of the most frequent patient complaints, but there is wide variability in how different patients or physicians define constipation. Acute episode of constipation most frequently is associated with poor habits and medication side effects (Table 4–9) with/without an additional problem site (anastomosis, anorectal pain, etc). Chronic constipation belongs to a category of functional disorders: defined as conditions comprising a variable combination of chronic and recurrent GI symptoms that lack a structural or biochemical abnormality:

- GI transit and waste evacuation are either too slow (constipation), too fast (diarrhea), or in wrong direction (GERD).

- Additional symptoms: pain/discomfort, urgency, gas production, nausea and vomiting.

- Frequently associated with personality disorders.

TABLE 4–9. Constipating Medications.

Class	Examples
Opioid analgesics	Morphine agonists, codeine
Antidepressants (tri-/tetracyclic, monoamine oxidase inhibitors)	Sertraline, bupropion tranylcypromine
Neuroleptics/antipsychotics	Paroxetine
Parkinson medications	Dopaminergic, anticholinergic
Anticonvulsants	Phenytoin, clonazepam
5-HT$_3$ antagonists	Alosetron
Antacids	Aluminum, calcium compounds
Antihypertensives	Calcium channel blockers, clonidine
Anticholinergics	Diphenoxylate, atropine, loperamide
Metal supplements	Iron, bismuth
Nonsteroidal anti-inflammatory drugs (NSAIDs)	Ibuprofen, diclofenac
Bile-acid binding resin	Cholestyramine
Chemotherapy	Vinca alkaloids
Long-term (ab-)use of stimulant laxatives	All laxatives

TABLE 4–10. Chronic Constipation Defining Criteria (Rome III Criteria, 2006).

	Mandatory Symptoms	Supportive Symptoms
Time factor:	≥2 of the following symptoms:	
> 3 days per month in past 3 months	< 3 unassisted bowel movements per week	Absence of loose stools (when not taking laxatives)
Symptom onset ≥6 months before diagnosis (when not taking a laxative)	Straining 25% of the time	Insufficient criteria for irritable bowel syndrome (IBS)
	Sensation of incomplete evacuation ≥25% of the time	< 2 bowel movements per week in > 6 months (when not taking a laxative)
	Lumpy/hard/pellet-like stools ≥25% of the time	
	Sensation of anorectal obstruction or blockage/prolonged time needed for defecation ≥25% of the time	
	Manual maneuvers ≥ 25% of the time	

Important to distinguish between short episode of constipation and chronic constipation: → defining criteria for chronic constipation: Table 4–10. Overlapping pathophysiologic entities: slow-transit constipation (45–50%), pelvic floor dysfunction/dyssynergia (50–60%), constipation-predominant IBS (50–60%). Ogilvie syndrome is a separate and independent entity.

Physician's task is to delineate the symptom "constipation" as:

• Result of a poor habits?
• Caused by local morphologic problem (obstruction, etc)?
• Caused by a systemic problem?
• True functional problem of the intestines?

High likelihood of increasing frustration for patients (lack of improvement), physicians (lack of "easy" treatment, unfavorable time/effort ratio for reimbursement, etc), insurers/employers (cost, absenteeism from work, indirect cost).

Epidemiology

Estimated US prevalence (including telephone survey): 12–20% (range 2–28%) or 63 million people; 40–50% of individuals with > 5-year history of constipation; 2% of respondents use laxative at least every other day. Gender: female/male ratio = 1.6 to 2.3:1.

Symptoms

Defecation:

- Decreased frequency of bowel movements: < 1 every 3 days.
- Increased consistency of stools: lumpy/hard stool or stool pellets.
- Need for straining or even manual disimpaction.
- Need for external /transvaginal digital support.
- Sense of incomplete evacuation; multiple/repetitive small bowel movements.

Abdominal symptoms: fullness, LLQ pain.

Secondary symptoms: depression, anal fissure, hemorrhoids, diverticulitis, overflow incontinence.

Absence of alarming symptoms: bleeding, weight loss, fever, etc.

Differential Diagnosis

Morphologic obstruction: partial or complete LBO.

Slow-transit constipation: absence of morphologic problem, intrinsic neuromuscular dysfunction with colonic inertia.

Pelvic floor dysfunction: functional outlet obstruction (anismus), intussusceptions, prolapse, rectocele.

IBS: absence of morphologic problem, normal-transit constipation, relief with defecation, ROME III criteria.

Secondary constipation: hypothyroidism, hyperparathyroidism, diabetes, renal failure, pregnancy, neurologic disorders (eg, Parkinson disease), drug side effects.

Ogilvie syndrome typically distinct entity.

Pathology

No primary colonic pathology.

Secondary pathology: melanosis coli (lipofuscin pigment in submucosal macrophages [no melanin]), colonic muscular hypertrophy, colonic diverticulosis.

Pathophysiology: factors affecting colonic transit and evacuation:

- Endoluminal factors (stool consistency).
- Intrinsic factors (neuromuscular network, pacer and distention receptor function, motility).
- Extrinsic factors (neural function, endocrine factors, drugs).
- Evacuatory function (pelvic neuromuscular coordination).

Evaluation

Required minimal standard
History:

- Exact analysis of patient's symptoms: number/ frequency/quality of bowel movements, supportive maneuvers for evacuation, dietary habits, past/current management (laxatives, enemas/suppositories, fibers, etc).
- Associated symptoms: bleeding, abdominal distention, weight loss, pain, nausea/vomiting, prolapse? Incontinence (fecal, gas, urine), fatigue.
- List of medications (drug-induced constipation).
- History of prior surgeries (adhesions, prolapse syndrome, etc).
- Previous colonic evaluations (flexible sigmoidoscopy, colonoscopy, barium enema)?
- Comorbidities (hypothyroidism, diabetes, coronary artery disease, COPD, liver/kidney disease, weight loss, etc).

Clinical examination: general appearance, habitus, emotional status? Abdominal exam: distention, mass, organomegaly, local tenderness? Anorectal exam: perineal descent, vaginal, rectal or bladder prolapse, sphincter tone, stricture, rectocele, rectal mass, fecal impaction?

Anoscopy/rigid sigmoidoscopy: morphologically distal obstruction?

Limited/full colonic evaluation: depending on risk factors and age, baseline exam prior to any other studies → rule out morphologic cause of constipation.

Colonic transit time study: Sitzmark (or scintigraphic) study → characteristic marker distribution patterns:

- Complete elimination → IBS.
- Diffusely dispersed throughout colon → slow-transit constipation (Figure 4–24).
- Distal accumulation → outlet obstruction → defecating proctogram/dynamic MRI.

Additional tests (optional)
Defecating proctogram (see above).

Dynamic MRI.

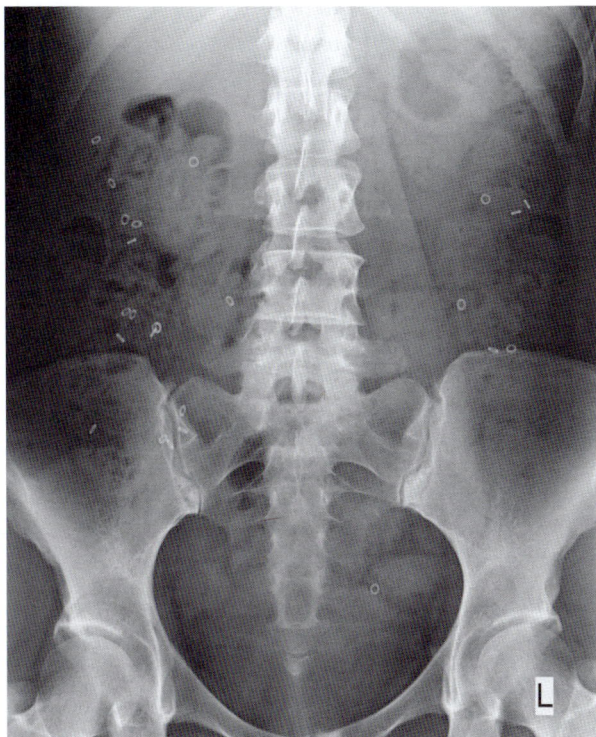

Figure 4–24. Sitzmark study in slow-transit constipation (colonic inertia).

Urogynecologic evaluation.

Anophysiology studies (including EMG and balloon expulsion test).

Contrast enema.

Blood work: only if suspicion of endocrine imbalance (hypothyroidism, hypercalcemia, etc).

Classification

- Temporary constipation without signs of chronicity.
- Poor habit constipation.
- Morphologic constipation.

• Functional chronic constipation: slow-transit constipation, normal-transit constipation, pelvic floor dyssynergia.

Nonoperative Treatment

General:

• Dietary modification and stool regulation: increase fiber (> 25–30 g/day), increase fluid intake (> 1.5–2 L/day); reserve sufficient time after meals for bowel movements (gastrocolic reflex); increase physical activity, avoid constipating medications (if possible).

• Laxatives (eg, polyethylene glycol [PEG], lubiprostone, lactulose, milk of magnesia, etc.)

• Stool softeners.

• Suppositories, enemas.

IBS: even if condition appears treatment-refractory, the management remains primarily nonoperative. Tegaserod maleate (prokinetic 5-HT$_4$ receptor agonist withdrawn from US market in 2007, never approved in Europe) may be beneficial in selected individuals.

Pelvic floor dyssynergia (anismus, levator ani syndrome, paradoxical pub-orectalis contraction): physical therapy/biofeedback training.

Operative Treatment

Indication

• Selected patients with treatment-refractory slow-transit constipation.

• Correctable pelvic floor dysfunction and/or morphologic outlet obstruction.

Operative approach

• Slow-transit constipation: (sub-)total colectomy, antegrade irrigational stoma (MACE).

• Rectocele: repair.

• Pelvic floor descent/pelvic organ prolapse syndrome: organ suspension (rectopexy with/without sigmoid resection, sacrocolpopexy, cystopexy), rectocele repair.

Outcome

Most active patients do well with medical management

Total abdominal colectomy: 85–90% satisfaction in properly selected patients, 50–60% if IBS and pelvic floor dysfunction included; morbidity:

10–15% unsatisfactory bowel frequency and/or incontinence, recurrent bowel obstruction, recurrent/persistent constipation.

Follow-up

Functional reassessment (constipation/diarrhea, continence for stool/gas and urine) after 3 and 6 months.

Cross-reference

FUNCTIONAL DISORDERS—IRRITABLE BOWEL SYNDROME (IBS, 564.1)

Overview

IBS ("visceral hypersensitivity") is the classical example of a functional disorder, defined as nonspecific abdominal symptoms (pain, gas formation, etc) in association with altered bowel habits (constipation, diarrhea, both), but absence of any morphologic or biochemical abnormalities.

Pathophysiology: disturbance of brain/gut interaction results in abnormal processing of physiologic stimuli, which triggers altered motility, increased contractility/spasticity, and visceral hypersensitivity/-algesia and is associated with a reduced intestinal volume tolerance.

Lacking any specific tests or markers, IBS remains a diagnosis of exclusion (the term *IBS* generally is overused!) → Rome III criteria (2006) are used for standardization of diagnostic criteria: Table 4–11. Important to

TABLE 4–11. IBS-Defining Criteria (Rome III Criteria, 2006).

	Mandatory Symptoms	Supportive Symptoms
Main complaint:	≥2 of the following symptoms:	
Abdominal discomfort or pain: ≥3 days per month in at least past 3 months	Improvement with defecation Association with change in frequency of bowel movements Association with change in form of stool	Urgency, bloating Abnormal frequency of bowel movements (≤3 per week or > 3 per day) Abnormal stool quality according to Bristol Stool Form Scale (see Table 4–12):
Symptom onset ≥6 months before diagnosis		• Lumpy/hard • Loose/watery stool • Passing of mucus Straining or feeling of incomplete evacuation

Subtype definition only based on stool consistency: see classification on page 437.

distinguish IBS from other benign or malignant causes of respective symptoms. Frequent overlap with other functional and personality disorders.

High probability of frustration on patient's (quality of life) and physician's side (lack of improvement), significant financial impact on health care system.

Epidemiology

US prevalence 8–20%, of which 65% have minor symptoms with no request for treatment, 30% sporadic physician's visit, 5% severe symptoms. Mostly female predominance, but some global variability of male/female gender ratio, eg, 1:2 (US) to 4:1 (India). All ages affected, peak 20–65 years.

Symptoms

Abdominal symptoms: pain/discomfort with relief upon defecation, bloating, heartburn, GERD, nausea, vomiting.

Stool habits: alteration with constipation, diarrhea, mixed symptoms; urgency, discharge of mucus or blood, sense of incomplete evacuation, straining.

Frequently associated but nondiagnostic symptoms: fibromyalgia, headache, backache, genitourinary symptoms.

Psychosocial symptoms: anxiety, panic attacks, mood disorder, sleep disturbance, etc.

Differential Diagnosis

Other benign/malignant causes of abdominal pain/discomfort, eg, partial obstruction (adhesions), diverticular disease, etc.

Other benign/malignant causes of morphologic constipation/obstruction.

Other causes of functional constipation, eg, slow-transit constipation, pelvic floor dysfunction, etc.

Coexistence of IBS with any of the above.

Pathology

No primary colonic pathology.

Evaluation

Required minimal standard
History:
• Exact analysis of patient's symptoms including stool characteristics (Table 4–12): temporal relationship between pain/discomfort and bowel habits.

TABLE 4–12. Bristol Stool Form Scale.

Type	Description of Stool	Label
1	Separate hard lumps (difficult to pass)	Constipation
2	Lumpy, sausage-shaped	
3	Sausage with cracks on surface	Normal
4	Smooth and soft sausage/snake	
5	Soft blobs with clear-cut edges (passed easily)	
6	Fluffy pieces (mushy)	Diarrhea
7	Watery/liquid without solid pieces	

- Identification of "alarm symptoms": fever, GI bleeding, weight loss, anemia, abdominal/pelvic mass.
- Identification of nonintestinal pain triggers: physical activity, urination, menstruation, trauma, etc.
- List of medications (drug-induced constipation).
- History of prior surgeries (adhesions, prolapse syndrome, etc).
- Previous colonic evaluations (flexible sigmoidoscopy, colonoscopy, barium enema)?
- Comorbidities (psychiatric, hypothyroidism, diabetes, coronary artery disease, COPD, liver/kidney disease, etc).

Clinical examination: general appearance, habitus, emotional status? Abdominal exam: unspecific findings, possibly tenderness to palpation (occasionally disproportionate emotional reaction to exam), absence of true morphologic pathology.

Anoscopy/rigid sigmoidoscopy: rule out distal morphologic pathology?

Limited/full colonic evaluation: depending on age and risk factors serves as baseline exam prior to any other studies to rule out morphologic cause of constipation.

Colonic transit time study: complete elimination of Sitzmark indicative of normal-transit constipation, consistent with IBS-C.

Additional tests (optional)

Stool examination: fecal occult blood, stool leukocytes, O&P (eg, *Giardia lamblia,* ameba, etc).

Other imaging modalities: defecating proctogram, dynamic MRI, small bowel follow-through, etc.

Anophysiology studies.

Classification

- IBS-C: IBS with constipation → hard/lumpy stools ≥ 25%, loose/watery stools < 25%.
- IBS-D: IBS with diarrhea → loose/watery stools ≥ 25%, hard/lumpy stools < 25%.
- IBS-M: IBS with mixed symptoms → hard/lumpy stools ≥ 25%, loose/watery stools ≥ 25%.
- IBS-U: undefined IBS → absence of sufficient abnormality in stool consistency.
- IBS-A: IBS with alternating symptoms → symptom fluctuance over time.

Nonoperative Treatment

General

Even treatment-refractory IBS → primarily nonoperative management:

- Reassurance, counseling, education.
- Dietary modification: elimination of triggers, increased fluid intake (> 1.5–2 L/day).
- Stool regulation: > 25–30 g bulking fibers per day, but risk of increased flatulence!
- Psychosocial "hygiene," psychological support.
- Acupuncture?
- Probiotics?

Pain

- Uncertain benefit from smooth muscle relaxants for pain relief?
- Potentially low-dose antidepressant medication.

Constipation

- Laxatives (eg, polyethylene glycol [PEG], lubiprostone, lactulose, milk of magnesia, etc).
- Stool softeners.
- Prokinetics, eg, tegaserod maleate (5-HT$_4$ receptor agonist, withdrawn from US market in 2007, never approved in Europe).

Diarrhea

- Drug therapy: loperamide, diphenoxylate/atropine, cholestyramine, alosetron (selective serotonin 5-HT$_3$ receptor antagonist, risk of intestinal ischemia).

Operative Treatment

Indication
- Almost never indicated, unless specific target with high probability of functional improvement (caveat: unnecessary operations!).
- Resective surgery for normal-transit constipation (eg, subtotal colectomy) associated with high probability of failure (patient satisfaction, quality of life, recurrent bowel obstructions, diarrhea).

Operative approach
Not applicable.

Outcome

Persistent or recurrent symptoms expected, but with guidance and supportive measures → most patients can be maintained in a functional condition.

Follow-up

Functional reassessment (pain, constipation/diarrhea, quality of life, triggering factors) at regular intervals.

Cross-reference

FUNCTIONAL ANORECTAL PAIN—LEVATOR ANI SYNDROME *(569.42)*

Overview

Levator ani syndrome comprises a not entirely homogenous collection of painful conditions (pain, pressure, discomfort, burning) in the rectum, sacrum, and/or anococcygeal area that is often aggravated by long periods sitting or upright position and is not associated with visible pathology. However, the condition may initially have been triggered by local pathology but now runs detached in an autonomous pain cycle.

Several synonyms: chronic proctalgia, levator ani spasm, puborectalis syndrome, pyriformis syndrome, pelvic tension myalgia, coccygodynia, proctodynia.

Definition by Rome III criteria (2006): three mandatory criteria (preferably but not necessarily for > 3 months):

- Chronic or recurrent rectal pain/aching.
- Duration of episodes > 20 minutes.
- Exclusion of other causes of rectal pain.

Epidemiology

Exact incidence unknown; estimated 3–6% of adults affected, one-third of whom are seeking medical attention.

Symptoms

Anorectal and (high) rectal discomfort, occasionally with radiation into gluteal muscles and lower extremities → dull ache, sensation of constant rectal pressure ("ball") or heaviness, occasional burning. Potential worsening with bowel movements.

Differential Diagnosis

Anal fissure, thrombosed external hemorrhoid, abscess and fistular disease, prostatitis, coccygodynia, proctalgia fugax, HIV-associated ulcer, malignancy-associated lesion (cancer, melanoma, leukemia, lymphoma, etc), ischemia, IBD, cryptitis.

Pathology

Lack of visible pathology.

Evaluation

Required minimal standard

History: onset/pattern of symptoms, lack of specific symptoms (prolapse, lump/bump, bleeding, fevers/chills, etc)? Previous evaluations and treatments? Stool quality, bowel habits? Emotional condition: psychological distress, tension, anxiety?

Clinical examination including anoscopy/rigid sigmoidoscopy: absence of any other painful lesions in anorectum, except laterally: tender levator muscles → local digital pressure triggering patient's discomfort.

Full/partial colonic evaluation as per general screening guidelines.

Additional tests (optional)

Anophysiology testing, including balloon expulsion test and EMG.

Defecating proctogram.

Classification

• Levator ani syndrome.

• Unspecified functional anorectal pain (lack of tenderness on levators).

Nonoperative Treatment

Maintaining stool regularity (supplemental fibers, fluid intake, stool softener, etc).

Warm sitz baths → general and pelvic floor relaxation.

Physical therapy, biofeedback training, digital massage of levator ani muscles.

Electrogalvanic stimulation (EGS): low-frequency oscillating current → induction of muscle fasciculation and fatigue → break and desensitization of spastic muscle contraction cycles.

Muscle relaxants: hyoscyamine, topical nitroglycerine, calcium antagonists.

Acupuncture?

Uncertain benefit: injection of botulinum toxin A.

Psychotherapy?

Operative Treatment

Indication

Surgery to be avoided.

Operative approach

Not applicable.

Outcome

Combined efforts should result in 50–75% improvement.

Follow-up

Recheck patient after 4–6 weeks of initiated treatment.

Cross-reference

FUNCTIONAL ANORECTAL PAIN—PROCTALGIA FUGAX *(569.42)*

Overview

Proctalgia fugax comprises sporadic sudden attacks of severe anorectal pain (acute muscle spasm) lasting several seconds or minutes with subsequent complete resolution. Attacks lack a morphologic pathology, may occur during sleep and wake the patient up. Occurrence overall infrequent with < 5 episodes per year in 50% of patients.

Definition by Rome III criteria (2006): 3 mandatory criteria (preferably but not necessarily for > 3 months):

• Recurrent episodes of anal or lower rectal pain.
• Duration of episodes: seconds to minutes.
• Absence of anorectal pain between episodes.

Epidemiology

Exact incidence unknown, estimated 5–15% of adults sporadically affected, of whom < 20% seek medical attention. Equal gender distribution.

Symptoms

Sharp and severe anorectal and low rectal pain.

Differential Diagnosis

Anal fissure, thrombosed external hemorrhoid, abscess and fistular disease, prostatitis, levator ani syndrome, coccygodynia, HIV-associated ulcer, malignancy-associated lesion (cancer, melanoma, leukemia, lymphoma, etc), ischemia, IBD, cryptitis.

Pathology

Lack of visible pathology.

Evaluation

Required minimal standard

History: characteristic description of attacks (time, duration, frequency)? Lack of specific anorectal/pelvic symptoms: prolapse, lump/bump, bleeding, fevers/chills, etc? Previous evaluations and treatments? Stool quality, bowel habits? Emotional condition: psychological distress, tension, anxiety?

Clinical examination including anoscopy/rigid sigmoidoscopy: intervals of complete absence of any pathology or pain.

Full/partial colonic evaluation as per general screening guidelines.

Additional tests (optional)
Only if clinical diagnosis is in doubt:
- Anophysiology testing, including balloon expulsion test and EMG.
- Defecating proctogram.

Classification
- Sporadic form.
- Familial form.

Nonoperative Treatment
Majority of patients with rare episodes: reassurance and explanation of symptom complex.

Patients with frequent symptoms: $\rightarrow$ uncertain benefit from:
- Nitroglycerine: interrupting acute episode?
- Calcium antagonists?
- Inhalation of salbutamol (β-adrenergic agonist): shortening of ≥ 20 minutes episodes of proctalgia.
- Clonidine (α-agonist).
- Acupuncture?

Operative Treatment
Indication
Surgery not indicated.

Operative approach
Not applicable.

Outcome
Generally benign and self-limited.

Follow-up
Recheck patients as needed.

Cross-reference

"INCIDENTALOLOGY"—APPROACH TO INCIDENTAL FINDINGS

Overview

More sophisticated imaging tools and systematic intraoperative evaluation will invariably reveal unexpected findings and pathologies that are (1) unrelated to the primary disease, (2) not consistent with, or (3) exceed the preoperative working hypothesis and treatment plan. While anticipated combinations of separate surgeries may be very rational, particularly in symptomatic patients, the decision to perform a potentially harmful extension of the primary procedure should be based on scientific evidence.

Classification

- Related to primary disease → worse than expected findings.
- Unrelated to primary disease → findings without immediate pathologic value.
- Unrelated to primary disease → findings with current or potential future pathologic impact.

Common Problems/Dilemmas

- Possible extension or change of the surgery not previously discussed with patient, lack of informed consent → decision "in the patient's best interest."
- Evidence about natural course potentially not available → "best guess" decision.
- Unnecessary prolongation of the procedure.
- Risk of possible additional complications to be considered.
- Final pathology might be at variance with intraoperative assessment: eg, tumor despite adherence not invading another organ, etc.

Specific Scenarios

Normal appendix

- Question: incidental appendectomy yes/no?
- Natural course without procedure: 6–10% lifetime risk of acute appendicitis → diagnosis remains difficult, access to appendix potentially more difficult after previous major abdominal surgery, morbidity not negligible.
- Attributable risk of complications: minimal (leak).

- Practical approach:
  - Appendectomy—yes: absence of contraindications, appendix after primary procedure in different location or difficult to access. In addition: appendectomy of abnormal-appearing appendix.
  - Appendectomy—no: otherwise clean operation with implant (eg, rectopexy), malnourished patient, poor intestinal condition (LBO, diffuse peritonitis), major extra effort to mobilize appendix.

Meckel diverticulum

- Question: incidental Meckel diverticulectomy yes/no?
- Natural course without procedure: 2% prevalence → 6–7% overall lifetime risk of complications: pain, bleeding, obstruction (intussusception, volvulus, fibrous band), morbidity/mortality of symptomatic Meckel diverticulum: 2% mortality, > 10% morbidity.
- Attributable risk of complications: risk < 2% (leak, obstruction).
- Practical approach:
  - Resection—yes: absence of contraindications, diverticulum > 2 cm, presence of fibrous band.
  - Resection—no: otherwise clean operation with implant (eg, rectopexy), malnourished patient, poor intestinal condition (LBO, diffuse peritonitis).

Cholelithiasis

- Question: incidental cholecystectomy yes/no?
- Natural course without procedure: 10–25% of gallstone carriers become symptomatic.
- Attributable risk of complications: < 3%.
- Practical approach:
  - Cholecystectomy—yes: symptomatic patient, gallbladder with signs of chronic or recurrent inflammation (despite lack of history), no disproportionate extension of incision—eg, RUQ intervention (eg, right hemicolectomy), laparoscopic procedure.
  - Cholecystectomy—no: if extension of incision needed only for this purpose, asymptomatic patient with absence of any inflammatory changes.

Adrenal mass

- Question: workup needed? Adrenalectomy yes/no?
- Natural course without procedure: depending on nature (endocrine active/inactive adenoma, metastasis, pheochromocytoma, hyperplasia, etc).
- Attributable risk of complications: endocrine crisis if inadequate perioperative priming.

- Practical approach:
  - Workup needed: < 3 cm → monitoring, 3–6 cm → endocrine evaluation, > 6 cm → evaluation and resection.
  - Adrenalectomy—yes: only if endocrine workup done, anesthesia management adjusted.

Normal-appearing ovaries

- Question: ovariectomy in postmenopausal women undergoing cancer operation?
- Natural course without procedure: 2–3% lifetime risk of ovarian cancer, 3–4% ovarian metastases from colorectal cancer (CRC), poor prognosis if CRC involving the ovaries (stage IV).
- Attributable risk of complications: ureteral injury 0.1–0.2%.
- Practical approach: theoretical benefit of prophylactic oophorectomy questionable → incidental adnexectomy increasingly abandoned by colorectal surgeons as it is more likely to avoid GYN malignancy than improve CRC survival.

Hernia

- Question: hernia repair yes/no? With or without mesh?
- Natural course without procedure: 5% lifetime risk of incarceration, enlargement, worse outcome for emergency procedure.
- Attributable risk of complications: infection of foreign body, recurrent hernia.
- Practical approach: additional incisions or extension of incision not recommended for just that purpose; repair with mesh not recommended in contaminated field → reinforcement with biologic material (collagen, etc).

Tumor involving other organs

- Question: more extensive resection? Ostomy? Abort procedure?
- Situations: rectal cancer invading the prostate → pelvic exenteration?; involvement of GYN organs → hysterectomy, adnexectomy?; involvement of ureter/kidney → nephrectomy yes/no? carcinomatosis → bypass/ostomy?, etc.
- Natural course without procedure: incomplete resection → clinical recurrence (adjuvant therapy does not make up for insufficient operation.
- Attributable risk of complications: depending on the type of operation.
- Practical approach:
  - Proceed: if more extensive surgery likely to improve chance of cure and not resulting in measurable impact on quality of life: eg, nephrectomy, adnexectomy, hysterectomy.

– Abort and discuss: if more extensive surgery associated with significantly increased morbidity/mortality or a potentially altered quality of life (eg, pelvic exenteration).

– Ostomy: yes if needed → routine preoperative discussion and marking avoids that conflict.

Cancer instead of expected diverticulitis

• Question: change in surgical approach yes/no?

• No because resection for diverticulitis should anyway follow oncological principles.

Sigmoid diverticulitis instead of expected appendicitis

• Question: definite surgical treatment for diverticulitis yes/no?

• Natural course without procedure: largely outdated data, 16–20% chance of recurrent attacks, up to 50% after complicated attack.

• Attributable risk of complications: anastomotic leak, recurrent diverticulitis, need for ostomy.

• Practical approach: if preoperative symptoms so significant that no time for imaging studies → definitive treatment with surgical resection favored (primary anastomosis with/without colonic lavage); potential alternative: lavage and drainage alone, followed by antibiotic treatment?

Right-sided diverticulitis instead of expected appendicitis

• Question: Ileocecal resection/right hemicolectomy yes/no?

• Natural course without procedure: overwhelming majority of cases responding to antibiotic treatment, low risk of recurrence.

• Attributable risk of complications: anastomotic leak, SBO.

• Practical approach: if preoperative symptoms so significant that no time for imaging studies → definitive treatment with surgical resection favored (primary anastomosis).

IBD instead of expected appendicitis

• Question: appendectomy yes/no? Ileocecal resection yes/no?

• Natural course without procedure: nearly 100% recurrent disease and risk of future surgical intervention; only 50% risk after ileocecal resection (in addition, benefit of having histologic confirmation).

• Attributable risk of complications: leak, recurrent disease, short bowel syndrome.

• Practical approach:

– Ileocecal resection—yes: if disease limited to ileocecal region.

– Ileocecal resection—no: if multisegmental involvement.
  • Appendectomy—yes: if access through McBurney incision.
  • Appendectomy—no: if access through midline and appendix normal.

Tumor instead of expected appendicitis

• Question: Oncologic resection (right hemicolectomy) yes/no?

• Natural course without extension of procedure (ie, appendectomy only): risk of lymph node metastases, increased risk of tumor recurrence, need for subsequent surgery for oncological resection.

• Attributable risk of complications: anastomotic leak, SBO, no relevant impact on bowel function.

• Practical approach: clinical evaluation of intraoperative findings and immediate pathologic assessment of specimen (including frozen section if available): if malignancy confirmed or very likely → definitive treatment with surgical resection favored (primary anastomosis).

Cross-reference

PEDIATRICS—CONGENITAL AGANGLIONIC MEGACOLON *(HIRSCHSPRUNG DISEASE, 751.3)*

Overview

Anorectal malformation with initially normal macroanatomy that results from incomplete population of the distal colon with neuronal elements. Development of enteric nervous system: migration of neuroenteric cells from neural crest to the GI tract from proximal to distal, first to myenteric (Auerbach) plexus, then to submucosal (Meissner) plexus.

Hirschsprung disease: incomplete migration results in a lack of neuroenteric network in the distal rectum and extending in continuity toward proximal rectum for varying lengths → lack of peristalsis and inability to relax muscle tone in aganglionic segment (including internal anal sphincter) + increased distal smooth muscle tone and spasticity → constipation and increasing dilation of colon proximal to aganglionic segment → necrotizing enterocolitis (acute) or megacolon (chronic). Severity of symptoms and untreated natural course with some variability. Increased incidence of other anomalies (Down syndrome, intestinal atresia).

Treatment consists of resecting the pathologic aganglionic distal segment with respective reconstruction. Decision-making process includes assessment of whether:

- Untreated condition is life-threatening (eg, acute necrotizing enterocolitis, perforation)?
- Other life-threatening anomalies that need priority attention are present (eg, cardiac)?
- Primary reconstruction (with/without defunctioning colostomy) or secondary reconstruction (bridging with colostomy) is needed?

Epidemiology

Incidence: 1 in 4400 to 1 in 7000 live births with male/female ratio of 4:1 (subgroup long-segment: 1:1). Incidence of familial cases: 6–10%.

Associated anomalies: Down syndrome 4–16%, anal/intestinal atresia 0.5–3.5%.

In adolescents and adults: variable incidence (3–20%).

Symptoms

Neonates (80–90%): symptomatic during first 24–72 hours of life → delayed passage of meconium > 24–48 hours, constipation, abdominal distention, poor feeding, emesis, failure to thrive. Complications: Hirschsprung-associated enterocolitis, cecal perforation. Variant: relatively asymptomatic.

After newborn period: history of severe constipation, cycles of constipation/distention with breakthrough episodes of explosive diarrhea, abdominal distention (chronic), enterocolitis (acute distention), failure to thrive. Variant: relatively asymptomatic.

Adulthood (3–20%): history of chronic constipation since childhood, abdominal distention.

Differential Diagnosis

Meconium plug.

Cystic fibrosis (meconium ileus).

Morphologic obstruction (atresia, anorectal malformations; caveat: possible combination of both).

Intestinal neuronal dysplasia: on biopsy neural hyperplasia and increased number of ganglia.

Total intestinal aganglionosis: entire GI tract involved.

Small left colon syndrome (transient dysmotility in children of diabetic mothers).

Endocrine imbalance: hypothyroidism, adrenal insufficiency.

Adulthood: Chagas disease.

Other causes of constipation.

Pathology

Macroscopic

- Depending on duration of symptoms: varying degrees of preaganglionic colonic distention.
- Acute complication of enterocolitis.

Microscopic

- Normal: paucity of ganglia within 1.5–2 cm proximal to dentate line.
- Hirschsprung: absence of ganglion cells in submucosal and myenteric plexus of distal large intestine > 2 cm from dentate line, possible neural hyperplasia (adrenergic, cholinergic), otherwise normal colonic architecture.

Evaluation

Required minimal standard

Diagnosis of Hirschsprung disease:

- Abdominal x-ray: megacolon? Small bowel dilation?

- Anorectal manometry (best to diagnose short-segment Hirschsprung, of limited practical use in infants and children): absence of RAIR (reflex relaxation with rectal distention).
- Barium enema: spastic distal segment with characteristic transition zone to dilated proximal bowel, retention of barium at 24 hours? May be false negative in short-segment Hirschsprung.
- Biopsy: diagnostic gold standard (accuracy 99%): serial biopsies that include a thickness of submucosa equal to the mucosa, starting 2 cm proximal to dentate line: → no submucosal plexus, but increased acetyl cholinesterase stain. (caveat: last 1.5–2 cm do not contain ganglia even in normal patients!)

Additional tests (optional)
Evaluation of associated anomalies.

Classification

- Classical form of Hirschsprung (80–90%): < 40 cm of distal colon affected.
- Long-segment Hirschsprung (7–10%): aganglionic segment extending proximally to hepatic flexure, or even total colonic aganglionosis, ie, complete involvement of colon.
- Ultrashort-segment Hirschsprung: only distal rectum involved.

Nonoperative Treatment

Colonic decompression, rectal irrigation through large-diameter tube: bridging to surgery.

Operative Treatment

Indication
- Neonatal/childhood period: any confirmed Hirschsprung disease (unless in combination with lethal anomalies).
- Adults: depending on presentation and failure of conservative management.

Operative approach
Poor condition: colostomy, secondary reconstruction later.

Good condition: primary reconstruction with/without diversion:

1. Modern approach: one-stage pull-through procedure normoganglionic bowel (frozen sections):
   a. Laparoscopic-assisted endorectal pull-through.
   b. Transanal endorectal pull-through in the newborn.
2. Classical operations: Rehbein, Swenson, Duhamel, Soave.

Massive megacolon: colonic contractility impairment persisting even after resection of aganglionic segment (decompensated Frank-Starling mechanism): proctocolectomy and ileoanal pull-through procedure.

Outcome

Mortality: 1–2%.

Anastomotic leak: 5–7%.

Postoperative enterocolitis: 6–20%.

Long-term good bowel function: 80–90%.

Other complications: stricture, perirectal fistula, incontinence, persistent constipation (particularly after Duhamel and Soave procedures).

Follow up

Functional reassessment in regular intervals.

Cross-reference

PEDIATRICS—CONGENITAL MALFORMATIONS
(751.2)

Overview

Anorectal malformations comprise a large number of macromorphologic anatomic anomalies that result from incomplete or incorrect embryologic development and fusion steps and manifest as abnormal number and form of orifices.

Timing of the genetic program errors and stops results in different levels and severities of anatomic defects: high (severe), intermediate (moderate), low (mild). Prognosis depends on (1) severity of the anorectal malformation and (2) impact of other anomalies.

Frequent association with chromosomal and other morphologic defects (cardiac, urogenital system, skeleton, etc).

For treatment planning → assessment whether:

• Untreated condition is life-threatening (eg, complete atresia without fistula)?

• Other life-threatening anomalies that need priority attention are present (eg, cardiac)?

• Primary reconstruction (with/without defunctioning colostomy) or a secondary reconstruction (bridging with colostomy) is needed?

Epidemiology

Incidence: 1 in 3500 to 1 in 5000 births with male preponderance (55–65%).

Associated malformations (in 60–65%):

• Chromosomal abnormalities (15%).

• VACTERL (10–15%): Vertebral anomalies, Anal atresia, Cardiac defect (eg, ventricular septum defect), Tracheo-Esophageal fistula, Renal abnormalities, Limb abnormalities.

• Cardiac: 15–30% (Fallot tetralogy, ventricular septal defect).

• GI: tracheoesophageal fistula 8–10%, Hirschsprung disease 3%, duodenal atresia 2%.

• Urogenital: vesicoureteral reflux 60%, renal agenesis/malformation.

• Vertebral: spinal dysraphism 15–35% (eg, tethered cord).

Symptoms

Asymptomatic unless not recognized and treated in time → obstructive symptoms, urinary tract infections.

Differential Diagnosis

Only with regards to different variants and associated morphologic and genetic defects.

Pathology

Macropathology of the various subforms of malformations (see classification).

Evaluation

Required minimal standard

Visible abnormality on first comprehensive examination at birth:

- Flat perineum, short sacrum, little muscle contraction → high anomaly.
- Females: single perineal opening → cloacal malformation.

After 24 hours → gas and meconium moving toward rectum:

- Males → urinalysis for meconium; females → meconium through vagina.
- Gas or meconium visible in perineal raphe → low anomaly.

Lateral pelvic radiograph ("babygram") in upside-down position (with marking of perineum/anus): distance of defect?

Ultrasound/MRI: assessment of pelvic floor anatomy.

Additional tests (optional)

Depending on conclusiveness of the presentation.

Search for associated anomalies: ultrasound → hydronephrosis? skeletal x-rays, etc.

Classification

Type of defect:

- Imperforate anus/rectal atresia/anal stenosis with/without fistula.
- Fistula (to perineum, urinary system, vestibulum/vagina).
- Cloaca.

Level of defect:

- High lesions (supralevator): 25%.
- Intermediate lesions: 30–35%.
- Low lesions (infralevator): 40–45%.

More detailed classifications: Wingspread classification, Pena classification.

Nonoperative Treatment

Temporarily only at initial presentation: NPO, insertion of NGT.

Long-term problems: management of incontinence, bowel regimen, etc.

Operative Treatment

Indication
Any anorectal malformation.

Operative approach
Temporizing measures
Colostomy in double-barrel technique: → complete diversion, reduced risk of urinary tract infection, access to mucus fistula, no risk of closed loop.

Reconstruction (primary or secondary)
• Posterior sagittal anorectoplasty (PSARP): preferred approach for majority of patients: prone-jackknife position, electrical stimulation device for evaluation/localizing of sphincter contraction:
  – Low anomalies: anoplasty or minimal PSARP without colostomy.
  – High and intermediate anomalies: colostomy → PSARP at 4–8 weeks.
• Abdominoperineal pull-through procedure: not needed in majority of patients.

Reoperations for persistent dysfunction (eg, incontinence)
• Muscle good, but bowel previously misplaced: relocation to correct site.
• Absent muscle function: artificial bowel sphincter, graciloplasty, MACE procedure. Permanent colostomy usually not needed unless patient miserable and above-mentioned local reconstructive efforts fail.

Outcome

Fecal continence: low anomalies 85–90%, high anomalies 30–40%. Manifest fecal incontinence: 25–40%.

Urinary incontinence: 2–18% (except cloaca → up to 60–70%).

Other complications: anal stenosis 30%, rectal mucosal prolapse, constipation 25% (more frequent in low anomalies with megarectum) → overflow incontinence.

Follow-up

Functional reassessment at regular intervals.

Persistent fecal incontinence → options: conservative management (scheduled enemas, antidiarrheals, etc), implantation of artificial bowel sphincter, MACE procedure, colostomy.

Cross-reference

PEDIATRICS—ACQUIRED COLORECTAL PROBLEMS

Overview

In addition to the problems of and around congenital anorectal malformations, children may present with a number of specific pediatric colorectal conditions, as well as with a wide array of colorectal problems that are known from but not limited to adult patients, eg, fissure, fistula/abscess, constipation. Most of these problems are dealt with in similar fashion, adjusted to the patient's age and ability to understand and participate in the treatment plan.

1. Constipation/encopresis:
    a. Dietary, social, and psychological issues.
    b. Rarely: morphologic problems.
2. Skin pathology:
    a. Diaper rash: toxic effect of stool/urine within occlusive confinement of diapers.
    b. Contact dermatitis: to ointments, creams, soap, etc.
    c. Candidiasis: inflammatory rash, frequently with enhanced margins.
    d. Erythrasma: bacterial infection (*Corynebacterium minutissimum*) → diagnosis made using the Wood lamp.
    e. Mollusca contagiosa: clusters of small round papulous lesions, viral infection (molluscum contagiosum virus, belongs to DNA Poxviridae).
3. Parasites:
    a. Pinworm infection (*Enterobius vermicularis*): perianal pruritus, particularly at night → tape test.
    b. Other worm/parasite infestation.
4. Anal pain/bleeding:
    a. Anal fissure: most commonly acute (constipation, transition to potty training) → resolution with stool management, glycerin suppositories, milk of magnesia.
    b. Hemorrhoids: rare in children but not impossible.
    c. Perirectal abscess/-fistula.
    d. Anal irritation: secondary to diarrhea, fissure, prolapse, etc.
5. Rectal prolapse:
    a. Risk factors: malnutrition, cystic fibrosis, chronic constipation.
6. GI /colonic pathology:
    a. Intussusception.

b. Meckel diverticulum: → bleeding, pain, intussusception.

c. Necrotizing enterocolitis.

d. Intestinal malrotation.

e. Polyps:

    (1) Hamartomatous polyps: juvenile polyps, Peutz-Jeghers, juvenile polyposis, etc.

    (2) Hyperplastic polyps.

    (3) Inflammatory polyps.

    (4) Adenomatous polyps.

7. Sexual abuse:

  a. Anal canal trauma.

  b. Condyloma acuminata?

Cross-reference

COMPLICATIONS—URETERAL INJURY *(997.5)*

Complication

Injury to the ureter may be recognized either during surgery or in the post-operative period (urine leak, urinoma, uremia, hydronephrosis, etc). Incidence ~0.2%.

Typical sites of the injury:

• Retroperitoneal in proximity to left colonic vascular stalk.

• Entry to the pelvis, crossing iliac vessels.

• Pelvis at anterolateral entry to the bladder.

Differential Diagnosis

Bladder injury, urethral injury.

Causes

• Inadequate visualization of course of the ureter, lack of verification of ureteral position prior to transecting the vascular stalk, scarred retroperitoneum after previous surgery or inflammatory process (eg, severe diverticulitis).

• Injury mechanism: transection, segmental resection, ligation or crushing with clamp (imprecise bleeding control), denudation of the ureter.

• Preventive measures: ureteral stent placement for anticipated intraoperative difficulties, lighted stents available for laparoscopic procedures.

Not discussed here: intentional transection of the ureter because of disease involvement (eg, cancer).

Evaluation

Required minimal standard

• Intraoperative suspicion/recognition: verification with indigo carmine extravasation → surgical clarification of anatomy, urology consult (if available).

• Recognition in postoperative period:

– Drain with suspicious output: → IV indigo carmine, elevation of creatinine in drain fluid (compared with serum).

– No drain and further investigation: → imaging studies to confirm and localize injury: ultrasound, CT, IV urogram, retrograde ureteropyelography.

Cofactors for Decision-Making Process

• Intra- or postoperative recognition? → time since last exploration: hostile abdomen?

- Retrospectoscope on intraoperative difficulties → clue about location of injury.
- Current patient condition: sepsis, hemodynamic stability?

Management

Timing
- Intraoperative: immediate repair.
- Postoperative early (< 7 days postoperatively): reexploration and post-primary repair.
- Postoperative late (> 7 days): temporizing measures (eg, percutaneous nephrostomy tubes, stent, etc) → secondary repair/reconstruction (either through laparotomy or through extraperitoneal access) after 6–12 weeks.

Operative approach
- Ureteral stenting alone: if minor injury without stenosis → reevaluation after 3–6 weeks.
- Ureteroureterostomy with/without limited ureteral resection: direct spatulated watertight ureteral anastomosis over double J-stent → removal of stent after 3–6 weeks.
- Ureteroneocystostomy: resection and reimplantation of ureter with appropriate antireflux technique into bladder.
- Ureteroneocystostomy with psoas hitch: transverse incision of ipsilaterally mobilized bladder dome → vertical closure to result in elongation of bladder, fixation of bladder in place by nonabsorbable sutures to tendinous part of psoas muscle, reimplantation of ureter.
- Transureteroureterostomy: if insufficient length to reach bladder → transposition and anastomosis of injured ureter to contralateral ureter.
- Further techniques: Boari flap (creation of conduit from bladder dome flap), intestinal conduit.

Cross-reference

COMPLICATIONS—POSTOPERATIVE ILEUS
(546.3)

Complication

Postoperative ileus is an expected motility disorder of the intestinal tract after an operation and general anesthesia. Prolonged postoperative ileus, however, is a dysmotility persisting beyond this expected time frame.

1. Delayed recovery of upper GI function (small bowel, stomach: normal 24–48 hours):

   a. Lack of appetite, inability to tolerate or advance oral intake, epigastric fullness or pressure, heartburn, burping, later progression to nausea and vomiting.

   b. If NGT already in correct position: persistent high output.

2. Delayed recovery of lower GI function (colon: normal 2–4 days):

   a. Increasing abdominal distention, diffuse rather than colicky discomfort, lack of passage of flatus or stool: progression to nausea and vomiting as late symptoms of lower GI dysfunction.

   b. It is not possible that upper GI function initially recovers timely, but that the patient subsequently experiences setback secondary to delayed recovery of lower GI function.

3. Systemic effects of prolonged postoperative ileus:

   a. Loss and third-spacing of fluids, electrolyte and acid-base abnormalities, tachycardia, later hypotension.

   b. Malnutrition if ileus persists beyond 5 days.

Differential Diagnosis

Local problem: anastomotic leaks, mechanical bowel obstruction (eg, kinking, volvulus, internal hernia, adhesions), persistent ischemia, interloop abscess, aspiration, etc.

Systemic problem: congestive heart failure; steroid deficiency → ileus may be the first and subtle symptom of a relative deficiency (particularly in patients with history of steroid medication, eg, IBD).

Causes

Exact pathogenesis for postoperative ileus unclear. Speculations: intrinsic vs extrinsic factors (Table 4–13):

• Any condition interfering with normal and relatively labile equilibrium of intestinal motility and propulsion → activation of central nervous system reflex pathways and sympathetic system → disorganized irregular electrical activity → paralysis of particular bowel segment.

TABLE 4–13. Triggers of Postoperative Ileus.

Category	Conditions
Peritoneal impact	Laparotomy, blunt/penetrating abdominal trauma
Infection	Peritonitis, sepsis, SIRS
Drugs	Anesthesia, exogenous/endogenous opiates, psychotropics, anticholinergics
Cardiopulmonary failure	Right ventricular failure, low cardiac output, hypoxia
Vascular	Underperfusion, portal hypertension, portal vein thrombosis
Retroperitoneal/ mediastinal pathology	Hematoma, infection
Spinal disorder	Vertebral fracture, spinal cord injury
Metabolic disorders	Hyponatremia, hypokalemia, hypomagnesemia, uremia, diabetic coma
Endocrine disorders	Adrenal insufficiency, diabetes, hypothyroidism

SIRS, systemic immune response syndrome.

- Focal morphologic alteration of bowel (injury, disease or inflammation) → interruption/reversal of antegrade propagation of coordinated contractions.
- Inflammatory cascade: release of active mediators (eg, nitric oxide) and proinflammatory cytokines which inhibit intestinal motility.
- Opiate-mediated (μ_2 receptors) inhibition of intestinal smooth muscle contractility.

Evaluation

Required minimal standard

Rule out evidence of leak: overall condition, tachycardia (may initially be the only symptom), fever, sepsis with organ dysfunction, hemodynamic stability, nutritional status, disproportional pain, etc.

Abdominal exam: diffuse peritoneal signs, wound infection.

Imaging studies:

- Abdominal series and chest x-ray: evidence of increasing rather than decreasing extraluminal air?

– Water-soluble contrast enema: leak?

– CT scan: abscess, fluid collection, transition point?

Cofactors for Decision-Making Process

• Retrospectoscope on nature of the disease, intraoperative findings and difficulties.

• Current patient condition (general, local)?

• Index of suspicion for problem other than dysmotility?

• Chance to surgically improve condition?

• Timing since last exploration?

Management

Prevention during index operation

• Emergency indication: aggressive and timely management to minimize exposure time of bowels to negative impacts (eg, fecal or purulent contamination).

• Elective surgery: optimization of patient's general condition and nutritional status.

• Surgeon- and surgery-related factors:

– Minimize extent and duration of intraoperative trauma, exposure to room air, lower body temperature.

– Need for adhesiolysis, enterotomies, devascularization, blood loss.

– Laparoscopic rather than open approach if feasible.

• Pain management:

– Exogenous opiates or endogenous opiate pathways → inhibitory effect on smooth muscle contractility.

– Preferential use of nonopiate drugs (eg, NSAIDs) → reduce opiate consumption, positive effect on ileus resolution by inhibition of prostaglandin-mediated inflammation and depression of smooth muscle contractility.

– Opiate antagonists reverse intestinal dysmotility: naloxone → unspecific (increased pain); alvimopan, methylnaltrexone → specific competitive μ-receptor antagonists not crossing blood-brain barrier.

– Thoracic epidural anesthesia: analgesia without intestinal/respiratory depression, pharmacologic sympathectomy → promoting intestinal motility.

• Fast-track postoperative management.

Conservative management

• Correction of electrolyte and acid-base imbalances, fluid resuscitation.

• History of steroid medication → stress dose of 100 mg hydrocortisone IV.

- Placement of NGT for decompression, prevention of repeated vomiting, and to reduce aspiration risk.
- Optimization of underlying comorbidities, eg, cardiopulmonary function, renal function, diabetes, adrenal insufficiency, hypothyroidism.
- Ileus > 5 days or preexisting malnutrition → parenteral nutrition.
- Pharmacologic treatment:
  - Nausea → metoclopramide, odansetron.
  - Prokinetics → erythromycin (no proven benefit), neostigmine, metoclopramide, tegaserod maleate (currently not available)?

Operative approach
- Early abdominal reexploration:
  - Evidence of surgical complication within 7–10 days.
  - Suspicion of mechanical SBO within 7–10 days.
- Late abdominal exploration:
  - Persistent ileus/SBO after 4 weeks.

Cross-reference

COMPLICATIONS—LEAK *(997.4)*

Complication

Postsurgical evidence (abscess, fistula, sepsis) for extravasation of enteric content or contrast from intestines, either from anastomotic dehiscence or unrecognized enterotomy. Diagnosis based on clinical symptoms (eg, peritonitis, sepsis), clinical suspicion (low-grade fever, elevated WBCs, unexplained tachycardia, persistent bowel dysfunction), or radiologic documentation in otherwise asymptomatic patient (eg, if proximally diverted). Incidence: rectum 5–10%, colon 2%, small bowel 1%, IPAA 4–5%, continent ileostomy 12%.

Differential Diagnosis

Abscess not in connection to intestines (eg, infected hematoma, postdiffuse peritonitis).

Causes

Technical error, insufficient blood supply, tension, poor tissue quality (postradiation, malnutrition, active infection), drug effect (steroids, bevacizumab, other chemotherapy agents), smoking.

Prophylactic proximal diversion does not prevent a leak but reduces septic sequelae.

Evaluation

Required minimal standard

Assessment of patient's overall condition: tachycardia (may initially be the only symptom), sepsis with organ dysfunction, hemodynamic stability, nutritional status, etc.

Abdominal exam: diffuse peritonitis, enterocutaneous fistula, wound condition.

Leak suspected but not confirmed: water-soluble contrast enema, CT scan.

Cofactors for Decision-Making Process

- Retrospectoscope on intraoperative difficulties.
- Current patient condition (general, local)?
- Leak confined or causing diffuse peritonitis?
- Chance for a better surgical anastomosis?
- Timing since last exploration?

Management

Conservative
- Confined leak → CT-guided abscess drainage → confined fistula.
- Diverted leak → reassessment after 6–12 weeks.
- Leak with sepsis → supportive measures in conjunction to surgery: NGT, antibiotics, cardiopulmonary optimization.

Operative approach
- Early symptomatic leak (< 7–10 days) → abdominal reexploration for damage control:
  – Diversion and drainage.
  – Takedown of anastomosis and ostomy (Hartmann type).
  – Redo-anastomosis (with/without diversion).
  – Often bowels rigid from inflammation → neither resection nor stoma possible → repair/drainage or placement of drain into the leak with goal to create confined fistula.
- Later recognition of leak (> 10 days) → hostile abdomen:
  – Proximal diversion (if possible).
  – Attempt to control sepsis → CT-guided or open drain placements → attempt to create confined fistula.
  – Diffuse peritonitis/sepsis → damage control laparotomy with wide drainage.

Cross-reference

COMPLICATIONS—STOMA NECROSIS *(569.60)*

Complication

Dusky appearance of newly created ostomy.

Differential Diagnosis

Traumatized stoma, hematoma, mucosal sloughing only.

Causes

Inadequate blood supply: insufficient mobilization of the intestine, inadequate opening in the abdominal wall ($\rightarrow$ strangulation), internal wrapping of bowel around stoma ($\rightarrow$ strangulation), morbid obesity with huge abdominal pannus and thickened mesentery, independent ischemic event (embolus, thrombus).

Evaluation

Required minimal standard

Assessment of patient's overall condition: septic, hemodynamic stability, etc.

Assessment of the extent of necrosis: insertion of test tube + illumination with flashlight:

- Dark mucosa limited to epifascial segment, pink mucosa visible below.
- Dark mucosa extending below the fascia level.

Cofactors for Decision-Making Process

- Retrospectoscope on intraoperative difficulties.
- Current patient condition?
- Ostomy intended as temporary or permanent? $\rightarrow$ initially intended time frame for reversal?
- Onset of complication compared with its creation: if > 2 weeks postoperatively $\rightarrow$ has the distal site (eg, anastomosis) already healed?

Management

Timing

- Subfascial $\rightarrow$ urgent revision, otherwise risk of intraperitoneal perforation: $\rightarrow$ abscess, enterocutaneous fistula, sepsis.
- Epifascial $\rightarrow$ acceptance of stricture $\rightarrow$ elective stoma revision or takedown.

Operative approach

Acute:

– Early after stoma creation: reexploration → better mobilization of intestine, wider abdominal wall opening, thinning of abdominal pannus, possible relocation, possible selection of different bowel segment (eg, transverse colon instead of ileum).

– > 2 weeks after stoma creation: consider exploration with definitive takedown of temporary ostomy, if healing of distal site confirmed (clinical, endoscopic, contrast enema).

Elective: stoma revision or relocation vs stoma takedown.

Cross-reference

COMPLICATIONS—DELAYED WOUND HEALING *(998.3)*

Complication

Failure of a wound to close in a timely manner, either defined by persistently unfavorable wound appearance or a time frame > 3 months.

Differential Diagnosis

Perirectal or enterocutaneous fistula, suture granulomata, decubitus ulcer.

Causes

Wound infection (5–10% incidence, particularly if multidrug-resistant bacteria involved, eg, MRSA, pseudomonas, etc), inadequate blood supply (eg, flaps), tension, formation of deeper pockets, persistent feeding of the wound from deeper abscess or fistula, continued fecal contamination, obesity, infected foreign body (eg, mesh), neglected wound care, diabetes, immunosuppression, malnutrition, immobility, drug effect (steroids, infliximab, bevacizumab, other chemotherapy agents).

Evaluation

Required minimal standard

Assessment of patient's overall condition: sepsis, hemodynamic stability, nutritional status, HIV status, etc.

Wound evaluation (if necessary under anesthesia): location (abdominal, perirectal, anal canal, other), size, configuration, depth (fistula?), unfavorable configuration, wound components (soft tissue, bone, foreign body, etc), culture results (MRSA, fungi, etc).

Cofactors for Decision-Making Process

• Retrospectoscope on intraoperative difficulties.
• Current patient condition (general, local)?
• Need for examination under anesthesia?
• Chance to surgically improve wound condition?

Management

Conservative

• Wound opening, debridement, wound irrigation (shower, bath), wet-to-dry dressing changes, povidone-iodine ointment mixed with granular sugar, perifocal hair removal (shaving, depilatory cream).

- Wound-VAC, ie, vacuum-assisted wound dressing (if anatomically suitable): goals are to achieve a clean, manageable wound and promote contraction of wound edges; reduced frequency of dressing changes (only every 2–4 days). Risks: vacuum damage on bowel causing enterocutaneous fistula; loss of foam in depth of wound resulting in foreign body.
- Antibiotics typically not indicated for adequate wound: only used to treat significant phlegmonous component or hidden sepsis.

Operative approach
- Reexploration of wound with reexcision of the wound, debridement of necrotic material, opening of pockets, better wound configuration.
- Combination with well-vascularized muscle or myocutaneous flaps.
- Creation of temporary colostomy (in selected cases).

Cross-reference

Chapter 5

Operative Techniques

Operative Techniques

TAMPONADE ANAL CANAL

Principle

Compression and tamponade of the anal canal in case of acute distal hemorrhage as bridging for stabilization until definitive assessment or procedure is possible (Figure 5–1).

Setting

Where needed, when no immediate access to OR.

Alternatives

Examination and surgical hemostasis in OR.

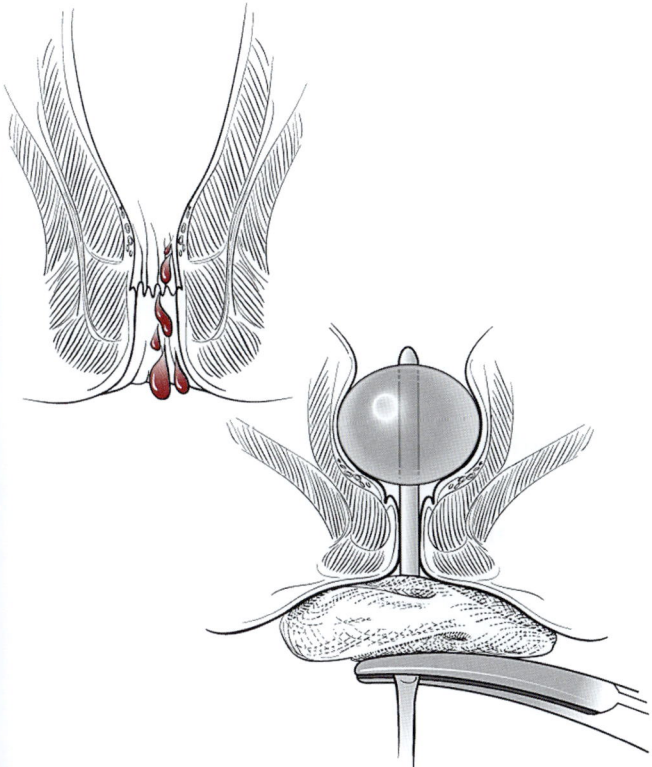

Figure 5–1. Balloon tamponade of the anal canal.

Indication

Massive hemorrhage (postsurgical, spontaneous hemorrhoidal, or Dieulafoy hemorrhage).

Preparatory Considerations

None.

Surgical Steps

1. Patient positioning: any position.
2. Insertion of largest available Foley catheter into anal canal.
3. Insufflation of balloon with 60 mL of water/saline.
4. External traction on catheter to allow balloon to exert pressure on anal canal.
5. Placement of external pad pack (gauze, towels) around catheter (external counter pressure).
6. Placement of hemostat clamp to catheter (under tension) at level of external packing.

Anatomic Structures at Risk

Anal canal.

Aftercare

Hemodynamic stabilization, monitoring.

Antibiotic coverage as long as balloon in place.

Maximal length of tamponade: 24 hours.

Plan for definitive surgical care.

Complications

Continued bleeding, anal canal necrosis, infection.

Cross-reference

Topic	*Chapter*
Bleeding per rectum	1 (p 4)
Liability in colorectal surgery	2 (p 56)
Clinical examination	2 (p 61)
Complications—delayed wound healing	4 (p 470)
Hemorrhoid procedures	5 (pp 506–512)
Perioperative management—anorectal	7 (p 688)
Comorbidities—liver disease	7 (p 696)

INCISION/DRAINAGE OF PERIRECTAL ABSCESS *(SIMPLE)*

Principle

Decompression of perirectal abscess to allow resolution of acute inflammation and pressure (pain!). Management of fistula only of secondary priority: if I&D is performed under general anesthesia, excision of the cryptoglandular origin and definitive fistula procedure may be reasonable, but there is increased risk of creating tracts that are not truly there (inflamed tissue).

Setting

Outpatient, office (or inpatient, bedside/OR procedure in selected cases).

Alternatives

Nonoperative management: generally not indicated except if abscess spontaneously perforated.

Modified Hanley procedure for horseshoe abscess.

Indication

Every perirectal abscess.

Preparatory Considerations

Clinical assessment, ie, pain and local inflammatory signs; do not wait for fluctuance in perirectal area. Neither WBC nor imaging studies are needed (except in very unusual circumstances).

In all patients receiving general anesthesia: at least rigid sigmoidoscopy.

Surgical Steps

1. Patient positioning: any position, but prone jackknife position has several advantages—access to all perianal compartments (including deep postanal space), superior view with comfortable access for surgeon/assistant, decreased congestion of the hemorrhoidal plexus.

2. Disinfection.

3. Unless general anesthesia: local anesthesia of the skin over the maximal swelling.

4. Identification of drainage site: maximum swelling/erythema/tenderness, but as close to the anal verge as possible (to keep possible fistula tract short).

5. Bovie available → excision of a skin disk; no Bovie available → cruciate incision of the skin with scalpel and excision of each corner. Pus has to flow, otherwise the correct site or level has not been reached.

6. Loculations: digital breaking is not indicated in an awake patient; but if under anesthesia provide active debridement and adequate drainage (possible counter-incisions and drain placement if large cavity is found).

7. Search for fistula: not indicated in an awake patient; if under anesthesia → gentle assessment (but avoid creating false tracts in altered tissue!): if positive → excision of cryptoglandular lesion and placement of seton (eg, vessel loop).

8. Hemostasis.

9. Loose insertion of iodoform gauze is acceptable but no major packing is needed.

10. Absorbing dressing.

Anatomic Structures at Risk

Anal sphincter muscle.

Aftercare

Antibiotics: Simple abscess in healthy patient—no; abscess with significant phlegmon—yes; abscess in immunosuppressed/diabetic patient—yes; signs of sepsis—yes (inpatient).

Open wound care: sitz baths or showers twice per day, after bowel movements.

Assessment of whether persistent fistula is present after 3–6 weeks. If absess was a recurrent one, fistula has to be postulated.

Complications

Bleeding, urinary retention (sign of sepsis?), progressive infection, pelvic/perineal sepsis, persistence of perirectal fistula (requiring subsequent surgery): ~50%.

Cross-reference

Topic	Chapter
Pain, perirectal	1 (p 38)
Perianal/-rectal abscess	4 (p 174)
Pilonidal disease	4 (p 182)
Modified Hanley procedure	5 (p 479)
Fistula surgery	5 (pp 483–488)
Perioperative management—anorectal	7 (p 688)

MODIFIED HANLEY PROCEDURE FOR HORSESHOE FISTULA/ABSCESS

Principle

Decompression and drainage of ischioanal fossae and deep postanal space of Courtney with excision of primary cryptoglandular origin and placement of drains/setons to allow resolution of acute inflammation and pressure (pain!): Figure 5–2. As these deep perirectal abscesses usually require general anesthesia, management of the fistula/primary fistula opening generally is indicated.

Setting

Outpatient or inpatient, OR, general anesthesia.

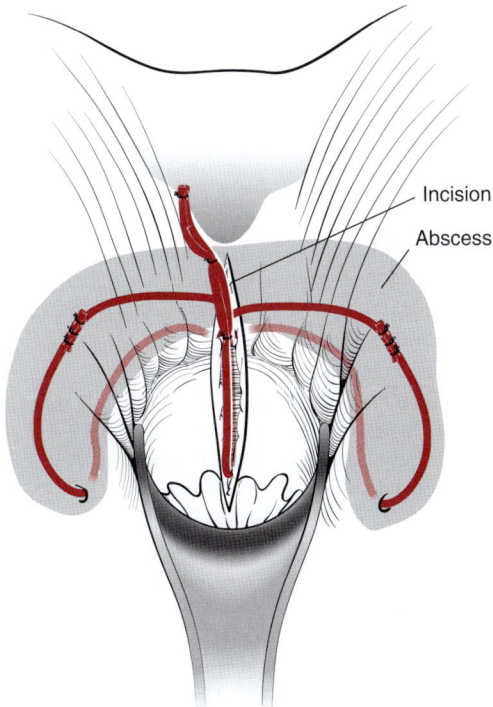

Figure 5–2. Modified Hanley procedure with two lateral draining and one midline cutting seton.

Alternatives

Nonoperative management: generally not indicated except if abscess spontaneously perforated.

Simple I&D for perirectal abscess(es): elective management.

Endorectal advancement flap.

Collagen plug for perirectal fistula.

Indication

Horseshoe abscess or fistula.

Preparatory Considerations

Clinical assessment: bilateral abscesses or fistula openings, primary commonly in posterior midline, invisible abscess but indurated/tender postanal space. Neither WBC nor imaging studies are needed (except in very unusual circumstances).

In all patients, at least rigid sigmoidoscopy once under anesthesia (emergency); in elective cases, prior colonic evaluation per guidelines.

Surgical Steps

1. Patient positioning: prone jackknife position.

2. In absence of previous colonic evaluation: at least rigid or flexible sigmoidoscopy.

3. For elective cases: pudendal/perianal nerve block with 15–20 cc of a local anesthetic in addition to general anesthesia to improve relaxation of anal sphincter muscles.

4. Midline incision of skin and mucosa extending from tip of coccyx to primary fistula opening in posterior midline at dentate line. Careful division of underlying connective tissue, just until muscle fibers become visible. Excision of primary crypt at dentate line.

5. Starting at tip of coccyx, dissection is carried deeper, ie, through anococcygeal ligament. Sphincter complex is pushed anteriorly and should not be divided.

6. Access to deep postanal space of Courtney: identification by anatomic location, presence of abscess (acute) or granulation tissue (chronic), guidance from probe through primary opening.

7. From deep postanal space, blunt lateral dissection toward both ischioanal fossae. Extension to anterior end of the acute inflammation/induration or to the preexisting fistula openings.

8. Secondary incisions (abscess) or excision/widening of secondary fistula openings. Debridement of abscess cavities or fistula tracts with curette or gauze.

9. Primary opening: insertion of vessel loop (as cutting seton) from primary opening to postanal space/posterior incision. Placement of three large silk ties to the loop such that it sits tight on the muscle but without tension. Approximation of muscle and mucosal layer around seton, particularly if primary opening is significantly larger than the loop.

10. Secondary openings: placement of Penrose drains (acute abscess) or also vessel loops (chronic fistula) from postanal space to secondary opening(s). Securing of individual loops with three large silk ties.

11. Hemostasis.

12. Absorbing dressing.

Anatomic Structures at Risk

Anal sphincter complex, rectum.

Aftercare

Antibiotics: abscess/fistula in healthy patient—no; abscess with significant phlegmon—yes; abscess/fistula in immunosuppressed/diabetic patient—yes; signs of sepsis—yes (inpatient).

Open wound care: sitz baths or showers twice per day, after bowel movements.

Removal of lateral drains in clinic after 2–4 weeks, possible prior downsizing before complete removal.

Once lateral drains are gone: tightening of cutting seton in monthly intervals.

Complications

Bleeding, urinary retention (sign of sepsis?), recurrent/progressing infection, pelvic/perineal sepsis, persistence of perirectal fistula (requiring subsequent surgery).

Recurrent/persistent fistula (10–15%). Fecal incontinence: anal disconfiguration, sphincter weakness.

Cross-reference

Operative Techniques

FISTULA-IN-ANO—FISTULOTOMY VS SETON

Principle

Fistulotomy (lay-open technique) for very superficial fistula with minimal resulting damage to sphincter muscle. Alternatively, placement of setons into the existing fistula tracts to allow for adequate drainage of active suppurations. Two different types of setons:

- Cutting seton: placed around sphincter portion involved in a transsphincteric fistula with intent to have the seton slowly erode through that sphincter portion (Figure 5–3).
- Draining seton (single, multiple, short-term/long-term): placed into existing fistula tract solely to avoid future pus accumulation and allow tract to close down onto seton. A draining seton may also be placed in preparation for future fistula procedures, eg, collagen plug placement.

Setting

Outpatient, OR, general anesthesia.

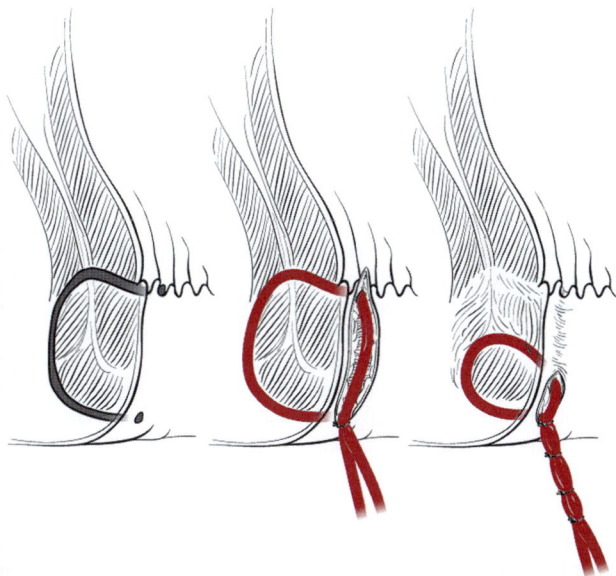

Figure 5–3. Seton management of transsphincteric fistula.

Operative Techniques

Alternatives

Nonoperative management: generally not indicated if fistula is symptomatic.

Fistulotomy/fistulectomy.

Endorectal advancement flap.

Collagen plug for perirectal fistula, fibrin glue injection.

Modified Hanley procedure.

Indication

Fistula-in-ano.

Preparatory Considerations

Clinical assessment: identification of secondary (external) opening, potentially of primary opening; presence of bilateral fistula openings or scars: horseshoe fistula; identification helpers—probing, peroxide injection, imaging (ERUS, MRI, etc).

Elective cases: partial/full colonic evaluation per guidelines.

Surgical Steps

1. Patient positioning: prone jackknife position.

2. For elective cases: pudendal/perianal nerve block with 15–20 cc of local anesthetic in addition to general anesthesia to improve relaxation of the anal sphincter muscles.

3. Insertion of anal retractor and circumferential examination of dentate line: identification of primary opening? If not visible: testing with injection of peroxide into secondary opening (avoid overflow spill) → appearance of bubbling at a primary opening?

4. Careful probing of fistula tract with curved silver probe taking care to avoid creating new tract by forceful advancement. If insertion is not easy: placement of Kocher clamp to external opening and centrifugal traction (ie, away from anus) to straighten fistula tract while trying to insert probe again. If still no success: partial external fistulotomy to reassess course vs fistuloscopy (using ureteroscope). If primary opening cannot be found despite all attempts: removal or wide drainage of sinus, but unfortunately high chance of failure and reopening of a fistula later.

5. Fistula tract successfully probed → assessment of the extent of sphincter involvement:

   a. Fistulotomy: very superficial tract without relevant sphincter involvement (< 20%) → fistulotomy from secondary to primary opening along the probe (eg, with electrocautery).

b. Cutting seton: > 20% sphincter involved → cutting seton: devision of mucocutaneous layer between two openings without cutting through muscle (caveat: no cutting seton over intact skin), pulling in a suture tied to edge of gauze, scrubbing out fistula tract (with gauze or brush) → pulling in seton (eg, an elastic vessel loop), which is tied down with three sutures such that it just sits on the muscle without strangulating it.

c. Draining seton: > 20% sphincter involved but seton placement only to cool off suppuration, prevent recurrent abscesses (eg, long-term setons in Crohn disease), or mature fistula without immediate plan to eliminate fistula (but, eg, later fistula surgery with collagen plug): seton pulled into tract and tied to itself without division of mucocutaneous layer between primary and secondary opening.

6. Hemostasis.

7. No dressing needed.

Anatomic Structures at Risk

Anal sphincter complex, anal configuration (→ risk of keyhole deformity).

Aftercare

Open wound care until complete healing (fistulotomy), skin closure except for seton (cutting/draining seton): sitz baths or showers twice per day, after bowel movements.

Cutting seton: tightening of cutting seton in monthly intervals until it has eroded through the involved sphincter complex (leaving a scar behind): (Figure 5–3).

Complications

Bleeding, urinary retention (sign of sepsis?), recurrent infection, pelvic/perineal sepsis, recurrent/persistent fistula (10–15%). Fecal incontinence (benchmark < 5%): anal disconfiguration, sphincter weakness.

Cross-reference

Operative Techniques

FISTULA-IN-ANO—ENDORECTAL ADVANCEMENT FLAP

Principle

Closure of the primary fistula opening by means of a plication of the muscle layer and an overlying advancement flap to cover the site of the opening to induce an obliteration of the fistula tract once it is not fed anymore.

Setting

Outpatient, OR, general anesthesia.

Alternatives

Nonoperative management: generally not indicated if fistula is symptomatic.

Fistulotomy/fistulectomy.

Seton management.

Collagen plug for perirectal fistula, fibrin glue injection.

Modified Hanley procedure.

Indication

Fistula-in-ano.

Preparatory Considerations

Clinical assessment: identification of secondary (external) opening, potentially primary opening; bilateral fistula openings or scars suggestive of horseshoe fistula; identification helpers—probing, peroxide injection imaging (ERUS, MRI, etc).

Elective cases: partial/full colonic evaluation per guidelines.

Surgical Steps

1. Patient positioning: prone jackknife position.
2. For elective cases: pudendal/perianal nerve block with 15–20 cc of a local anesthetic in addition to general anesthesia to improve relaxation of anal sphincter muscles.
3. Insertion of anal retractor and identification of primary opening.
4. Careful probing of fistula tract with silver probe.
5. Insertion of anal retractor and reassessment of the fistula. Depending on local anatomy, placement of Lone Star retractor may prove advantageous.
6. Limited excision of primary opening, removal of epithelialized tract within muscle layer, widening/excision of secondary opening.

7. Closure of muscular defect with interrupted Vicryl sutures.

8. Marking of U-shaped broad-based flap, base starting distal to primary fistula opening, extending laterally and proximally (one quarter to one-third of anterior circumference). Atraumatic raising of flap: after adequate mobilization, flap should cover defect without any tension. Careful hemostasis; avoid traction or diffuse cautery damage to flap.

9. Suturing flap in place in two layers: deeper muscular layer (Vicryl), maturation of mucosal anastomosis with interrupted sutures (eg chromic).

Anatomic Structures at Risk

Anal sphincter complex, anal configuration (keyhole deformity).

Aftercare

Open wound care until complete healing of secondary opening: sitz baths or showers twice per day, after bowel movements.

Complications

Bleeding, urinary retention (sign of sepsis?), recurrent infection, pelvic/perineal sepsis, recurrent/persistent fistula (20–30%), creation of an ectropion, fecal incontinence.

Cross-reference

Operative Techniques

FISTULA-IN-ANO—INSERTION OF COLLAGEN PLUG

Principle

Obliteration of the fistula tract by inserting and suturing in place a manufactured collagen plug through the primary fistula opening in the rectum. More durable than the fibrin glue injection, long-term data on this new method are pending.

Setting

Outpatient, OR, general anesthesia.

Alternatives

Nonoperative management: generally not indicated if fistula is symptomatic.

Fistulotomy/fistulectomy.

Seton management.

Fibrin glue injection.

Endorectal advancement flap.

Modified Hanley procedure.

Indication

• Transsphincteric fistula-in-ano.

• Not indicated: very superficial tract, very short tract, very large diameter tract, active suppuration.

Preparatory Considerations

Clinical assessment: identification of secondary (external) opening, potentially primary opening; bilateral fistula openings and scars suggestive of horseshoe fistula; identification helpers—probing, peroxide injection, imaging (ERUS, MRI, etc).

Elective cases: partial/full colonic evaluation per guidelines.

Surgical Steps

1. Patient positioning: prone jackknife position.
2. Disinfection.
3. For elective cases: pudendal/perianal nerve block with 15–20 cc of a local anesthetic in addition to general anesthesia to improve relaxation of anal sphincter muscles.
4. Insertion of anal retractor and identification of primary opening.

5. Careful probing of fistula tract with silver probe.

6. Limited excision/enlargement of secondary opening to facilitate drainage.

7. Irrigation of tract with peroxide, otherwise no debridement or curettage.

8. If internal opening is recessed: limited mobilization of mucosal edge.

9. Rehydration of collagen plug for 2 minutes in antibiotic solution.

10. Insertion of silver probe through secondary opening and pulling in a suture that is tied to end of rehydrated collagen plug.

11. Pulling in plug from primary toward secondary opening until plug sits snugly.

12. Transmuscular absorbable fixation suture to fix plug at primary opening, trimming of excess plug.

13. Trimming of excess plug at secondary opening flush at skin level, no plug fixation.

Anatomic Structures at Risk

Anal sphincter complex.

Aftercare

Open wound care until complete healing of secondary opening: sitz baths or showers twice per day, after bowel movements.

Avoidance of strenuous activity, exercise, heavy lifting, intercourse for 2 weeks.

Avoidance of constipation or diarrhea.

Complications

Bleeding, urinary retention (sign of sepsis?), loss of the collagen plug, infection, pelvic/perineal sepsis, recurrent/persistent fistula (25–50%).

Cross-reference

Operative Techniques

EXCISION OF PILONIDAL CYST

Principle

Elective excision of the pilonidal cyst and its associate fistulous tracts and pits. Multiple approaches are described with varying degrees of radicality, primarily open (Figure 5–4) vs primarily closed techniques.

Setting

Outpatient, OR procedure.

Alternatives

Nonoperative expectant approach: quiescent disease, < 2 episodes.

I&D for acute flare-up with abscess.

Flap procedures.

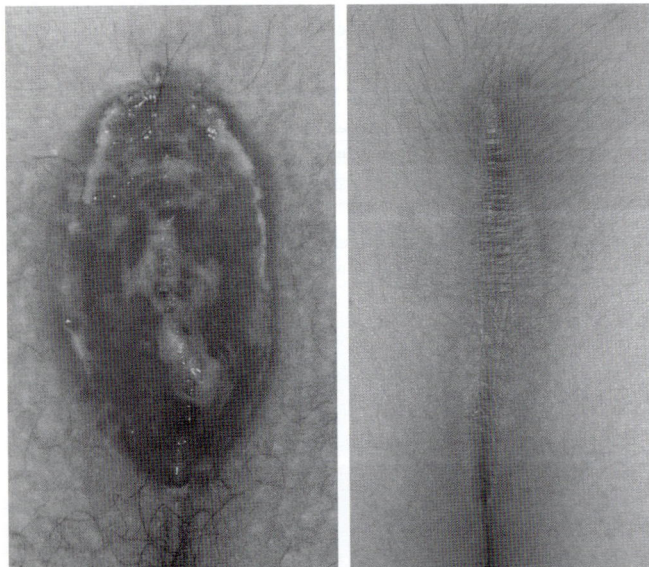

Figure 5–4. Primarily open excision of pilonidal cyst.

Indication

- History of recurrent acute pilonidal disease ($\geq$ 2 episodes).
- Chronic pilonidal sinus/fistula.
- Cancer ($\rightarrow$ combined-modality treatment).

Preparatory Considerations

None except digital rectal exam.

Surgical Steps

1. Patient positioning: prone jackknife or prone position, lateral taping of buttocks is not indicated.

(A) Primarily open technique

2. Marking of symmetric elliptical skin incision, which incorporates all openings. Avoid proximity to anus (sphincter injury!).

3. Incision of skin.

4. Extirpation of whole specimen in such a way that a flat funnel-shaped wound results without undermining of wound edges.

5. Marsupialization of wound edges is possible, but not needed if shape of wound is as required (see above).

6. Hemostasis.

7. Petroleum jelly gauze and absorbing dressing, no packing needed.

(B) Closed technique with lateral approach

2. Curved lateral incision, potentially with incorporation of eccentric secondary fistula opening.

3. Undermining of subcutaneous tissue toward midline.

4. Debridement of cyst and fistula tracts: it is not necessary to remove all indurated parts, just fistula as such.

5. Excision of midline pits (eg, using punch biopsy).

6. Debridement of fistulous tracts.

7. Hemostasis.

8. Closure of lateral incision and midline wounds with absorbable suture.

(C) Closed technique with midline approach

2. Marking of symmetric elliptical skin incision, which incorporates all openings. Avoid proximity to anus (sphincter injury!)

3. Incision of skin.

Operative Techniques

4. Extirpation of whole specimen in such a way that a flat funnel-shaped wound results without undermining of wound edges.

5. Hemostasis.

6. Laying of 3–4 strong retention sutures from lateral, through the fascia at bottom of wound, to other side.

7. Closure of wound in midline with interrupted sutures.

8. Compression roll of a few gauzes over which lateral retention sutures are tied.

Anatomic Structures at Risk

Anal sphincter complex (at caudad end).

Aftercare

(A) Primarily open excision
No limit to physical activity. Daily showers/sitz baths, scrubbing of wound with cloth, removal of hair around wound (hair removal cream or razor).

(B) Closed technique with lateral approach
Limited physical activity for 2–3 weeks.

(C) Closed technique with midline approach
Strict limitation of physical activity for 2–3 weeks. Removal of compression roll after 7–10 days. Removal of stitches after 3 weeks.

Complications

Bleeding, infection, dehiscence (of closed wounds), recurrent fistula/sinus formation, delayed wound healing.

Cross-reference

Topic	Chapter
Pilonidal disease	4 (p 182)
Perioperative management—anorectal	7 (p 688)

EXCISION/FULGURATION OF ANAL WARTS

Principle

Surgical removal and/or destruction of anogenital condylomata. Electro-cautery and laser are equally effective in terms of recovery time, pain, and scar formation, but laser is more expensive and associated with higher recurrence rate. Relatively limited number of warts can be treated with local anesthesia in the office; a larger extent requires systemic or regional anesthesia.

Setting

Outpatient, office or OR.

Alternatives

Nonoperative management: small extent, accessible (ie, typically external).

Wide excision with flap reconstruction: almost never primarily indicated, even in presence of confluent warts.

Laser destruction: more expensive equipment, no perioperative advantage, higher recurrence rates.

Indication

- Larger extent and/or number of external condylomata.
- Internal condylomata.
- Treatment-refractoriness with nonsurgical management.

Preparatory Considerations

Clinical assessment of all possible sites.

HIV status.

Rigid or flexible sigmoidoscopy to rule out concomitant STDs; full colonic evaluation per guidelines.

Surgical Steps

1. Patient positioning: any position (prone jackknife, lithotomy, lateral) that allows access to affected sites, intraoperative change of position may be necessary.
2. Disinfection.
3. Safety precautions: small-pore surgical masks, suction-equipped electrocautery to minimize anecdotally reported hazard of HPV transmission to surgeon's upper airways.

Operative Techniques

4. Even if general anesthesia: preemptive injection of long-lasting local anesthetic.

5. Insertion of anal retractor, assessment of internal involvement.

6. Excision: careful grasping of individual warts with forceps and excision at their base with scissors or needle-tip Bovie. Process all removed tissues for pathology. Even primarily large and confluent-appearing warts often have multiple individual stalks and healthy skin areas may be preserved in between (Figures 5–5A and 5–5B).

7. Fulguration with needle-tip Bovie: cauterization of smaller and flat warts, scratching off eschar, followed by repeat treatment.

8. If fistula present, tract often colonized by condylomata → appropriate fistula treatment in conjunction with complete wart removal.

9. Verification that all foci eliminated (internal and external).

10. Hemostasis.

11. Injection of 5 million units of interferon alfa (suspended in 5 mL of saline) diffusely into anoderm.

12. No dressing needed.

Anatomic Structures at Risk

Anal sphincter muscle. Anoderm → risk of stenosis.

Aftercare

Open wound care: sitz baths or showers twice per day and after bowel movements.

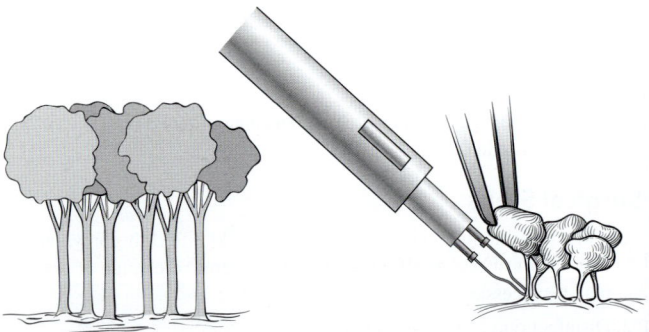

A

Figure 5–5A. Excision of confluent-appearing warts (separate stems as in a forest).

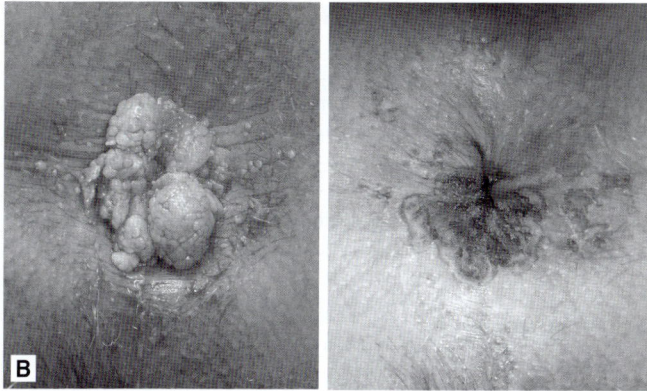

Figure 5–5B. Excision/fulguration of warts.

Operative Techniques

Review of pathology: 10–20% incidence of carcinoma in situ → watchful waiting vs rebiopsy; rarely invasive cancer → wider reexcision vs other treatment modalities.

Follow-up in clinic every 3–6 weeks, every 3 months after wound healing.

Complications

Bleeding, infection (rare), delayed wound healing, recurrent wart formation (30–50%), incontinence to stool/gas, anal stenosis. Dyspigmentation.

Cross-reference

Topic	Chapter
HIV-associated anorectal diseases	4 (p 206)
STDs	4 (p 210)
Anal condylomata	4 (p 215)
AIN	4 (p 220)
Buschke-Lowenstein giant condylomata	4 (p 228)
Anal cancer	4 (p 230)
Perioperative management—anorectal	7 (p 688)

LATERAL INTERNAL SPHINCTEROTOMY *(LIS)*

Principle

Radial incision of internal sphincter muscle (open or closed technique) to achieve reliable reduction of the resting anal sphincter tone. LIS is the most successful of all treatment options for chronic anal fissures, but carries a risk of incontinence.

Sphincterotomy may be combined with excision of sentinel skin tag (external end of fissure) and/or hypertrophic anal papilla (internal end of fissure), or formal fissurectomy.

Setting

Outpatient, OR or office procedure.

Alternatives

Conservative management: stool management, topical nitroglycerin/calcium antagonist.

Botulinum toxin A injection.

Fissurectomy with/without midline sphincterotomy.

Fissurectomy with injection of Botulinum toxin A.

Fissurectomy with anal advancement flap.

Indication

Chronic anal fissure.

Contraindication: preexisting fecal incontinence. Caveat: careful decision for patients with underlying diarrhea (higher probability of fecal incontinence).

Preparatory Considerations

Trial of nonsurgical management unless incapacitating symptoms.

In elective cases, colonic evaluation per guidelines (before or with procedure).

Administration of 2 enemas before operation. Single shot IV antibiotic prophylaxis. Disinfection of rectum with povidone-iodine solution.

Surgical Steps

1. Patient positioning: any position, but prone jackknife position with buttocks taped aside has several advantages—superior view with comfortable access for surgeon/assistant, decreased congestion of hemorrhoidal plexus.

2. Pudendal/perianal nerve block with 15–20 cc of a local anesthetic alone (office sphincterotomy), or in addition to general anesthesia to improve relaxation of the anal sphincter muscles.

3. Visualization and assessment of fissure (posterior or anterior midline): bare sphincter muscle fibers, signs of chronicity, eg, deep central aspect, elevated wound edges, formation of a sentinel skin tag, hypertrophic anal papillae.

(A) Open technique

4. Right lateral radial incision (ie, in between hemorrhoidal piles) from the anal verge, 1–1.5 cm in length, division of connective tissue overlaying the sphincter complex.

5. Identification of internal anal sphincter clearly (white fibers, internal to intersphincteric groove).

6. Loading of IAS fibers onto clamp, division of fibers with electrocautery between clamp's branches, slowly to avoid bleeding.

7. Proximal extent of sphincterotomy should not exceed level of proximal end of fissure in anal canal.

8. Careful hemostasis

9. Wound irrigation and closure with running 2-0 chromic suture.

(B) Closed technique

4. Identification of intersphincteric groove at right lateral quadrant (ie, in between hemorrhoidal piles).

5. Tangential insertion of Beaver-blade knife into intersphincteric groove.

6. Once inserted, the knife is turned 90 degrees to the inside.

7. Division of internal sphincter (blind or guided by digital exam). Avoid mucosal injury (risk of fistula).

8. Massaging of divided sphincter should reveal a submucosal gap.

9. Closure of the lancing site.

Both techniques—possible combination with fissurectomy or skin tag excision

10. Readjusting of anal retractor to fissure site.

11. Radial excision of fissure or fissure edges with inclusion of external sentinel skin tag.

12. Lateral mobilization of mucosa to allow sufficient mobility.

13. Closure of inside up to anal verge with running 2-0 chromic suture, making sure to achieve good hemostasis.

14. The most external part of the wound is left open for possible drainage.

Operative Techniques

Anatomic Structures at Risk

External anal sphincter, hemorrhoidal plexus.

Aftercare

Stool softeners, fibers, pain medication, sitz baths.

Complications

Bleeding, urinary retention, infection, pelvic/perineal sepsis, delayed wound healing, persistent fissure, incontinence to stool/gas: 5(–15)%.

Cross-reference

Topic	*Chapter*
Pain, perirectal	1 (p 38)
Anal fissure	4 (p 161)
Anorectal flaps	5 (p 516)
Perioperative management—anorectal	7 (p 688)

OVERLAPPING SPHINCTEROPLASTY

Principle

Repair of a sphincter defect in a patient with symptoms of fecal incontinence and sphincter defect identified clinically or ERUS (Figure 5–6A). Depending on the size of the defect, closing the muscle circle is necessary to allow translation of axial muscle contraction into a centripetal narrowing force to the anal canal. Scar tissue at the muscle ends should not be excised as it is the better tissue for holding the repair stitches than the actual muscle itself. Important not only to recreate the muscle ring but to also reconstitute the length of the high-pressure zone. No advantage to separate suturing of IAS and EAS.

Setting

Inpatient (possible outpatient in selected cases), OR procedure.

Alternatives

Conservative management: elimination of other incontinence-triggering factors if possible; stool management, fibers, antidiarrheals, scheduled enemas, physical therapy.

Colostomy, Malone antegrade colonic enema (MACE), gracioplasty, ABS, sacral nerve stimulation.

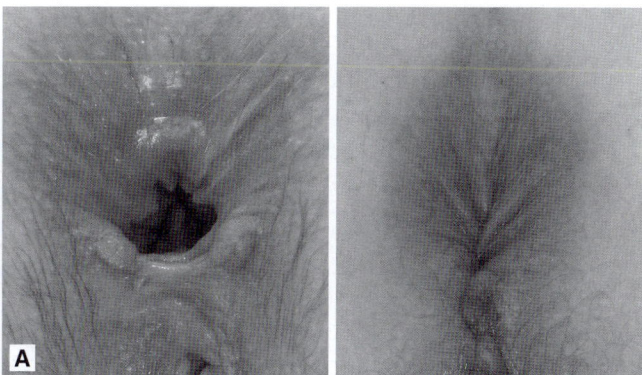

Figure 5–6A. Overlapping sphincteroplasty: preoperatively patulous, postoperatively closed.

Acute sphincter injury: direct repair with end-to-end approximation without overlap.

Indication

Fecal incontinence and identified sphincter defect. Impact of pudendal neuropathy controversial.

Preparatory Considerations

Colonic evaluation per guidelines, as well as in patients with altered stool quality (with biopsies).

Anophysiology studies for objective preoperative assessment.

Administration of full bowel cleansing vs two enemas only before operation. IV antibiotic prophylaxis, continued postoperatively for 3–5 days. Disinfection of rectum with povidone-iodine solution.

Surgical Steps

1. Patient positioning: any position, but prone jackknife position with buttocks taped aside has several advantages: superior view with comfortable access for surgeon/assistant, decreased congestion of hemorrhoidal plexus.

2. Pudendal/perianal nerve block with 15–20 cc of local anesthetic in addition to general anesthesia to improve relaxation of anal sphincter muscles.

3. Careful examination of area including anoscopy and vaginal palpation to rule out preexisting/hidden rectovaginal fistula.

4. Transverse incision to perineum (as anterior as possible).

5. Dissection of rectovaginal septum to level of puborectalis muscle. Injury to rectum and/or vagina must be avoided.

6. Ends of sphincter muscle are identified on both sides and mobilized as much as necessary, as little as possible. Too lateral dissection should be avoided to limit pudendal denervation: bleeding may indicate proximity to pudendal nerve branches. Residual muscle contractility can be checked by direct muscular stimulation with cautery.

7. Overlap repair using three interrupted 2-0 Vicryl sutures that are first prelaid (Figure 5–6B), then consecutively tied such that one sphincter end moves in front of the other. Free overlapping edge of anterior sphincter end is approximated to rest of reconstructed circle with a running 2-0 Vicryl suture. Possible reapproximation of puborectalis muscles with interrupted sutures toward center.

8. Irrigation of wound with diluted povidone-iodine (1:10). Hemostasis.

9. Repair should result in a concentric appearance of anus with radial folding all the way around. After overlap, digital rectal exam must be avoided: anus is never (!) too tight.

10. Closure of wound in a transverse direction: a few interrupted Vicryl stitches for adaptation of subcuticular tissue and 4-0 Monocryl to close off skin. Alternatively: sagittal closure of transverse incision to rebuild some perineal body.

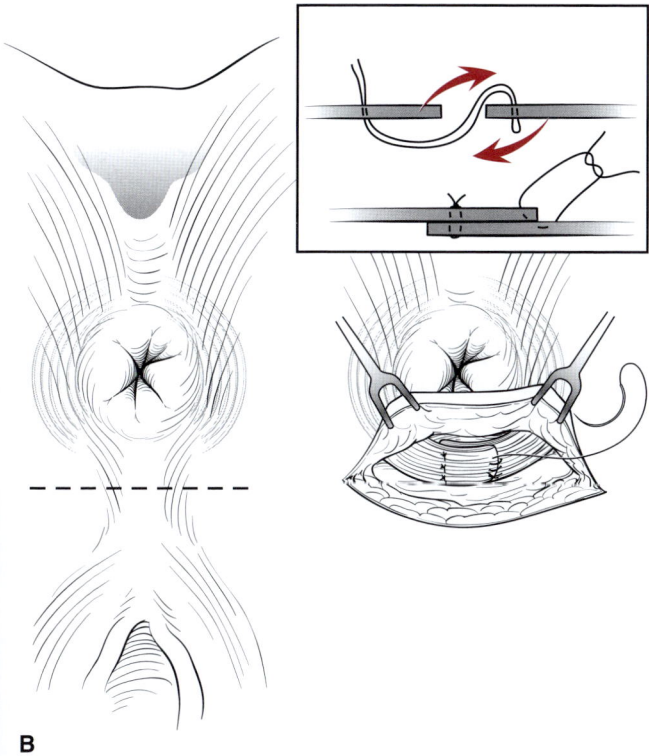

B

Figure 5–6B. Overlapping sphincteroplasty: direction of sutures to achieve nice overlap.

Anatomic Structures at Risk

Pudendal neurovascular bundle, sphincter muscle.

Aftercare

Stool softeners, fibers, pain medication, potentially mild laxative. After bowel movement: wiping to be avoided, rather rinsing, short sitz baths. Area to be kept dry, unless managed with open wound care.

After 6 weeks, consider supportive physical therapy.

Complications

Bleeding, urinary retention, infection, pelvic/perineal sepsis, formation of rectovaginal fistula, delayed wound healing, inability to provide improvement of fecal control or recurrent fecal incontinence, need for colostomy.

Cross-reference

IMPLANTATION OF THE ARTIFICIAL BOWEL SPHINCTER *(ABS)*

Principle

Implantation of an ABS device is a possible option for patients with treatment-refractory incontinence in whom the sphincter muscle cannot be repaired or otherwise optimized. It is the only truly dynamic functional solution allowing a patient to decide when or when not to move the bowels. Successful implantation is associated with a dramatic improvement in quality of life.

Challenge: risk of infection or device erosion (acute, chronic) which originally resulted in a nearly 40% explantation rate, but increasing experience, standardization of the technique, and antibiotic prophylaxis have reduced the risk to < 10%.

Setting

Inpatient, OR procedure.

Alternatives

Continuation of conservative treatment.

Sphincter repair: repeat sphincteroplasty.

Sphincter replacement: graciloplasty.

Neuromodulation: sacral nerve stimulation.

Reduction of stool load: irrigational stoma (eg, appendicostomy) for Malone antegrade colonic enema (MACE).

Diversion: colostomy.

Indication

Treatment-refractory incontinence with sufficient tissue quality and perianal space to take and embed device.

Absolute contraindications: any active inflammation, any open wound, lack of sufficient tissue (eg, rectovaginal septum), poor tissue quality (eg, very rigid and indurated tissue).

Relative contraindications: history of radiation therapy.

Preparatory Considerations

Colonic evaluation per guidelines.

Complete bowel cleansing.

Discussion of better side for valve implantation: typically opposite to patient's dominant hand.

Triple antibiotic prophylaxis: vancomycin, levofloxacin or cefoxitin, metronidazole.

Disinfection of vagina and rectum with povidone-iodine solution.

Sterile in-and-out bladder catheterization at beginning of case.

Surgical Steps

1. Back table preparation: sterile filling of system components with normal saline, complete removal of air bubbles → placement of device in antibiotic solution until implantation.
2. Patient positioning: modified lithotomy. Meticulous prepping and draping.

(A) Cuff implantation

3. Insertion of povidone-iodine–soaked vaginal pack into rectum.
4. Perianal incision: preferably two small anterolateral incisions (alternatively: one anterior transverse incision; bilateral vertical incisions).
5. Nontraumatic careful dissection around anal canal: damage to rectum or vagina to be avoided.
6. Cuff sizer for measurement of approximate circumference and length of anal canal.
7. Cuff placement: using large curved clamp, air-free cuff is inserted around anal canal with pillow facing toward canal: start at incision on side of planned valve implantation → posterior hemicircumference → anterior hemicircumference → locking cuff by threading tubing through adapter hole and pulling adapter hole over cuff button.
8. Connect tubing with tunneling instrument and pass along inguinal fold to suprapubic incision.
9. Subcutaneous sutures (avoid damage to cuff), subcuticular skin closure, skin glue.
10. Removal of anal pack.

(B) Balloon implantation

11. Suprapubic incision, transverse division of rectus fascia, separation at linea alba to access and free up prevesical space using blunt dissection.
12. Placement of prepared balloon in prevesical space and filling with 55 mL of recommended filling solution (saline).

(C) Cuff pressurization

13. Temporary connection of cuff and balloon tubing using a straight connector.
14. Removal of tubing clamps → wait 60 seconds for cuff to pressurize.

15. Reclamp tubing to the cuff and the balloon with silicone-shod mosquito clamps, followed by aspiration of all remaining fluid from balloon: → calculation of volume in cuff and tubing.

16. Refill balloon with 40 mL of filling solution and reclamp tubing.

(D) Implantation of control pump

17. Use of Hegar dilators to create a dependent pocket in soft tissue of labium or subdartos pouch of scrotum (opposite to patient's dominant hand).

18. Place pump in the pouch with deactivation button facing outward such that it is easily palpable.

19. Connection of all components.

20. Closure of suprapubic incision.

Anatomic Structures at Risk

Rectovaginal septum, vagina, anal canal.

Aftercare

Antibiotics per prophylaxis protocol.

Stool regularity, avoidance of fecal impaction. No need for sitz baths, but rinsing off of stool smearing. Preemptive skin care.

Avoidance of (longer) sitting, intercourse, digital rectal exam.

Depending on intraoperative tissue quality, device remains in deactivated state (ie, empty cuff) for 6–12 weeks to allow complete resolution of operative edema and formation of fibrotic capsule.

Complications

Infection, device erosion with external or rectovaginal perforation and fistula formation → need to remove device, risk to need temporary colostomy.

Perianal skin maceration while deactivated.

After activation: high incidence of constipation until patient become used to new management.

Cross-reference

Operative Techniques

HEMORRHOID OFFICE PROCEDURES
(BANDING, SCLEROSING, INFRARED COAGULATION)

Principle

Local office treatment to achieve shrinkage of engorged hemorrhoidal piles (right anterior and posterior, left lateral) tissue.

Setting

Outpatient, office procedure.

Alternatives

Excisional or stapled hemorrhoidectomy PPH.

Whitehead hemorrhoidectomy.

Conservative management.

Indication

Symptomatic internal hemorrhoids grades I, II and III. Caution: ASA medication, anticoagulation, immunosuppression.

Preparatory Considerations

In elective cases, prior colonic evaluation per guidelines.

Administration of enemas if rectum is full of stool. Single shot antibiotic prophylaxis in high-risk patients.

Surgical Steps

1. Patient positioning: any position, but prone jackknife position with best view and access.
2. Insertion of oblique-angle anoscope and consecutive exposure of hemorrhoidal piles.

(A) Banding

3. Verification of dentate line.
4. Positioning of loaded hemorrhoid ligator at proximal base (apex) of hemorrhoid.
5. Application of suction, traction (depending on device).
6. Firing of gun while suction/traction is maintained.
7. Verification of correct rubber band position proximal to dentate line.
8. Repeat procedure for remaining hemorrhoidal piles: simultaneous banding of three piles is acceptable.

9. Patient observation for 15–30 minutes: if development of pain → rubber band removal with hook-blade.

(B) Sclerosing

3. Verification of dentate line.

4. Syringe filled with sclerosing agent: 5% ethanolamine oleate, 1% ethoxysclerol, 5% phenol in oil, etc.

5. 25 G spinal needle (length factor!).

6. Submucosal injection of 1–2 cc into each hemorrhoid (caveat: intramucosal or deep injection may result in ulceration/sloughing).

7. Repeat procedure for remaining hemorrhoidal piles.

8. Patient observation for 15–30 minutes.

(C) Infrared coagulation

3. Verification of dentate line.

4. Pointing infrared coagulator to proximal base of hemorrhoid.

5. Delivery of 3–4 applications for 1.0–1.5 seconds.

6. Repeat procedure for remaining hemorrhoidal piles.

7. Patient observation for 15–30 minutes.

Anatomic Structures at Risk

Anoderm (below dentate line).

Aftercare

Stool softeners, fibers, pain medication, sitz baths.

Complications

Bleeding (immediately, after 4–7 days), urinary retention, infection, pelvic/perineal sepsis, delayed wound healing (persistent ulceration), recurrent hemorrhoids.

Cross-reference

EXCISIONAL HEMORRHOIDECTOMY
(FERGUSON, MILLIGAN-MORGAN)

Principle

Radial mucocutaneous excision of enlarged hemorrhoidal piles (right anterior and posterior, left lateral) with proximal suture ligature of vascular pedicle. Mucocutaneous defect closed (Ferguson) or left open (Milligan-Morgan). In very large and circumferential hemorrhoids, it may be preferable to combine the right anterior and posterior pedicle into one lateral excision,

For thrombosed external hemorrhoid: diminutive form of excision.

Setting

Outpatient, OR procedure (office procedure may be safe in selected cases).

Alternatives

Stapled hemorrhoidectomy PPH.

Whitehead hemorrhoidectomy.

Hemorrhoid banding and other office procedures.

Indication

Internal hemorrhoids:

- – Grade (II–)III with significant external component.
- – Irreducible, ie, grade IV hemorrhoids.
- – Involvement of less than all three piles.
- – Hemorrhoidectomy in patients with anoreceptive intercourse.

Thrombosed external hemorrhoid (< 72 hours postonset, occasionally longer if particularly large).

Preparatory Considerations

In elective cases, prior colonic evaluation per guidelines.

Administration of two enemas before operation. Single shot IV antibiotic prophylaxis. Disinfection of rectum with povidone-iodine solution.

Surgical Steps

1. Patient positioning: any position, but prone jackknife position with buttocks taped aside has several advantages—superior view with comfortable access for surgeon/assistant, decreased congestion of hemorrhoidal plexus.

(A) Classical excision of internal/external hemorrhoids (Figure 5–7A)

2. Pudendal/perianal nerve block with 15–20 cc of a local anesthetic in addition to general anesthesia to improve relaxation of anal sphincter muscles.

3. Insertion of dry sponge followed by slow traction on sponge will reveal tissue prolapse.

4. Insertion of Hill-Ferguson retractor.

5. Proximal suture ligature of vascular pedicle, suture not cut, but tagged.

6. Grasping of hemorrhoid and external component with two clamps.

7. V-shaped incision at base of hemorrhoid, beyond anal verge, dotting of line with electrocautery toward ligated pedicle. Important to retain adequate tissue bridge between various excision sites, otherwise risk of stricture.

8. Careful dissection to edge of sphincter muscle. All muscle fibers need to be carefully pushed away from hemorrhoidal tissue. Staying in correct plane will limit bleeding. Which dissection tool is used (scissors, electrocautery, harmonic knife, laser) is a matter of preference, not of scientific superiority.

9. Once level of pedicle is reached, suture ligature is again tied around base and specimen is subsequently amputated. Completion of hemostasis.

10. Milligan-Morgan: wound left open. Ferguson: wound closed with running absorbable suture, burying stump of vascular pedicle in proximal end, leaving only very last little segment on the outside open for possible drainage.

11. The other hemorrhoid piles are address in analogous fashion. It is most important to leave enough tissue in-between: as long as wounds can be closed while medium-size retractor is in place, the risk for a stricture seems minimal.

(B) Excision of thrombosed external hemorrhoid (Figure 5–7B)

2. Local injection just underneath/around the thrombosed hemorrhoid.

3. Elliptic excision (rather than just incision) of external component (no extension into anal canal): enucleation of thrombosed material.

4. Wound either left open or closed.

Anatomic Structures at Risk

Anal sphincter complex, anoderm.

Aftercare

Stool softeners, fibers, pain medication. Sitz baths.

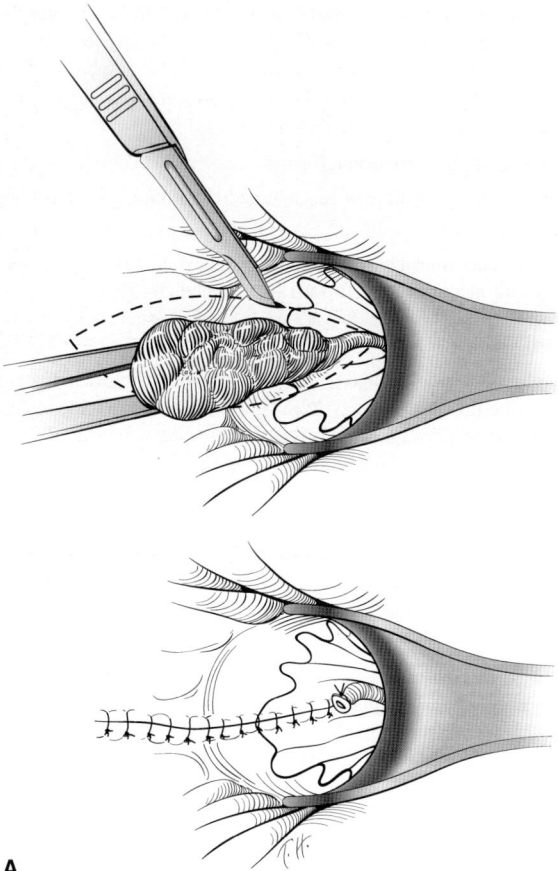

A

Figure 5–7A. Excisional hemorrhoidectomy (Ferguson technique).

Complications

Bleeding (1–6%), urinary retention (5–25%), infection (5–10%), pelvic/perineal sepsis, delayed wound healing, recurrent hemorrhoids, incontinence to stool/gas (2–10%), anorectal stricture (up to 6%). Risk of needing colostomy: ~0.1%.

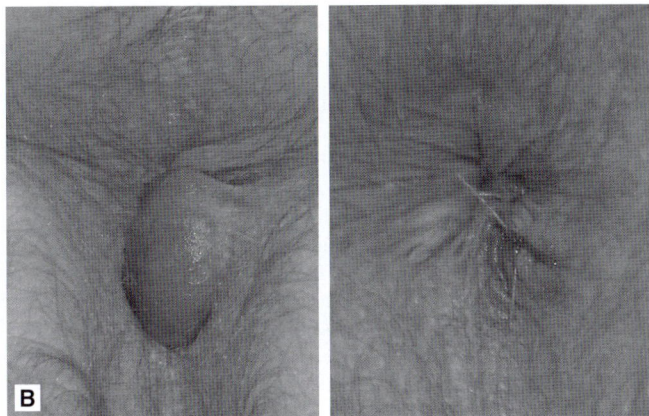

Figure 5–7B. Excision of thrombosed external hemorrhoid.

Cross-reference

STAPLED HEMORRHOIDECTOMY/-OPEXY—PPH

Principle

Stapled hemorrhoidectomy/-opexy, also referred to as Procedure for Prolapse and Hemorrhoids (PPH), has evolved as the preferred surgical option for most symptomatic internal hemorrhoids. In contrast to the excisional hemorrhoidectomy (Ferguson, Milligan-Morgan), this technique does not result in an external wound in the highly sensitive anoderm. Using a circular stapler, a 2-cm tissue ring of mucosa is excised with simultaneous reanastomosis above the dentate line. The primary goal is not to remove the hemorrhoids, but rather to lift the anorectal mucosa and reposition the hemorrhoidal cushions (Figures 5–8A and 5–8B). The improved venous outflow in combination with the interrupted submucosal blood supply decreases the hemorrhoidal congestion.

Setting

Outpatient, OR procedure.

Alternatives

Excisional hemorrhoidectomy (Ferguson, Milligan-Morgan).

Hemorrhoid banding and other office procedures.

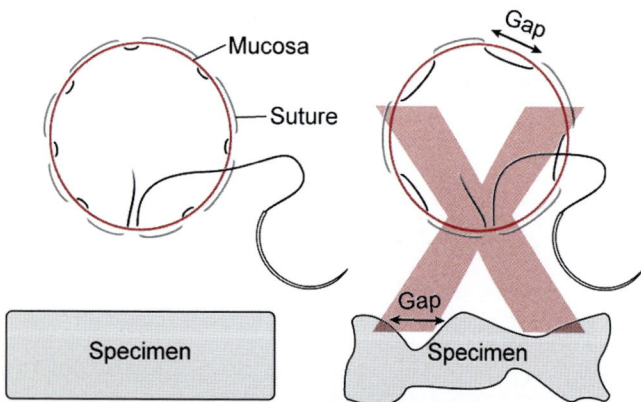

A

Figure 5–8A. PPH stapled hemorrhoidectomy: impact of suture placement on resulting specimen.

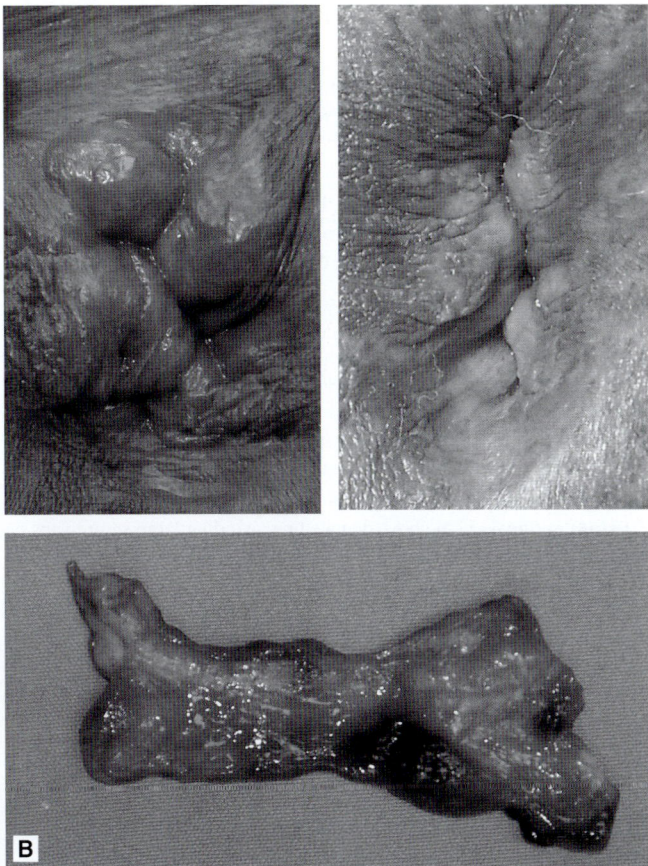

B

Figure 5–8B. PPH stapled hemorrhoidectomy: before and after, and rectangular specimen.

Indication

Circumferential internal hemorrhoids grade III, confluent grade II/I with relevant symptoms that are refractory to banding.

Not indicated for grade IV (incarcerated) hemorrhoids, if patient is primarily concerned about external hemorrhoid component, or for patients with anoreceptive intercourse (risk of injury from residual staples).

Preparatory Considerations

Colonic evaluation per guidelines.

Administration of two enemas before operation. Single shot IV antibiotic prophylaxis. Disinfection of rectum with povidone-iodine solution.

Surgical Steps

1. Patient positioning: any position, but prone jackknife position with buttocks taped aside has several advantages—superior view with comfortable access for surgeon/assistant, decreased congestion of hemorrhoidal plexus.

2. Pudendal/perianal nerve block with 15–20 cc of a local anesthetic in addition to general anesthesia to improve relaxation of anal sphincter muscles. Insertion of circular anal dilator facilitated without the (obsolete) manual stretch.

3. Insertion of anal dilator with transparent anal retractor. The latter serves to protect dentate line and is sutured to the skin.

4. Insertion of suture anoscope for placement of a mucosa-only purse-string suture 4–5 cm above dentate line, avoiding large suture gaps on luminal surface (Figure 5–8A), ie, new stitch starts right where previous stitch exits.

5. Digital rectal exam to check that purse string tightens easily, smoothly and circumferentially around finger.

6. Careful insertion of fully deployed circular stapler through staple line. Any resistance requires reassessment.

7. Purse-string suture is tied down to rod, and sutures ends are carried through lateral openings in stapler.

8. Closure of stapler to maximum while moderate traction on purse-string sutures aims at pulling a maximal amount of tissue into stapler chamber. No force should be necessary for closure.

9. Safety steps before the maximally closed stapler is actually fired:

   a. Sutures holding transparent circular anal retractor are divided and a thorough circumferential inspection around stapler is performed to ensure that dentate line has not accidentally been incorporated into stapler.

   b. In females, a vaginal examination is mandatory to ensure that posterior vaginal wall has not been incorporated/tethered into staple line.

10. Stapler is fired and kept in place in closed position for 5 minutes to ensure good hemostasis: often, no further intervention is needed; occasionally bleeding from staple line requires electrocautery or insertion of hemostatic suture.

11. Removal of stapler and examination of specimen (Figure 5–8B).

12. Although anal skin tags can be removed separately, the benefit of stapled hemorrhoidectomy will be gradually diminished.

Anatomic Structures at Risk

Vagina, rectum, sphincter complex/dentate line.

Aftercare

Stool softeners, fibers, pain medication. No need for sitz baths.

Complications

Bleeding, urinary retention, infection, pelvic/perineal sepsis, thrombosed external hemorrhoids, recurrent hemorrhoids, incontinence to stool/gas. Rectal perforation or rectovaginal fistula is rare if proper technique is used. Risk of needing colostomy: ~0.1%.

Cross-reference

Operative Techniques

ANORECTAL FLAPS

Principle

Relocation of healthy and elastic vascularized tissue from a donor site to the anorectal area in order to replace, augment, or cover areas of pathology.

Setting

Inpatient (selected outpatient?), OR procedure.

Alternatives

Direct coverage.

Open wound care.

Indication

- Anal stricture.
- Mucosal ectropion.
- Cloaca-like deformity.
- Defect closure after wide local excision.

Preparatory Considerations

Complete bowel cleansing.

Prophylactic antibiotics.

Most flaps do not need preemptive colostomy → creation in selected cases only.

Surgical Steps

1. Patient positioning: prone jackknife position; buttock taping depending on planned flap configuration.
2. Management of local pathology: eg, radial incision of stricture, excision of ectropion to level of dentate line, wide local excision, etc.

(A) House flap (single or multiple) for limited pathology in anal canal (stricture, ectropion): Figures 5–9A and 5–9B.

3. Marking of planned house flap(s) with a pen: care to achieve sufficient width (> 1.5 cm, up to 3–4 cm).
4. Incision and mobilization with preservation of blood supply (ie, no undermining): flaps have an automatic tendency to drop toward anal canal.
5. Fixation in receiver site with interrupted absorbable sutures and complete maturation internally and on flap sides.
6. Radial closure of harvest site(s); alternatively leave harvest site open.

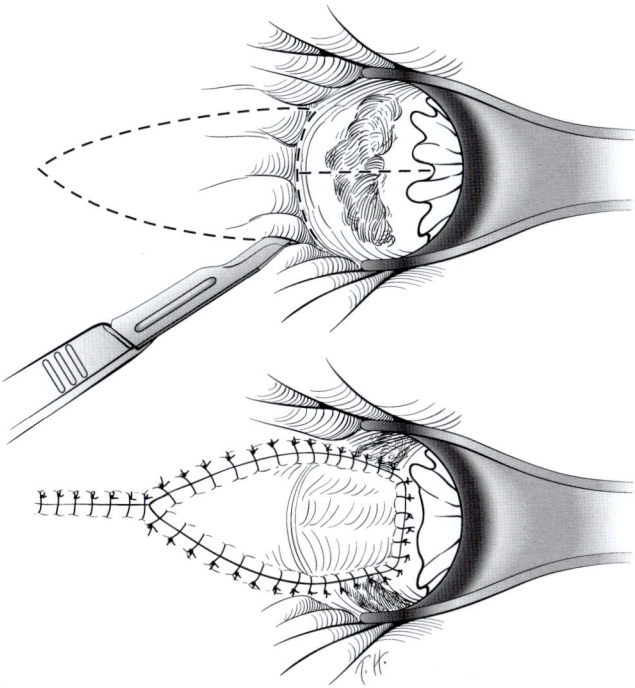

A

Figure 5–9A. Anal stricturoplasty with house flap.

(B) Rotational S-flaps for extensive defect closure (eg, after wide local excision)

3. Marking of planned large S-flaps with a pen with turning point in anus, care to extend sufficiently onto buttocks (8–10 cm diameter).

4. Incision and mobilization with preservation of adequate tissue layer for blood supply.

5. Rotation of flaps toward anal canal.

6. Fixation in most remote corner at receiver site with interrupted absorbable sutures and complete maturation of internal circumference.

7. Closure of radial side of flap using interrupted absorbable sutures with larger advancement steps on external side than on flap side, which results in closure of donor site.

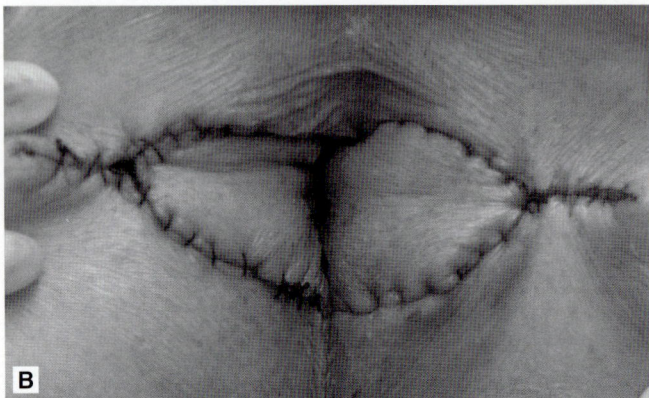

Figure 5–9B. Bilateral anal house flaps.

(C) Large bilateral gluteal skin advancement flaps for extensive defect closure (eg, after wide local excision)

3. Marking of planned large gluteal skin flaps (> 15 cm lateral length) with vertical length of medial side equal to half the circumference of a large anoscope.

4. Incision and mobilization with preservation of adequate tissue layer for blood supply.

5. Advancement of flaps toward anal canal.

6. Fixation of ends of medial side anteriorly and posteriorly at anal canal, symmetric approximation of contralateral flap, followed by complete circumferential maturation of mucocutaneous contact zone with interrupted absorbable sutures.

7. Closure of radial side of flap using interrupted absorbable sutures with larger advancement steps on external side than on flap side.

(D) Bilateral X-flaps for reconstruction of perineal body in cloaca-like deformity

3. Marking of planned flaps on skin with two cruciate lines to intercept in remnant of rectovaginal septum: care to obtain bilateral triangular skin flaps with wide enough angle (~40 degrees) to avoid ischemic changes at tips.

4. Separation of rectovaginal septum and reconstruction of anterior side anal canal, posterior side of vagina, sphincteroplasty.

5. Moving X-flaps toward opposite side (beyond midline), which results in augmentation of perineum.

6. Securing flaps in place with interrupted absorbable sutures.

Anatomic Structures at Risk

Sphincter complex, blood supply to the flaps, sufficient mobility.

Aftercare

Regular diet as tolerated 6 hours postanesthesia. Maintenance of soft stools (fibers, antidiarrheal medication, etc) as before surgery.

Limitation of activity.

Complications

Bleeding (surgeon-dependent).

Infection, abscess/fistula formation.

Flap necrosis, flap dehiscence → stricture formation.

Need for colostomy in case of unmanageable situation.

Cross-reference

Topic	Chapter
Constipation	1 (p 9), 4 (p 427)
Anal fissure	4 (p 161)
Fecal incontinence	4 (p 189)
Bowen disease	4 (p 224)
Paget disease	4 (p 224)
Complication—delayed wound healing	4 (p 470)
Perioperative management—anorectal	7 (p 688)

Operative Techniques

RECTOVAGINAL FISTULA REPAIR—ADVANCEMENT FLAP

Principle

Excision of the primary opening, reapproximation of the underlying muscular layer, mobilization of flap to cover the opening. Since the rectum is the high-pressure compartment (compared with vagina), the repair from a physics standpoint should be performed on the rectal side; rare circumstances may justify a repair from the vagina. Local repair is appropriate for low to mid-level fistulae. High fistula (colovaginal) needs to be ruled out or managed through an abdominal approach. Fecal diversion commonly is not necessary unless patient is very symptomatic.

Alternatives

Placement of a cutting seton.

Rectovaginotomy with layered closure of defect.

Insertion of collagen plug.

Interposition of muscle flap (bulbocavernosus, gracilis).

Indication

Symptomatic low to mid-level rectovaginal fistula.

Preparatory Considerations

Fecal diversion if patient is very symptomatic and local area is not ready for repair (< 3–6 months after formation).

In elective cases, prior colonic evaluation per guidelines.

Clinical examination often sufficient; combination with imaging studies if anatomy is unclear.

Administration of full bowel cleansing before operation. Single shot IV antibiotic prophylaxis, depending on findings, to be continued for 5 days. Disinfection of rectum and vagina with povidone-iodine solution.

Surgical Steps

1. Patient positioning: any position, but prone jackknife position with buttocks taped aside has several advantages—superior view with comfortable access for surgeon/assistant. Lithotomy position for transvaginal approach.
2. Pudendal/perianal nerve block with 15–20 cc of local anesthetic in addition to general anesthesia to improve relaxation of anal sphincter muscles.
3. Insertion of anal retractor and reassessment of fistula. Depending on local anatomy, placement of Lone Star retractor may prove advantageous.

4. Limited excision of primary opening, removal of epithelialized tract within muscle layer.

5. Closure of muscular defect with interrupted Vicryl sutures.

6. Marking of U-shaped broad-based flap, with base starting distal to primary fistula opening, extending laterally and proximally (one quarter to one third of anterior circumference). Atraumatic raising of flap: after adequate mobilization, flap should cover defect without any tension. Careful hemostasis; avoid traction or diffuse cautery damage to flap.

7. Suturing flap in place in two layers: deeper muscular layer (Vicryl), maturation of mucosal anastomosis with interrupted sutures (chromic).

8. Vaginal side left open.

Anatomic Structures at Risk

Sphincter muscle, rectovaginal septum, dentate line.

Aftercare

Stool management with softeners, fibers to avoid too soft/too hard bowel movements.

Pain medication.

Sitz baths.

Complications

Bleeding, urinary retention, infection, flap dehiscence with reopening of potentially larger fistula, need for colostomy, incontinence to stool/gas, delayed wound healing, pain. Rare: pelvic/perineal sepsis.

Cross-reference

Operative Techniques

RECTOVAGINAL FISTULA REPAIR— RECTOVAGINOTOMY WITH LAYERED CLOSURE

Principle

Complete transection of the perineal body between the rectal and vaginal fistula opening with excision of the epithelialized fistula tract and layered closure and reconstruction. Advantage: better exposure and more controlled closure of the various layers; disadvantage: more serious defect in cases of infection/dehiscence. Since a relevant rectovaginal fistula results in functional incontinence, transection/reconstruction of the sphincter muscle typically is well tolerated and not noticed as a disadvantage.

Method is appropriate for low- to mid-level fistulae. High fistula (colo-vaginal) needs to be ruled out or managed through an abdominal approach. Fecal diversion commonly is not necessary unless patient is very symptomatic before the repair or as a result of complications with dehiscence.

Alternatives

Placement of a cutting seton.

Endorectal advancement flap.

Insertion of collagen plug.

Interposition of muscle flap (bulbocavernosus, gracilis).

Indication

Symptomatic low to mid-level rectovaginal fistula, preferably preexisting sphincter defect.

Preparatory Considerations

Fecal diversion if patient is very symptomatic and local area is not ready for repair (< 3–6 months postformation).

In elective cases, prior colonic evaluation per guidelines.

Clinical examination often sufficient; combination with imaging studies if anatomy is unclear.

Administration of full bowel cleansing before operation. IV antibiotic prophylaxis with continuation for 5 days. Disinfection of rectum and vagina with povidone-iodine solution.

Surgical Steps

1. Patient positioning: any position, but prone jackknife position with buttocks taped aside has several advantages—superior view with comfortable access for surgeon/assistant. Lithotomy position for transvaginal approach.

2. Pudendal/perianal nerve block with 15–20 cc of local anesthetic in addition to general anesthesia to improve relaxation of anal sphincter muscles.

3. Insertion of anal retractor and reassessment of fistula.

4. Insertion of probe into fistula and division of whole perineal body with electrocautery. As various tissue levels are divided, marking corresponding tissues (eg, sphincter muscle) on either side with sutures.

5. Excision of epithelialized fistula tract and mucosal mobilization on rectal and vaginal side.

6. Layered closure, making sure both mucosal edges evert rather than invert. Reconstruction of sphincter muscle with 3-4 interrupted Vicryl sutures.

7. Maturation of mucosal sides, closure of skin with subcuticular sutures.

Anatomic Structures at Risk

Sphincter muscle.

Aftercare

Stool management with softeners/fibers to avoid too soft/too hard bowel movements.

Pain medication.

Sitz baths.

Complications

Bleeding, urinary retention, infection, flap dehiscence with reopening of potentially larger fistula, need for colostomy, incontinence to stool/gas, delayed wound healing, pain.

Rare: pelvic/perineal sepsis.

Cross-reference

Operative Techniques

RECTOVAGINAL FISTULA REPAIR—MUSCLE FLAP INTERPOSITION

Principle

Perineal repair of the rectovaginal fistula with interposition of well-vascularized tissue to achieve separation of the two compartments and improve local wound healing. Typically indicated when local tissue quality is less than optimal (postradiation, postsurgical, recurrent fistula). Muscle generally is well suited as long as it can be adequately mobilized while maintaining its blood supply. Options for muscle flap include:

- Bulbocavernosus muscle (Martius flap).
- Gracilis muscle.
- Gluteus muscle.

Access through the perineum, separation of rectum and vagina with layered closure of each of them. Tunneled insertion of the muscle flap from its harvest site and interposition to keep the two sutured mucosal layers separate from each other. This type of local repair typically is reserved for high risk low- to mid-level fistulae. High fistula (colovaginal) typically is manageable without a flap. Fecal diversion commonly is not necessary unless the patient is very symptomatic.

Alternatives

Repair with endorectal advancement flap.

Placement of a cutting seton.

Rectovaginotomy with layered closure of defect.

Insertion of collagen plug.

Interposition of a collagen sheet.

Indication

Symptomatic low- to mid-level rectovaginal fistula.

Preparatory Considerations

Fecal diversion if patient is very symptomatic and local area is not ready for repair (< 3–6 months postformation).

In elective cases, prior colonic evaluation per guidelines.

Administration of full bowel cleansing before operation. Single shot IV antibiotic prophylaxis, depending on findings to be continued for 5 days. Disinfection of rectum and vagina with povidone-iodine solution.

Surgical Steps

1. Patient positioning: any position, but prone jackknife position with buttocks taped aside has several advantages—superior view with comfortable access for surgeon/assistant. Lithotomy position for transvaginal approach.

2. Pudendal/perianal nerve block with 15–20 cc of local anesthetic in addition to general anesthesia to improve relaxation of anal sphincter muscles.

3. Insertion of anal retractor and reassessment of fistula.

4. Transverse incision to perineum (as anterior as possible).

5. Dissection of rectovaginal septum to level of puborectalis muscle. Injury to rectum and/or vagina must be avoided, but obviously both sides will end up with a defect once rectovaginal fistula is transected.

6. Limited excision of primary opening, removal of remnants of epithelialized tract within muscle layer.

7. Layered closure and maturation of both mucosal sides, making sure both mucosal edges rather evert toward their lumen than invert.

8. Muscle mobilization:

   a. Bulbocavernosus muscle: paralabial longitudinal incision, dissection through relatively vascular tissue layer, identification and mobilization of bulbocavernosus muscle. Anterior transection, verification of preserved blood supply.

   b. Gracilis muscle: three longitudinal medial incisions (or one complete incision), identification of muscle through proximal incision. Careful mobilization toward proximal neurovascular pedicle. Distal muscle mobilization. Disconnection of tendon as distally as possible.

   c. Gluteus muscle: curved lateral parasacral incision, identification of posterior edge of gluteus muscle and its broad insertion to sacrococcygeal junction. Mobilization of a portion of muscle. Avoid avulsion of neurovascular pedicle near ischial tuberosity.

9. Creation of tunnel from harvest site to perineum.

10. Interposition of mobilized muscle flap and fixation of its tip on opposite side; loose fixation of muscle body in perineum to avoid shifting of its position.

11. Irrigation of wound with diluted povidone-iodine (1:10). Hemostasis.

12. Subcutaneous approximation sutures.

13. Closure of skin incision(s).

Operative Techniques

Anatomic Structures at Risk

Integrity of rectovaginal septum. Vascular pedicles.

Aftercare

Stool management with softeners/fibers to avoid too soft/too hard bowel movements.

Pain medication.

Sitz baths.

Mobilization depending on harvest site.

Complications

Bleeding, urinary retention, infection, flap necrosis and/or dehiscence with reopening of potentially larger fistula, need for colostomy, incontinence to stool/gas, delayed wound healing, pain. Rare: pelvic/perineal sepsis.

Cross-reference

RECTOCELE REPAIR

Principle

Elective correction and reinforcement of anterior rectal wall herniation using one of three different approaches: transanal, transperineal, or transvaginal. Reinforcement of rectovaginal septum either with plication of muscle layer or implantation of collagen sheet. Selection of approach is primarily a matter of the surgeon's preference. Transanal approach overall is very well tolerated, with low pain level and low infection risk.

Setting

Inpatient (selected outpatient?), OR procedure.

Alternatives

Transabdominal pelvic floor suspension.

Indication

- Symptomatic rectocele.
- Not indicated: "innocent bystander" rectocele (incidental finding).

Preparatory Considerations

Full/partial colonic evaluation for all elective cases according to guidelines.

Bowel cleansing: full or at least two Fleet enemas.

Prophylactic antibiotics.

Surgical Steps

1. Patient positioning: any position, but prone jackknife position with buttocks taped aside has several advantages for approaches A and B—superior view with comfortable access for surgeon/assistant, decreased vascular congestion; lithotomy position for approach C.

(A) Transanal approach

2. Pudendal/perianal nerve block with 15–20 cc of local anesthetic in addition to general anesthesia to improve relaxation of anal sphincter muscles.

3. Insertion of Lone Star retractor.

4. Electrocautery marking of dotted line outlining broad-based U-flap in anterior circumference with apex near dentate line, and circumferential incision of mucosa.

5. Careful dissection of mucosa off underlying white muscular layer using cautery and traction on mucosa: if in correct plane there should be virtually no bleeding.

6. Placement of clamps on mobilized mucosa and distal traction, continuation of mucosal mobilization with continuous change of working site back and forth to where most tension.

7. Dissection to be continued until upper edge of rectocele reached.

8. Laying of 3–5 absorbable proximodistal sutures to muscular layer to obtain transverse plication of proximal to distal edge of rectocele.

9. Stepwise resection of mobilized mucosa (typical > 6 cm length) while performing full-thickness tension-free reapproximation of proximal end to distal edge. Maturing of mucosa.

10. Removal of Lone Star retractor.

(B) Transperineal approach

2. Transverse incision to perineum.

3. Careful dissection of rectovaginal plane, making sure not to injure rectum and/or vagina; dissection continued until past proximal edge of rectocele.

4. Reinforcement of anterior rectal wall/rectovaginal septum:

 a. Lateral approximation of puborectalis muscle with several interrupted stitches.

or

 b. Placement of collagen sheet, attaching it with a series of interrupted sutures to keep it in position.

5. Irrigation and perfect hemostasis.

6. Closure of incision in layers.

(C) Transvaginal approach

2. Insertion of vaginal retractor for exposure of posterior wall.

3. Longitudinal insertion of posterior vaginal wall mucosa (electrocautery) and lateral mobilization.

4. Maintenance of good hemostasis.

5. Placement of collagen sheet, attaching it with a series of interrupted sutures to keep it in position.

6. Resection of redundant vaginal wall/mucosa.

7. Longitudinal closure of incision.

Anatomic Structures at Risk

Rectovaginal septum, sphincter complex.

Aftercare

Regular diet as tolerated 6 hours postanesthesia. Maintenance of soft stools (fibers, stool softener, etc).

Complications

Recurrent rectocele.

Bleeding (surgeon-dependent).

Anastomotic dehiscence.

Infection, abscess/fistula formation, infected foreign body (particularly if nonbiologic material used).

Formation of rectovaginal fistula → need for colostomy.

Stricture formation.

Worsening fecal incontinence.

Dyspareunia (vaginal approach).

Cross-reference

Topic	*Chapter*
Constipation	1 (p 9)
Defecating proctogram	2 (p 114)
MRI	2 (p 124)
Pelvic floor dysfunction	4 (p 420)
Rectal prolapse repair	5 (pp 530–540)
Perioperative management—anorectal	7 (p 688)

Operative Techniques

RECTAL PROLAPSE—PERINEAL DELORME REPAIR

Principle

Elective resection of redundant distal rectal mucosa and reanastomosis with plication of preserved muscular layer (Figure 5–10). Considered the least invasive procedure, but carries the overall highest recurrence risk. In incontinent patients, Delorme may potentially provide a theoretical benefit of bulking up the muscle complex (plication). However, successful correction of prolapse alone is expected to improve sphincter function in 70% of patients.

Setting

Inpatient (selected outpatient?), OR procedure.

Alternatives

Sigmoid resection with/without rectopexy—laparoscopic or open.

Rectopexy only—laparoscopic or open.

Perineal Altemeier repair.

Thiersch procedure.

Indication

Full-thickness (or mucosal) rectal prolapse.

Preparatory Considerations

Full colonic evaluation for all elective cases.

Bowel cleansing: full or at least two Fleet enemas.

Prophylactic antibiotics.

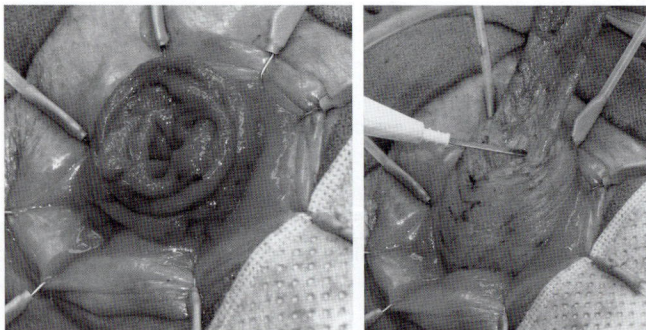

Figure 5–10. Rectal prolapse repair in Delorme technique.

Surgical Steps

1. Patient positioning: any position, but prone jackknife position with buttocks taped aside has several advantages—superior view with comfortable access for surgeon/assistant, decreased vascular congestion.

2. Pudendal/perianal nerve block with 15–20 cc of local anesthetic in addition to general anesthesia to improve relaxation of anal sphincter muscles.

3. Insertion of dry sponge, followed by slow traction on sponge, will reveal tissue prolapse.

4. Insertion of Lone Star retractor.

5. Electrocautery marking of dotted line 1 cm proximal to dentate line and circumferential incision of mucosa.

6. Slow dissection of mucosa off underlying white muscular layer using cautery and traction on mucosa (Figure 5–10): if in correct plane there should be virtually no bleeding.

7. Placement of clamps on mobilized mucosa and distal traction with continuation of mucosal mobilization with continuous change of working site circumferentially around where most tension.

8. Dissection to be continued until no further protrusion.

9. Simultaneous stepwise resection of mobilized mucosa while eight muscle-plicating absorbable mucomuscular sutures are laid but not yet tied: important to take same number of steps (eg, 3–4) for all individual sutures.

10. Removal of Lone Star retractor and sequential tying of sutures.

11. Complete maturation of mucosal anastomosis using one to three interrupted chromic sutures in between each Vicryl suture.

Anatomic Structures at Risk

Hemorrhoidal plexus, rectovaginal septum, muscularis propria/rectal wall with accidental full-thickness resection (Altemeier) instead of mucosal resection.

Aftercare

Regular diet as tolerated 6 hours postanesthesia. Maintenance of soft stools (fibers, stool softener, etc).

Complications

Recurrent prolapse.

Bleeding (surgeon-dependent).

Operative Techniques

Anastomotic dehiscence.

Abscess/fistula formation.

Formation of rectovaginal fistula → need for colostomy.

Stricture formation.

Worsening fecal incontinence.

Cross-reference

RECTAL PROLAPSE—PERINEAL ALTEMEIER REPAIR

Principle

Perineal proctectomy with full-thickness resection, including vascular ligation of redundant distal rectum, reanastomosis with coloanal anastomosis. Procedure of choice as emergency operation for incarcerated prolapse. Disadvantage: interruption of blood flow from the distal to the proximal rectum. Higher recurrence risk than in abdominal procedures. In incontinent patients, may be combined with levatorplasty. However, correction of prolapse alone is expected to improve sphincter function in 70% of patients.

Setting

Inpatient, OR procedure.

Alternatives

Sigmoid resection with/without rectopexy—laparoscopic or open.

Rectopexy only—laparoscopic or open.

Perineal Delorme repair.

Thiersch procedure.

Indication

• Full-thickness (or mucosal) rectal prolapse.
• Incarcerated prolapse.

Preparatory Considerations

Full colonic evaluation for all elective cases.

Bowel cleansing: full or at least two Fleet enemas.

Prophylactic antibiotics.

Surgical Steps

1. Patient positioning: any position, but prone jackknife position with buttocks taped aside has several advantages—superior view with comfortable access for surgeon/assistant, decreased vascular congestion.
2. Pudendal/perianal nerve block with 15–20 cc of local anesthetic in addition to general anesthesia to improve relaxation of anal sphincter muscles.
3. Insertion of dry sponge, followed by slow traction on sponge will reveal tissue prolapse.

4. Insertion of Lone Star retractor.
5. Electrocautery marking of dotted line in viable tissue roughly 1 cm proximal to dentate line (appears "more distal" in prolapsed rectum) and circumferential transection of rectal wall.
6. Delivering of all redundant bowel (elective procedure); avoid excessive resection in emergency situation.
7. Creation of mesenteric window at level of anal verge and mesenteric/mesorectal devascularization with clamps and ligatures.
8. Possible plication of levator muscles.
9. Coloanal anastomosis: stepwise transection of delivered/prolapsed bowel at level of anal verge while securing bowel in place with interrupted seromuscular sutures and subsequent complete maturation of mucosal layer.

Anatomic Structures at Risk

Hemorrhoidal plexus, rectovaginal septum, colonic blood supply (watershed areas).

Aftercare

Regular diet as tolerated 6 hours postanesthesia. Maintenance of soft stools (fibers, stool softener, etc).

Complications

Recurrent prolapse.

Bleeding (surgeon-dependent).

Anastomotic dehiscence.

Abscess/fistula formation.

Formation of rectovaginal fistula → need for colostomy.

Stricture formation.

Worsening fecal incontinence.

Cross-reference

Topic	*Chapter*
Prolapse	1 (p 40)
Defecating proctogram	2 (p 114)
MRI	2 (p 124)
Hemorrhoids	4 (p 167)

Operative Techniques

RECTAL PROLAPSE—RECTOPEXY
(LAPAROSCOPIC VS OPEN)

Principle

Elective complete posterior mobilization of rectum down to pelvic floor with subsequent posterior resuspension to presacral fascia, typically with implantation of mesh or collagen sheet (Figure 5–11). Commonly amenable to laparoscopic approach. This is the procedure of choice for recurrent rectal prolapse after previous perineal resection (Altemeier, or unknown perineal technique), in which abdominal resection would carry a risk of creating an avascular segment.

Setting

Inpatient, OR procedure.

Alternatives

Sigmoid resection, posterior rectal mobilization, with/without rectopexy (unless resection contraindicated).

Abdominal LAR with coloanal anastomosis.

Vascularity-sparing sigmoid resection.

Perineal rectal prolapse repair: Delorme, Altemeier, Thiersch procedure.

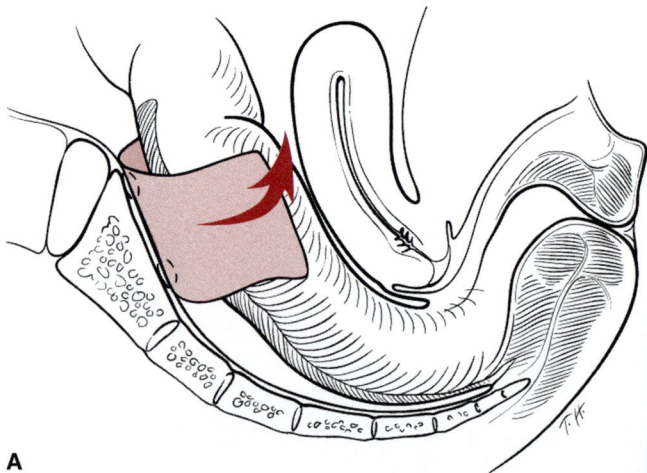

A

Figure 5–11A. Rectopexy: posterior mobilization to rectal floor and mesh placement.

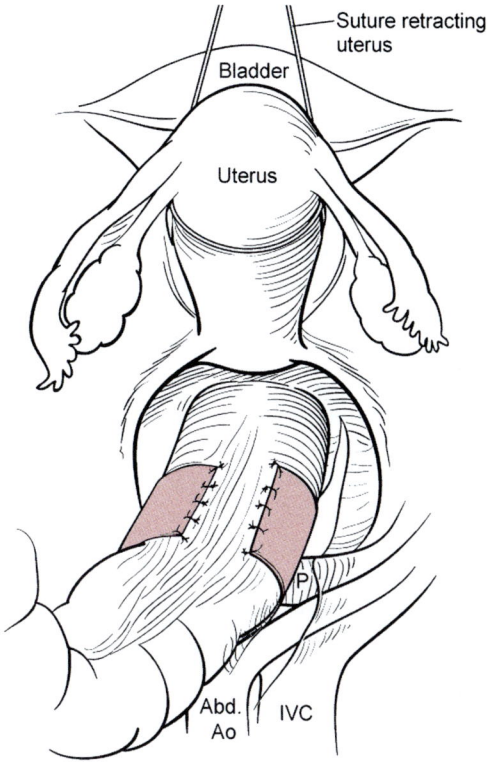

Figure 5-11B.   Rectopexy: view into pelvis with suspended uterus and posterior mesh-fixation of mobilized rectum.

Indication

- Full-thickness rectal prolapse,
- Recurrent rectal prolapse postperineal resection ($\rightarrow$ risk of ischemic segment with abdominal resection).

Preparatory Considerations

Full colonic evaluation for all elective cases.

Bowel cleansing (traditional) vs no bowel cleansing (evolving concept).

Prophylactic antibiotics.

Surgical Steps

1. Patient position: modified lithotomy position.

(A) Laparoscopic approach

2. Creation of pneumoperitoneum (Veress or Hasson technique).

3. Placement of 3(–4) trocars: periumbilical 10–12 mm, bilateral 5 mm, possibly one RUQ 5 mm trocar for retraction.

(B) Open approach

2. Laparotomy: lower midline, transverse suprapubic (transection of rectus muscle), Pfannenstiel incision (transverse incision to skin and anterior rectus sheath with midline rectus-saving celiotomy).

3. Placement of abdominal wall retractor or wound protector to expose left portion of colon.

Both techniques

4. Abdominal exploration: characteristic deep peritoneal reflection, secondary pathology (liver/gallbladder, colon, female organs, small bowel), other abnormalities.

5. Female patients (in laparoscopic approach): fixation of uterus to anterior abdominal wall—percutaneous insertion of long straight needle through avascular portion of lateral ligaments, guided around corpus uteri back through contralateral lateral ligament to abdominal wall and tied outside over gauze.

6. Opening of right-sided peritoneal surface along base of mesosigmoid, extension to pelvis.

7. Incision of left-sided peritoneal surface along white line of Toldt toward pelvis, no mobilization toward splenic flexure.

8. Identification of inferior mesenteric vessels. The space right behind vascular stalk is entered and a window created. Developing plane below sigmoid mesentery vessels to bluntly reflect retroperitoneal tissues and expose left ureter.

9. Hypogastric nerves are identified and protected by pushing them toward the back. Blunt dissection behind vascular stalk (avascular plane) to entry of pelvis and complete posterior mobilization along Waldeyer fascia to pelvic floor. Avoidance of extensive bilateral mobilization to minimize risk of autonomic nerve dysfunction.

10. Positioning of implant: 6 × 10 cm implant (Marlex mesh, collagen sheet) inserted for laparoscopic procedure; mesh is rolled up and pushed through camera port, unwrapped internally, and positioned posterior to mobilized rectum.

11. Fixation of implant to presacral fascia with interrupted nonabsorbable sutures (or hernia stapler) to promontory and presacral fascia (caveat: presacral veins!).

12. Rectopexy wrap: sides of implant are bilaterally wrapped around rectum, leaving anterior one-third of rectum free and fixed with bilateral series of 3–4 sutures.

13. Removal of temporary uteropexy.

14. Drains according to surgeon's preference. No need for NGT.

15. Closure of incision(s).

Anatomic Structures at Risk

Left ureter, presacral veins, gonadal vessels, hypogastric nerves.

Aftercare

Fast-track recovery: in absence of nausea or vomiting, oral liquids are started on POD1 and advanced as tolerated. Maintenance of soft stools.

Complications

Recurrent prolapse.

Bleeding (surgeon-dependent): presacral veins, gonadal vessels.

Ureteral injury (0.1–0.2%).

Mesh infection or mesh migration/erosion.

Cross-reference

RECTAL PROLAPSE—SIGMOID RESECTION AND RECTOPEXY

Principle

Elective resection of sigmoid redundancy, complete posterior mobilization of the rectum down to the pelvic floor with subsequent resuspension to the presacral fascia. Considered the procedure with the lowest recurrence rate. Colon resection is desirable in patients with underlying constipation, but should be avoided in case of underlying diarrhea.

Setting

Inpatient, OR procedure.

Alternatives

Laparoscopic approach.

Rectopexy only—laparoscopic or open.

Perineal rectal prolapse repair: Delorme, Altemeier, Thiersch procedure.

Indication

Full-thickness rectal prolapse.

Preparatory Considerations

Full colonic evaluation for all elective cases.

Bowel cleansing (traditional) vs no bowel cleansing (evolving concept).

Prophylactic antibiotics.

Surgical Steps

1. Patient position: modified lithotomy position.
2. Laparotomy: lower midline, transverse suprapubic (transection of rectus muscle), Pfannenstiel incision (transverse incision to skin and anterior rectus sheath with midline rectus-saving celiotomy).
3. Placement of abdominal wall retractor or wound protector to expose left portion of colon.
4. Abdominal exploration: characteristic deep peritoneal reflection, secondary pathology (liver/gallbladder, colon, female organs, small bowel), other abnormalities.
5. Opening of right-sided peritoneal surface along base of mesosigmoid, extension to pelvis.

6. Incision of left-sided peritoneal surface along white line of Toldt toward pelvis, no mobilization toward splenic flexure. Opening of retroperitoneum, identification of areolar tissue. Firm pressure against sigmoid mesentery to bluntly reflect retroperitoneal tissues and expose left ureter.

7. Identification of inferior mesenteric vessels. The space right behind vascular stalk is entered and a window created. Hypogastric nerves are identified and protected by pushing them toward the back. Blunt dissection behind vascular stalk (avascular plane) to entry of pelvis and complete posterior mobilization along Waldeyer fascia to pelvic floor. Avoidance of extensive bilateral mobilization to minimize risk of autonomic nerve dysfunction.

8. Defining resection margins:

    a. Distal: upper rectum so that anastomosis is roughly at promontory.

    b. Proximal: as much as is needed to eliminate sigmoid redundancy.

9. Stepwise division (between clamps and ligatures) of mesentery to proximal point of resection.

10. Devascularization:

    a. Majority of patients: standard devascularization at vascular stalk (superior hemorrhoidal)—before tissue division verification of ureter location. Creation of a window in mesorectum at distal point of resection (see above). Division of mesorectum between clamps/ligatures.

    b. Patient with history of perineal resection: risk of avascular segment with standard devascularization → correct operations:

        (1) Rectopexy only.

        (2) Vascular arcade-sparing sigmoid resection, ie, devascularization close to bowel while preserving vasculature to bowel distal to transection.

        (3) Bowel transection at level of former anastomosis, elimination of redundancy and respective blood supply.

11. Division of bowel by means of linear stapler.

12. Retrieval of specimen and gross examination by pathologist and/or surgeon.

13. Anastomosis:

    a. Stapled: purse-string suture to proximal end, circular stapler anvil inserted, stapler body through anus, and tension-free anastomosis.

    b. Hand-sewn: one-layer vs two-layer.

14. Testing of anastomosis: submerging under water, finger compression of bowel proximal to anastomosis, and insufflation of air through proctoscope.

15. Rectopexy:

    a. Suture rectopexy: series of three to four bilateral sutures to fix edge of rectum to presacral fascia.

    b. Rectopexy with 6×10 cm implant (Marlex mesh, collagen sheet) after posterior mobilization of rectum—fixation of implant with interrupted nonabsorbable sutures to promontory and presacral fascia (caveat: presacral veins!) and bilateral wrapping around and series of three to four bilateral sutures to fix it to edge of rectum, leaving anterior one- third of rectum free. Caveat: with resective procedure preferetial use of a biological implant rather than a Marlex mesh to avoid mesh infection.

16. Drains according to surgeon's preference. No need for NGT.

17. Closure of incision.

Anatomic Structures at Risk

Left ureter, gonadal vessels, hypogastric nerves, presacral veins.

Aftercare

Fast-track recovery: in absence of nausea or vomiting, oral liquids are started on POD1 and advanced as tolerated. Maintenance of soft stools.

Complications

Recurrent prolapse.

Bleeding (surgeon-dependent): presacral veins, inadequate ligature of vascular stalk, gonadal vessels.

Anastomotic leak (2%): most commonly due to technical error, tension, inadequate blood supply.

Ureteral injury (0.1–0.2%).

Mesh infection or mesh migration/erosion.

Cross-reference

Topic	*Chapter*
Prolapse	1 (p 40)
Defecating proctogram	2 (p 114)
MRI	2 (p 124)
Hemorrhoids	4 (p 167)

Operative Techniques

SIGMOID RESECTION
(OPEN, ANASTOMOSIS VS HARTMANN)

Principle

Oncologic resection of the sigmoid colon with ligation of the vascular pedicle and corresponding lymphadenectomy. Primary anastomosis is the reconstruction of choice but may not be suited to the individual patient. In that case, a discontinuous Hartmann resection with blind distal stump and end-colostomy would be effectuated.

Setting

Inpatient, OR procedure.

Alternatives

Laparoscopic approach.

On-table lavage with primary anastomosis.

Colonoscopic stent placement as bridge to (semi-)elective surgery.

Indication

• Sigmoid cancer, diverticulitis, volvulus, rectal prolapse.
• LBO.

Preparatory Considerations

Full colonic evaluation for all elective cases, tattooing of small lesions is advisable.

Bowel cleansing (traditional) vs no bowel cleansing (evolving concept).

Ureteral stents for redo cases or extensive disruption of anatomy (eg, inflammation).

Marking of possible stoma sites.

Prophylactic antibiotics.

Surgical Steps

1. Patient position: modified lithotomy position.
2. Laparotomy: lower midline, transverse suprapubic (transection of rectus muscle), Pfannenstiel incision (transverse incision to skin and anterior rectus sheath with midline rectus-saving celiotomy).
3. Placement of abdominal wall retractor or wound protector to expose left portion of colon.

4. Abdominal exploration: local resectability, secondary pathology (liver/gallbladder, colon, female organs, small bowel), other abnormalities.

5. Defining resection margins:

    a. Distal: at least upper rectum (confluens of teniae).

    b. Proximal: oncologic margin, normal bowel wall texture (does not require absence of diverticula).

6. Retrograde dissection from sigmoid toward splenic flexure along white line of Toldt. Opening of retroperitoneum, identification of areolar tissue. Firm pressure against sigmoid mesentery to bluntly reflect retroperitoneal tissues and expose left ureter. Incision of peritoneum is continued into pelvis.

7. Opening of right-sided peritoneal surface along base of mesosigmoid, extension to pelvis.

8. Identification of inferior mesenteric vessels. The space right behind vascular stalk is entered and a window created. Hypogastric nerves are identified and protected by pushing them toward the back. Dissection of redundant adipose tissue around vessels is carried out under direct vision.

9. Clamps are placed to vascular stalk (either inferior mesenteric or superior hemorrhoidal). Before tissue is divided, ureter is again checked! Stalk is then divided and addressed with double ligatures and/or a suture ligature.

10. Stepwise division (between clamps and ligatures) of mesentery to proximal point of resection.

11. Blunt dissection behind vascular stalk (avascular plane) to entry of pelvis. In case of rectal prolapse: complete posterior mobilization along Waldeyer fascia to pelvic floor.

12. Creation of window in mesorectum at distal point of resection (see above). Division of bowel by means of linear stapler. Division of mesorectum between clamps/ligatures.

13. Retrieval of specimen and gross examination by pathologist and/or surgeon.

(A) Reconstruction with primary anastomosis

    a. Anastomosis:

        (i) Stapled: purse-string suture to proximal end, circular stapler anvil inserted, stapler body through anus and tension-free anastomosis.

        (ii) Hand-sewn: 1-layer vs 2-layer.

    b. Testing of anastomosis: submerging under water, finger compression of bowel proximal to anastomosis, and insufflation of air through proctoscope.

Operative Techniques

(B) Hartmann: no reconstruction but end-colostomy

    c. Creation of end colostomy: site preferably marked preoperatively or by educated guess, maturing only after main incision closed.

    d. Closure of lateral aspect between ostomy-bearing segment and abdominal wall (to avoid internal wrapping of small bowel around that segment).

Both techniques

14. Drains according to surgeon's preference. No routine need for NGT (unless obstructed).

15. Closure of incision.

16. Maturation of ostomy (in case of Hartmann).

Anatomic Structures at Risk

Left ureter, gonadal vessels, hypogastric nerves.

Aftercare

Fast-track recovery: in absence of nausea or vomiting, oral liquids are started on POD1 and advanced as tolerated.

In case of Hartmann resection: planning of takedown after complete recovery.

Complications

Bleeding (surgeon-dependent): presacral veins, inadequate ligature of vascular stalk, gonadal vessels.

Anastomotic leak (2%): most commonly due to technical error, tension, inadequate blood supply.

Ureteral injury (0.1–0.2%).

Cross-reference

Topic	*Chapter*
LBO	1 (p 27), 4 (p 355)
Pain—abdominal	1 (p 35)
Colorectal cancer	4 (p 252)
Colonic volvulus	4 (p 364)
Diverticular disease	4 (p 368)
Colonoscopic stent placement	5 (p 585)
On-table lavage	5 (p 588)
Creation of end-ileostomy or -colostomy	5 (p 592)
Perioperative management—abdominal	7 (p 684)
Fast-track recovery	7 (p 714)

LEFT HEMICOLECTOMY *(OPEN)*

Principle

Oncologic resection of left colon with ligation of vascular pedicle and corresponding lymphadenectomy.

Setting

Inpatient, OR procedure.

Alternatives

Laparoscopic approach.

Extended right hemicolectomy (inclusion of both flexures, part of descending colon).

Subtotal or total colectomy (inclusion of part of or whole sigmoid colon).

Long Hartmann stump and end ileostomy.

Indication

Left-sided colon cancer/polyps (splenic flexure, descending colon).

Preparatory Considerations

Full colonic evaluation for all elective cases, tattooing of small lesions advisable.

Bowel cleansing (traditional) vs no bowel cleansing (evolving concept).

Ureteral stents for redo cases or extensive disruption of anatomy (eg, inflammation).

Marking of possible stoma sites.

Prophylactic antibiotics.

Surgical Steps

1. Patient position: modified lithotomy position (surgeon's preference).
2. Laparotomy: periumbilical midline incision.
3. Placement of abdominal wall retractor or wound protector vs dynamic abdominal wall retraction with hand-held retractor to expose right side of colon.
4. Abdominal exploration: local resectability, secondary pathology (liver/gallbladder, colon, female organs, small bowel), other abnormalities.
5. Defining resection margins: mid transverse colon (left branch of mid colic artery), splenic flexure, descending colon with/without inclusion of sigmoid colon (left colic artery only vs IMA).

6. Mobilization of left colon from its retroperitoneal attachments, starting at sigmoid along white line of Toldt, moving along colonic gutter to splenic flexure. Landmarks: ureter, gonadal vessels, omentum, spleen (avoid injury).

7. Development of lesser sac: oncologic resection requires at least half omentectomy—division of gastrocolic ligament in several steps (alternative in proven benign disease: omental sparing with dissection of omentum off the transverse colon).

8. Identification of left branch of mid colic artery.

9. Oncologic devascularization of left colon with clamping and transecting major vascular stalks (ligature, suture ligatures): either taking IMA at aortic run-off + vein at inferior edge of pancreas or taking only left colic artery while leaving superior hemorrhoidal artery. Caveat: before dividing tissue, remote location of ureters to be verified.

10. Transection of bowel colocolonic (sigmoid left) or colorectal (sigmoid taken) anastomosis: preferably end-to-end anastomosis (stapled vs hand-sewn); functional end-to-end (side-to-side) anastomosis suboptimal for left-sided colon because it results in "giant diverticulum," may cause constipation/stool trapping, and makes colonoscopy more difficult.

11. Resection of specimen and macroscopic assessment of specimen: verification of pathology and resection margins.

12. Oversewing of staple lines with interrupted sutures.

13. Closure of mesenteric window.

14. Drains not indicated (unless specific indication). No need for NGT.

15. Closure of incision.

Anatomic Structures at Risk

Left ureter, gonadal vessels, spleen, pancreas tail, mid colic artery.

Aftercare

Fast-track recovery: in absence of nausea or vomiting, oral liquids are started on POD1 and advanced as tolerated.

Complications

Bleeding (surgeon-dependent): traction on spleen, inadequate ligature of vascular stalk, mid colic artery.

Anastomotic leak (2%): most commonly due to technical error, tension, inadequate blood supply.

Ureteral injury (0.1–0.2%).

Cross-reference

Operative Techniques

RIGHT HEMICOLECTOMY *(OPEN)*

Principle

Oncologic resection of the right colon with ligation of the vascular pedicle and corresponding lymphadenectomy.

Setting

Inpatient, OR procedure.

Alternatives

Laparoscopic approach.

Extended right hemicolectomy (inclusion of distal transverse colon and splenic flexure).

Long Hartmann stump and end-ileostomy.

Indication

Right colon cancer, right-sided diverticulitis, cecal volvulus.

Preparatory Considerations

Full colonic evaluation for all elective cases, tattooing of small lesions is advisable.

Bowel cleansing (traditional) vs no bowel cleansing (evolving concept).

Ureteral stents for redo cases or extensive disruption of anatomy (eg, inflammation).

Marking of possible stoma sites.

Prophylactic antibiotics.

Surgical Steps

1. Patient position: supine or modified lithotomy position (surgeon's preference).
2. Laparotomy: periumbilical or epigastric midline, right transverse (from umbilicus), right subcostal incision.
3. Placement of abdominal wall retractor or wound protector vs dynamic abdominal wall retraction with hand-held retractor to expose right side of colon.
4. Abdominal exploration: local resectability, secondary pathology (liver/gallbladder, colon, female organs, small bowel), other abnormalities.
5. Defining resection margins:

    a. Cecum/ascending colon: right branch of mid colic artery.

    b. Hepatic flexure: extended right hemicolectomy.

6. Mobilization of right colon from its retroperitoneal attachments, starting at ileocecal junction, moving along colonic gutter to hepatic flexure. Landmarks: ureter, duodenum (avoid injury).

7. Development of lesser sac: oncologic resection requires at least half omentectomy—division of gastrocolic ligament in several steps (alternative in proven benign disease: omental sparing with dissection of omentum off he transverse colon).

8. Identification of ileocolic vascular stalk: becomes evident through slight traction of cecum to RLQ.

9. Oncologic devascularization of right colon with clamping and transecting major vascular stalks (ligature, suture ligatures). Before dividing tissue, remote location of ureters to be verified.

10. Stepwise continuation toward right branch of mid colic artery.

11. Transection and ileotransverse anastomosis may either be performed in individual steps or combined through one side-to-side linear stapler and one transverse closure/resection of specimen.

12. Macroscopic assessment of specimen: verification of pathology and resection margins.

13. Oversewing of staple lines with interrupted sutures.

14. Closure of mesenteric window.

15. Drains not indicated (unless specific indication). No need for NGT.

16. Closure of incision.

Anatomic Structures at Risk

Right ureter, duodenum, superior mesenteric vein, mid colic artery.

Aftercare

Fast-track recovery: in absence of nausea or vomiting, oral liquids are started on POD1 and advanced as tolerated.

Complications

Bleeding (surgeon-dependent): traction on superior mesenteric vein, inadequate ligature of vascular stalk, mid colic artery.

Anastomotic leak (2%): most commonly due to technical error, tension, inadequate blood supply.

Ureteral injury (0.1–0.2%).

Operative Techniques

Cross-reference

(SUB-)TOTAL COLECTOMY, ILEORECTAL ANASTOMOSIS *(OPEN)*

Principle

Resection of the whole (or most of the) colon while preserving the rectum (and a portion of the sigmoid colon) and avoiding pelvic dissection:

- Cancer/polyps: oncologic resection + reduction of mucosa at risk, facilitation of surveillance (flexible sigmoidoscopy in the office), acceptable bowel function.
- Slow-transit constipation: either total abdominal colectomy with IRA or subtotal colectomy with anastomosis to the mid sigmoid: too little → constipation; too much → 15% of unacceptable diarrhea.
- IBD: total abdominal colectomy with IRA in highly selected cases depending on circumstances (30–60% requiring later completion proctectomy).

Setting

Inpatient, OR procedure.

Alternatives

Laparoscopic approach.

Total abdominal colectomy with end-ileostomy.

Proctocolectomy with IPAA or end-ileostomy.

Indication

- HNPCC with colorectal cancer proximal to rectum.
- FAP and AFAP with relative rectal sparing (< 20 polyps in rectum).
- Multiple synchronous colon cancers and/or polyps.
- Treatment-refractory slow-transit constipation.
- Ulcerative colitis with relative rectal sparing and preserved rectal compliance.
- Crohn colitis: rectal sparing, good sphincter function, lack of active perianal manifestations.

Preparatory Considerations

Full colonic evaluation and histologic documentation for all elective cases, tattooing of most distal polyp site, rigid sigmoidoscopy to rule out rectal cancer.

Bowel cleansing (traditional) vs no bowel cleansing (evolving concept).

Ureteral stents for redo cases or extensive disruption of anatomy (eg, inflammation).

Marking of possible stoma sites.

Prophylactic antibiotics.

IBD cases: Anophysiology studies for rectal compliance; small bowel follow-through or CT enterography to rule out small bowel involvement, steroid stress dose (if needed), discontinuation of other immunosuppressives.

Surgical Steps

1. Patient position: modified lithotomy position.
2. Laparotomy:
   a. Periumbilical or lower midline: infraumbilical incision sufficient if stomach can be reached, otherwise extension above umbilicus.
   b. Alternative access: transverse suprapubic (transection of rectus muscle), Pfannenstiel incision (transverse incision to skin and anterior rectus sheath with midline rectus-saving celiotomy).
3. Dynamic abdominal wall retraction to expose right side, then left side of colon.
4. Abdominal exploration: local resectability, secondary pathology (liver/gallbladder, colon, female organs, small bowel), other abnormalities.
5. Defining distal resection margin:
   a. Total abdominal colectomy: upper rectum (confluence of teniae).
   b. Subtotal colectomy (HNPCC, slow-transit constipation): sigmoid colon, ie, either proximal sigmoid or where most distal polyp tattooed (HNPCC), or mid sigmoid colon (slow-transit constipation).
6. Mobilization of right colon from its retroperitoneal attachments, starting at ileocecal junction, moving along colonic gutter to hepatic flexure. Landmarks: ureter, duodenum (avoid injury).
7. Development of lesser sac: oncologic resection requires at least half omentectomy on side of tumor: division of gastrocolic ligament in several steps (alternative in proven benign disease: omentum-sparing, ie, dissection of omentum off transverse colon).
8. Retrograde dissection from sigmoid toward splenic flexure along white line of Toldt. Opening of retroperitoneum, identification of areolar tissue. Firm pressure against sigmoid mesentery to bluntly reflect retroperitoneal tissues and expose left ureter. Incision of peritoneum is continued into pelvis.
9. Completion of splenic flexure mobilization by retraction of distal transverse and proximal descending colon and conjoining the two in stepwise ligation. Avoid splenic tear.
10. Once retroperitoneal mobilization is complete from ileum to sigmoid:

stepwise devascularization of colon with clamping and transecting of major vascular stalks (ligature, suture ligatures). Before dividing tissue, remote location of ureters to be verified.

11. Transection of terminal ileum with 75-mm linear stapler.

12. Distal resection point: stepwise division of mesentery or mesorectum between clamps and ligatures.

13. Transection at distal resection point: depending on exposure and mobility either with reload of 75-mm linear stapler or transverse cutter/stapler.

14. Removal of complete specimen, macroscopic examination: confirm diagnosis. Frozen sections if uncertain pathology or margin.

15. (A) Stapled end-to-end ileorectal anastomosis (IRA) or ileosigmoidal anastomosis (ISA): purse-string (hand-sewn, device with Keith needle, or all-in-one device). Insertion of largest possible circular stapler anvil. Insertion of stapler through anus and tension-free anastomosis. Assessment of donut completeness.

   (B) Functional end-to-end ISA: parallel alignment of distal ileum and mid sigmoid. Small antimesenteric enterotomy on both sides, insertion of 75-mm linear stapling device. Closure of residual opening: hand-sewn, reload of linear stapler, transverse (cutting) stapler.

16. Testing of anastomosis: submerging under water, finger compression of bowel proximal to anastomosis, and insufflation of air through proctoscope.

17. Drains or NGT commonly not needed.

18. Closure of laparotomy incision.

Anatomic Structures at Risk

Both ureters, duodenum, spleen, mesenteric blood supply, gonadal vessels.

Aftercare

Fast-track recovery: in absence of nausea or vomiting, oral liquids are started on POD1 and advanced as tolerated. Steroid taper if needed.

Complications

Bleeding (surgeon-dependent): inadequate ligature of vascular stalks, splenic tear, gonadal vessels.

Anastomotic leak (2%): most commonly due to technical error, tension, inadequate blood supply, high-dose steroids, malnutrition.

Ureteral injury (0.1–0.2%).

Cross-reference

TOTAL ABDOMINAL COLECTOMY WITH END-ILEOSTOMY *(OPEN)*

Principle

The operation of choice for all nonelective cases of colitis regardless of underlying etiology (IBD, infectious, ischemic, etc): ie, (emergency) resection of the whole colon while preserving the rectum and avoiding complex pelvic dissection. This approach is fast, eliminates the majority of diseased bowel, avoids anastomosis, avoids difficult pelvic dissection, and preserves pelvic space for later reconstruction, ie, "it does not burn any bridges."

Setting

Inpatient, OR procedure.

Alternatives

Proctocolectomy with IPAA or end-ileostomy.

Total colectomy with end-ileostomy and distal mucous fistula.

Turnbull blowholes: only extremely rarely indicated.

Indication

- Fulminant colitis or toxic megacolon.
- Colitis with complication, eg, spontaneous or iatrogenic perforation.
- Colitis with severe malnutrition.
- Treatment with high-dose steroids, possibly with infliximab.
- Smoldering *C difficile* colitis, refractory to conservative treatment.

Preparatory Considerations

Toxic patient: short-term adequate resuscitation and monitoring.

All others: worsening or lack of improvement within 72 hours of optimal medical management, advance definition by involved teams of deadline and criteria when to declare failure of conservative treatment.

Marking of possible stoma sites: may be impossible in emergency setting and severe abdominal distention.

Therapeutic antibiotics, possibly steroid stress dose.

Surgical Steps

1. Patient position: modified lithotomy or supine position.
2. Long midline laparotomy: good exposure needed, distended/diseased bowels often friable and not tolerating any traction (risk of perforation).

3. Installation of abdominal wall retractor to expose whole abdomen.

4. Quick gentle abdominal exploration: additional pathology (liver/gallbladder, colon, female organs, small bowel), other abnormalities.

5. Mobilization of right colon from its retroperitoneal attachments, starting at ileocecal junction, moving along colonic gutter to hepatic flexure. Landmarks: ureter, duodenum (avoid injury).

6. Entry into lesser sac and division of gastrocolic ligament in several steps (alternative: omentum-sparing, ie, more time-consuming dissection of omentum off transverse colon).

7. Retrograde dissection from sigmoid toward splenic flexure along white line of Toldt. Opening of retroperitoneum, identification of areolar tissue. Firm pressure against sigmoid mesentery to bluntly reflect retroperitoneal tissues and expose left ureter. Incision of peritoneum is continued into pelvis.

8. Completion of mobilization of splenic flexure by retraction of distal transverse and proximal descending colon and conjoining the two in stepwise ligation. Avoid splenic tear.

9. Once retroperitoneal mobilization is complete from ileum to sigmoid: stepwise devascularization of colon with clamping and transecting major vascular stalks (suture ligatures). Before dividing tissue, remote location of ureters to be verified.

10. Transection of terminal ileum with 75-mm linear stapler.

11. Distal resection point: stepwise division of mesentery or mesorectum between clamps and ligatures.

12. Transection at distal resection point either with reload of 75-mm linear stapler or transverse cutter/stapler: depending on tissue quality: higher risk of stapling failure, need for hand-sewn closure of distal stump (or creation of mucous fistula).

13. Careful removal of complete specimen, macroscopic examination: confirm diagnosis. Frozen sections if uncertain pathology or margin.

14. Marking of rectal stump with long nonabsorbable colored monofilament suture (for later identification).

15. Creation of end ileostomy. Excision of skin disk at preoperatively marked site for ileostomy. Dissection of fat, incision of anterior rectus sheath, splitting of muscle to create gap. Small bowel loop carried through abdominal wall.

16. Closure of the laparotomy incision.

17. Maturation of ileostomy to 3 cm nipple. Appliance.

18. Washout of rectal stump with povidone-iodine, temporary rectal drain placement (to avoid rectal blow-out).

Anatomic Structures at Risk

Both ureters, duodenum, spleen, mesenteric blood supply, gonadal vessels.

Aftercare

ICU monitoring and stabilization. Extubation per respiratory and hemodynamic parameters.

Intestinal recovery: in absence of nausea/vomiting (extubated patient) or lack of residuals in NGT → start liquids by mouth or via enteral feeding tube, advance as tolerated.

Therapeutic antibiotics.

Steroid taper if needed.

Ileostomy takedown > 3–6 months when patient nutritionally and physically recovered and if steroids tapered off.

Complications

Bleeding (surgeon-dependent): inadequate ligature of vascular stalks, splenic tear, gonadal vessels.

Ongoing infection, sepsis, ARDS, multiorgan system failure, death.

Rectal blow-out.

Ureteral injury (0.1–0.2%).

Cross-reference

Operative Techniques

PROCTOCOLECTOMY, ILEAL J-POUCH ANAL ANASTOMOSIS *(OPEN)*

Principle

Restorative proctocolectomy: oncologic resection of the whole colon and rectum with a restorative ileoanal pull-through procedure, ie, creation of a new storage area (Figures 5–12A and 5–12B).

- Two-stage: with temporary ileostomy.
- One-stage: without ileostomy possible if technically perfect and no malnutrition or high-dose steroids

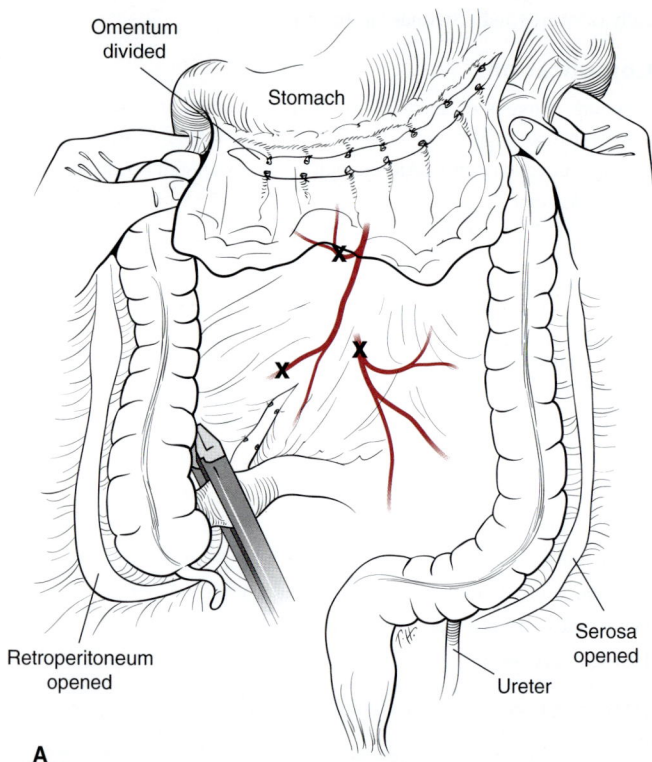

A

Figure 5–12A. Proctocolectomy: mobilization of the colon.

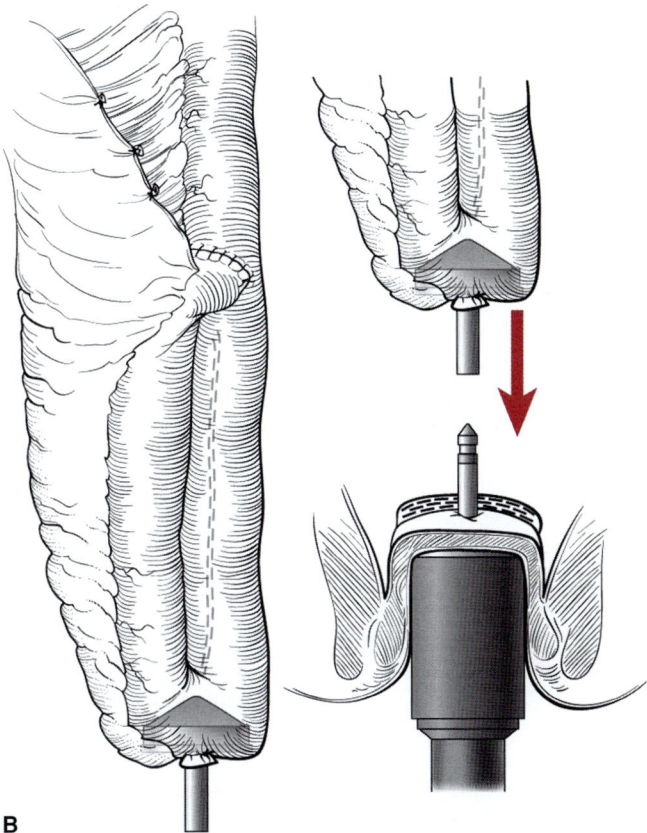

B

Figure 5–12B. Ileal J-pouch anal anastomosis.

Setting

Inpatient, OR procedure.

Alternatives

Laparoscopic approach.

Proctocolectomy with permanent ileostomy.

Indication

- Ulcerative colitis (except fulminant colitis).
- FAP.
- Rarely: multiple synchronous cancers and/or polyps.
- Crohn colitis: ileoanal pull-through procedure may be considered if there is no evidence of small bowel disease or perianal manifestations.

Preparatory Considerations

Full colonic evaluation and histologic documentation for all elective cases, rigid sigmoidoscopy to rule out rectal cancer.

Small bowel follow-through or CT enterography to rule out small bowel involvement.

Bowel cleansing (traditional) vs no bowel cleansing (evolving concept).

Ureteral stents for redo cases or extensive disruption of anatomy (eg, inflammation).

Marking of possible stoma sites.

Steroid stress dose, discontinuation of other immunosuppressives. Prophylactic antibiotics.

Surgical Steps

1. Patient position: modified lithotomy position.
2. Laparotomy:
   a. Lower midline: infraumbilical incision sufficient if stomach can be reached, otherwise extension above umbilicus.
   b. Alternative access: transverse suprapubic (transection of rectus muscle), Pfannenstiel incision (transverse incision to skin and anterior rectus sheath with midline rectus-saving celiotomy).
3. Dynamic abdominal wall retraction to expose right side, then left side of colon.
4. Abdominal exploration: small bowel (evidence of Crohn disease?), liver (PSC cirrhosis, gallstones?), colon (mass, covered perforation?), other abnormalities.
5. Mobilization of right colon from its retroperitoneal attachments, starting at ileocecal junction, moving along colonic gutter to the hepatic flexure. Landmarks: ureter, duodenum (avoid injury): Figure 5–12A.
6. Development of lesser sac: either dissection of omentum off transverse colon (omentum sparing), or division of gastrocolic ligament in several steps (resection of omentum).

7. Retrograde dissection from sigmoid towards splenic flexure along white line of Toldt. Opening of retroperitoneum, identification of areolar tissue. Firm pressure against sigmoid mesentery to bluntly reflect retroperitoneal tissues and expose left ureter. Incision of peritoneum is continued into pelvis.

8. Completion of mobilization of splenic flexure by retraction of distal transverse and proximal descending colon and conjoining the two in stepwise ligation (Figure 5–12A). Avoid splenic tear.

9. Once retroperitoneal mobilization is complete from ileum to sigmoid: stepwise devascularization of colon with clamping and transecting of major vascular stalks (ligature, suture ligatures). Before dividing tissue, remote location of ureters to be verified.

10. Transection of terminal ileum with 75-mm linear stapler.

11. Installation of abdominal wall retractor (eg, Bookwalter retractor) for pelvic dissection.

12. Continuation of serosal incision on both sides of mesosigmoid toward peritoneal reflection.

13. Developing avascular plane posterior to superior hemorrhoidal vessels but anterior to hypogastric nerve plexus leads to avascular plane anterior to Waldeyer fascia. Continuation of nerve-sparing dissection under direct visualization, no blunt dissection (avoid presacral veins!).

14. Sharp anterior and lateral dissection all the way to pelvic floor, identification of seminal vesicles (males), careful dissection of rectovaginal plane (females).

15. (A) Double-stapling technique: transection of distal rectum at puborectalis muscle, ie, ~2–3 cm proximal to dentate line with transverse linear stapler/cutter.

    (B) Hand-sewn technique: switch to perineal approach, installation of Lone Star retractor, incision of mucosa at dentate line, and mucosectomy up to puborectalis muscle where connection is made to presacral space.

16. Removal of complete specimen, macroscopic examination: confirm diagnosis. Frozen sections of margins in case of cancer.

17. Creation of pouch (Figure 5–12B): folding of distal ileum, apical enterotomy. Firing of 2–2$\frac{1}{2}$ cartridges of 75-cm linear stapler to create ~12 cm pouch. Free end of J to be shortened flush to inlet, approximated to afferent limb with a series of interrupted sutures.

18. (A) Stapled ileoanal anastomosis (Figure 5–12B): purse-string suture to apical enterotomy and insertion of largest possible circular stapler

anvil. Insertion of stapler through anus and tension-free anastomosis. Assessment of donuts and digital assessment of anastomosis.

(B) Hand-sewn ileoanal anastomosis: switch to perineal approach, guiding Babcock clamp through anus to grasp tip of pouch, pulling through and fixation with six seromuscular anchoring stitches, maturing mucosal junction. Removal of retractor.

19. Presacral drains according to surgeon's preference. No need for NGT.

20. For two-stage procedure: creation of loop ileostomy. Excision of skin disk at preoperatively marked site for ileostomy. Dissection of fat, incision of anterior rectus sheath, splitting of muscle to create gap. Small bowel loop (distal limb marked) wrapped with Seprafilm and carried through abdominal wall.

21. Closure of the laparotomy incision.

22. Maturation of loop ileostomy to 3 cm nipple. Appliance.

Anatomic Structures at Risk

Both ureters, duodenum, spleen, mesenteric blood supply, gonadal vessels, hypogastric nerves, presacral vein plexus, posterior vaginal wall.

Aftercare

Fast-track recovery: in absence of nausea or vomiting, oral liquids are started on POD1 and advanced as tolerated. Steroid taper if needed. Ileostomy takedown > 6 weeks if clinical/radiologic evidence that pouch is healed, and if steroids are tapered off.

Complications

Bleeding (surgeon-dependent): presacral veins, inadequate ligature of vascular stalks, splenic tear, gonadal vessels.

Anastomotic leak (4–10%): most commonly due to technical error, tension, inadequate blood supply, high-dose steroids, malnutrition.

Pouch-anal stricture (10–14%).

Ileoanal dysfunction.

Sexual dysfunction (1–3%) and infertility (25–40%).

Ureteral injury (0.1–0.2%).

Cross-reference

Operative Techniques

MUCOSECTOMY OF ANAL TRANSITIONAL ZONE *(ATZ)*

Principle

Elective excision of the residual ATZ cuff in patients with status post-ileoanal reconstruction in double-stapling technique for ulcerative colitis. The pouch is advanced and sutured to the dentate line. Despite some inflammatory changes in the ATZ in the majority of patients, only a minority requires excision (highly symptomatic, dysplasia).

Setting

Inpatient (selected outpatient?), OR procedure.

Alternatives

Conservative treatment of pouchitis or cuffitis.

Major revision or removal of ileoanal pouch.

Indication

- ATZ cuffitis.
- Ileoanal dysfunction (uncertain whether pouchitis or cuffitis): elimination of variable.
- ATZ dysplasia.

Preparatory Considerations

Bowel cleansing: stay on clear liquids the day before, two Fleet enemas prior to procedure.

Prophylactic antibiotics.

Surgical Steps

1. Patient positioning: any position, but prone jackknife position with buttocks taped aside has several advantages—superior view with comfortable access for surgeon/assistant, decreased vascular congestion.
2. Pudendal/perianal nerve block with 15–20 cc of local anesthetic in addition to general anesthesia to improve relaxation of anal sphincter muscles.
3. Placement of Lone Star retractor.
4. Incision of mucosa right at dentate line and circumferential dissection and mobilization of mucosa.
5. Continuation until stapled anastomosis reached.

6. Placement of full-thickness holding sutures to pouch proximal to staple line.

7. Resection of mucosa.

8. Placement of 4–8 full-thickness absorbable sutures from end of pouch to dentate line, consecutive tying.

9. Maturing of mucosa.

10. Removal of Lone Star retractor.

Anatomic Structures at Risk

Sphincter complex, pouch, rectovaginal septum.

Aftercare

Regular diet as tolerated 6 hours postanesthesia. Maintenance of soft stools (fibers, antidiarrheal medication, etc) as before the surgery.

Zinc-oxide based barrier cream regularly to perianal skin.

Complications

Bleeding (surgeon-dependent).

Infection, abscess/fistula formation.

Anastomotic dehiscence.

Stricture formation.

Formation of rectovaginal fistula → need for colostomy.

Worsening fecal incontinence.

Cross-reference

Operative Techniques

STRICTUROPLASTY

Principle

Restitution of unobstructed intestinal passage for symptomatic solitary or multisegmental strictures without bowel resection to minimize the risk of immediate or long-term short-bowel syndrome. The typical scenario is for Crohn disease or recurrent adhesions. In the presence of multiple strictures, different techniques may have to be employed during the same procedure.

Setting

Inpatient, OR procedure.

Alternatives

Laparoscopic-assisted approach.

Segmental resection.

Indication

• Crohn disease with symptomatic stricture(s).

• Adhesions with symptomatic stricture(s).

Preparatory Considerations

Small bowel evaluation: small bowel follow-through, CT enterography.

Evaluation of distal bowel to rule out hidden sites of obstruction.

Bowel cleansing if tolerated.

Suppression of disease activity (eg, infliximab → 4–6-week interruption prior to elective surgery).

Steroid stress dose?

Surgical Steps

1. Patient position: supine position (alternative: modified lithotomy).
2. Laparotomy, lysis of adhesions and assessment of entire intestines to define target lesions.
3. Assessment of hidden strictures: running marble (or artificial eye ball) via enterotomy through intestines.

(A) Heinecke-Mikulicz stricturoplasty for for short-segment stricture
4. Placement of holding sutures on both sides of stricture: not proximal/distal but along circumference.
5. Longitudinal antimesenteric incision of bowel through strictured area.
6. Lateral traction on holding sutures and transverse closure of enterotomy.

(B) Finney stricturoplasty for long-segment stricture (risk: creation of large atonic pocket)

4. Longitudinal antimesenteric incision of bowel through whole length of strictured area.

5. Folding of opened bowel: may be difficult in indurated, thickened/fore-shortened mesentery/bowel.

6. Closure of posterior bowel wall with continuation toward anterior wall.

(C) Isoperistaltic side-to-side stricturoplasty for very long or multisegmental strictures

4. Mobilization/division of mesentery at midpoint of diseased segment and transection of bowel.

5. Moving of two ends alongside in side-to-side fashion (for as much as 30–40 cm).

6. Approximation of two loops with interrupted seromuscular sutures.

7. Longitudinal antimesenteric enterotomy on both loops, spatulation of intestinal ends to avoid blind stumps.

8. If suspicious areas of disease: biopsy and frozen sections of to rule out malignancy.

9. Two-layer closure of two bowel segments.

Anatomic Structures at Risk

Small bowel mesentery.

Aftercare

Fast-track recovery: in absence of nausea or vomiting, oral liquids are started on POD1 and advanced as tolerated.

Complications

Bleeding (surgeon-dependent), tearing of mesentery, anastomotic leak, recurrent stricture.

Cross-reference

Topic	*Chapter*
IBD—Crohn disease	4 (p 327)
Creation of ileostomy	5 (pp 592, 596)
Medical management of Crohn disease	6 (p 672)
Perioperative management—abdominal	7 (p 684)
Fast-track recovery	7 (p 714)

Operative Techniques

ADHESIOLYSIS *(LAPAROSCOPIC VS OPEN)*

Principle

Laparoscopic vs open lysis of peritoneal adhesions, either as independent procedure or as part of larger operation. Adhesions are common after previous abdominal procedures and may result in acute or recurrent SBOs, recurrent/chronic abdominal pain, infertility, and difficult reoperative surgery. Whether a procedure is started laparoscopically or open should be based on the surgeon's personal knowledge of an individual's extent of adhesions and the current extent of abdominal distention.

Setting

Inpatient, OR procedure.

Alternatives

Conservative management.

Indication

- Complete SBO.
- Acute nonresolving partial SBO.
- Recurrent SBOs (elective setting).

Caveat: pain alone is usually not a sufficient indication for surgery and has a high likelihood of failure.

Preparatory Considerations

All
- Prophylactic antibiotics.
- Consenting process: making sure that patient understands that there is potential risk of an ostomy.

Emergency
- Fluid resuscitation
- NGT decompression.

(Semi-)Elective
- Full colonic evaluation (barium enema vs colonoscopy) to rule out colonic site of obstruction.
- Full bowel cleansing.

Surgical Steps

1. Patient position: modified lithotomy position, beanbag, strapped to table, both arms tucked.

   a. Laparoscopic: initial laparoscopic port placement in Hasson technique off previous scars—eg, midclavicular line at level of umbilicus; camera insertion and assessment of density of adhesions—camera lysis until sufficient space is developed to insert 2nd/3rd port above and below also on midclavicular line under direct visual control. If adhesions are too dense or space too limited—conversion to open procedure.

   b. Open: access through previous scar or new incision if it will provide better exposure; avoid electrocautery entry until confirmed that no bowel loops are attached underneath fascia.

2. Takedown of adhesions with ultrasonic shears, scissors, careful wiping: extreme care has to be taken (a) to improve and maintain good visibility and (b) to avoid enterotomy; if adhesions are very dense: use of saline injection to develop plane between loops of bowel.

3. If enterotomy/ies have occurred → always repair immediately to minimize risk of leaving enterotomy unclosed.

4. Definition of surgical goals:

   a. Identification of transition point → local lysis, possible resection/anastomosis.

   b. Running whole small bowel → freeing up of adhesions.

   c. Laparoscopy: adequate visibility and progress with time if (1) adhesions too dense, (2) bowel too distended, or (3) for other reasons no progress is made → conversion to open procedure.

5. After completion of mobilization: assessment of situation and appropriate resolution of problem areas; limited resection/anastomosis, bypass, ostomy, etc.

6. Reevaluation of peritoneal cavity and running of whole small bowel to check for and repair possible enterotomies.

7. Port removal and/or closure of abdominal incisions.

Anatomic Structures at Risk

Enterotomies.

Aftercare

Fast-track recovery: in absence of nausea or vomiting, oral liquids are started on POD1 and advanced as tolerated. Continuation of NGT decompression if bowels are very distended or if extensive adhesiolysis.

Operative Techniques

Complications

Bleeding (surgeon-dependent), anastomotic leak 1–3% ($\rightarrow$ abscess or enterocutaneous fistula formation), SBO up to 25%.

Cross-reference

LAPAROSCOPIC COLORECTAL SURGERY

Principle

Laparoscopic surgery—once a rarity and exceptional approach—has become an established and accepted standard approach for almost any abdominal problem. With a generation of surgeons who were brought up with laparoscopy as a routine component of their training and more sophisticated tools, there are virtually no contraindications anymore. Even for colon cancer, at least equivalency in oncologic outcomes has been documented after selected procedures. The only exception is rectal cancer where data are still inadequate and to some degree of concern (higher risk of positive radial margins).

- The laparoscopic approach should satisfy exactly the same principles as an open procedure but be even more meticulous about maintaining hemostasis. One approach is to laparoscopically follow the same steps with lateral mobilization, followed by vascular transection (lateral-to-medial approach). Because of the limited space and to take advantage of lateral attachments for retraction, however, the opposite direction may be chosen for the dissection, ie, medial-to-lateral approach.

- The technique may be straight laparoscopically, hand-assisted laparoscopic surgery, or a hybrid surgery (eg, laparoscopic mobilization of splenic flexure, open LAR).

- Conversion rates are irrelevant (except from a financial standpoint); they are not a measure of quality.

- Beginners should start with easy cases: eg, creation of colostomy, or skinny patient with palliative segmental sigmoid resection for cancer. Diverticulitis (even though a benign condition) may occasionally be extremely challenging.

Setting

Inpatient, OR procedure.

Alternatives

Open approach.

Indication

- Novice: laparoscopic creation of colostomy, sigmoid resection, ileocecal resection, right hemicolectomy.

- Advanced: left hemicolectomy, resections involving mid colic artery (eg, extended right hemicolectomy), subtotal colectomy, Hartmann reversal, rectopexy.

- Experts only: proctocolectomy, rectal dissection.

Operative Techniques

Preparatory Considerations

Identical to open procedures.

Specifically for laparoscopic approach:

- Tattooing of lesions for intraoperative identification.
- Avoidance of colonoscopy immediately prior to procedure (because gas-filled bowels limit the view).

Instrumentation:

- 5- and 10–12-mm ports (check with diameter of stapling device).
- Laparoscope, 1–2 insufflators.
- Atraumatic graspers, Babcocks, needle drivers, scissors, anvil grasper.
- Suction/irrigation device.
- Energy ligation device (eg, ultrasonic shears), clip applier, laparoscopic roticulating linear stapling devices.
- Wound protector, hand-assist port.
- Open instruments and staplers.

Surgical Steps

1. Patient position: lesion on left side → modified lithotomy position; lesion on right side → supine or modified lithotomy. Patient tightly secured on the table (eg, beanbag, tapes), both arms tucked, hips straight or in 0–10 degrees of flexion: "flight test" prior to draping—patient placed in extreme Trendelenburg and lateral position to verify adequate stabilization.

2. Equipment position such that surgeon, pathology, and monitor all are in line; adequate monitor position for assistants.

3. Access:

   a. Open Hasson technique.

   b. Alternative: Veress needle technique + optical port—if no previous laparotomies.

4. Visualization and placement of working ports under visual guidance.

(A1) Right lateral-to-medial approach

5. Mobilization of right colon from its retroperitoneal attachments, starting at ileocecal junction, moving along colonic gutter to hepatic flexure. Landmarks: ureter, duodenum (avoid injury).

6. Development of lesser sac: either dissection of omentum off transverse colon (omentum sparing), or division of gastrocolic ligament in several steps (resection of omentum).

7. Elevation of cecum and identification of ileocolic vascular stalk. Creation of window and clipping/division of individual vessels or stapling/cutting of whole stalk.

8. Enlargement of umbilical port to 4 cm, placement of wound protector, delivery of mobilized colon.

9. Open completion of mobilization of ileal mesentery.

10. Functional end-to-end anastomosis with total of two stapler cartridges. Closure of mesenteric gap.

11. Closure of incision and ports.

(A2) Right medial-to-lateral approach

5. Elevation of cecum and identification of ileocolic vascular stalk. Creation of window with clipping/division of individual vessels or stapling/cutting of whole stalk.

6. Retroperitoneal mobilization in avascular plane up to duodenum/pancreas, mobilization of hepatic flexure from underneath.

7. Development of lesser sac: either dissection of omentum off transverse colon (omentum sparing), or division of gastrocolic ligament in several steps (resection of omentum).

8. Mobilization of remaining hepatic flexure and lateral colon attachments, free ileal mesentery.

9. Enlargement of umbilical port to 4 cm, placement of wound protector, delivery of mobilized colon.

10. Open completion of mobilization of ileal mesentery.

11. Functional end-to-end anastomosis with total of two stapler cartridges. Closure of mesenteric gap.

12. Closure of the incision and ports.

(B1) Left lateral-to-medial approach

5. Mobilization of left colon from its retroperitoneal attachments: incision of white line of Toldt at sigmoid colon junction, moving along colonic gutter to splenic flexure. Landmarks: ureter, gonadal vessels (avoid injury).

6. Development of lesser sac: either dissection of omentum off transverse colon (omentum sparing), or division of gastrocolic ligament in several steps (resection of omentum).

7. Complete mobilization of splenic flexure.

8. Elevation of sigmoid colon and identification of vascular stalk. Creation of window: verification of ureter in remote location, clipping/division of individual vessels or stapling/cutting of whole stalk: IMA/IMV (at origin) vs superior hemorrhoidal stalk.

Operative Techniques

9. Continuation of serosal incision on both sides of mesosigmoid toward peritoneal reflection.

10. Blunt dissection behind vascular stalk (avascular plane) to entry of pelvis.

11. Creation of window in mesorectum at distal point of resection. Division of bowel by means of reticulating linear stapler (as many firings as needed). Division of mesorectum with energy ligation device.

12. Enlargement of umbilical port to 4 cm, placement of wound protector, delivery of mobilized colon.

13. Open completion of mobilization of proximal colon mesentery and bowel resection.

14. Purse-string suture to proximal end and insertion of circular stapler anvil.

15. Bowel returned to abdomen, sealing of wound protector and reinsufflation.

16. Anvil grasper to anvil and controlled anastomosis under direct visual control.

17. Testing of anastomosis: submerging under water, finger compression of bowel proximal to anastomosis, and insufflation of air through proctoscope—oversewing and retesting if needed (laparoscopic suturing skills).

18. Drains according to surgeon's preference. No need for NGT.

19. Closure of incision and ports.

(B2) Left medial-to-lateral approach

5. Elevation of sigmoid colon and identification of vascular stalk. Incision of serosa and creation of window: identification of ureter, followed by clipping/division of individual vessels or stapling/cutting of whole stalk after verifying ureter in remote location: IMA/IMV (at origin) vs superior hemorrhoidal stalk.

6. Retroperitoneal mobilization in avascular plane up to pancreas, mobilization of splenic flexure from underneath.

7. Development of lesser sac: either dissection of omentum off transverse colon (omentum sparing), or division of gastrocolic ligament in several steps (resection of omentum).

8. Completion of mobilization of splenic flexure and left colon from its retroperitoneal attachments.

9. Continuation of serosal incision on both sides of mesosigmoid toward peritoneal reflection.

10. Blunt dissection behind vascular stalk (avascular plane) to entry of pelvis.

11. Creation of window in mesorectum at distal point of resection. Division of bowel by means of reticulating linear stapler (as many firings as needed). Division of mesorectum with energy ligation device.

12. Enlargement of umbilical port to 4 cm, placement of wound protector, delivery of mobilized colon.

13. Open completion of mobilization of proximal colon mesentery and bowel resection.

14. Purse-string suture to proximal end and insertion of circular stapler anvil.

15. Bowel returned to abdomen, sealing of wound protector, reinsufflation.

16. Anvil grasper to anvil and controlled anastomosis under direct visual control.

17. Testing of anastomosis: submerging under water, finger compression of bowel proximal to anastomosis, and insufflation of air through proctoscope—oversewing and retesting if needed (laparoscopic suturing skills).

18. Drains according to surgeon's preference. No need for NGT.

19. Closure of incision and ports.

Anatomic Structures at Risk

Ureters, duodenum, pancreas, gonadal vessels, hypogastric nerves, fascial planes, presacral vein plexus.

Aftercare

Fast-track recovery: in absence of nausea or vomiting start of liquids on POD1, rapidly advance as tolerated.

Complications

Trocar injuries, injuries related to manipulation of small bowel or colon, collateral injuries (ureter, iliac vessels).

Conversion to open procedure is not a complication, but good judgment if lack of adequate view or progress.

Cross-reference

Topic	*Chapter*
Rectopexy—laparoscopic vs open	5 (p 536)
Sigmoid resection	5 (p 544)

Operative Techniques

LAPAROSCOPIC PORT PLACEMENT

Principle

Adequate laparoscopic exposure and surgery depends on rational placement of the ports. If there is a need to reestablish tactile sensation, insertion of a hand-port may facilitate and speed up the dissection.

- Number of ports is irrelevant: place as many as needed to have good retraction.
- Umbilicus: the mere fact that there is that anatomic structure in the center of the abdomen by no means mandates its use as a port site; it is often better to locate the port at more of a distance.
- Plan ports such that working instruments do not get into each other's way: use a semi-circle with target as the center. Retraction ports may be off that circle.
- Hand-port: select a location not too close to target but "wrist-to-fingertip" distance away from it; place such that the remaining bowel end will reach.
- Closure of ports: anything ≥ 10 mm.

Examples

(A1) Right hemicolectomy (Figure 5–13A)
1. Supraumbilical optical port → later enlargement for specimen delivery.
2. RLQ midclavicular line working port.
3. LUQ midclavicular line working port.
4. Additional ports: right side, level of umbilicus.

(A2) Right hemicolectomy
1. Supraumbilical hand-port → specimen delivery.
2. RUQ camera port.
3. RLQ working port.
4. LUQ midclavicular line working port.
5. Additional ports: LLQ.

(A3) Right hemicolectomy
1. Suprapubic Pfannenstiel incision for hand port → specimen delivery.
2. Umbilical optical port.
3. LUQ midclavicular line working port.

4. LLQ working port.

5. Additional ports: RLQ.

(B1) Sigmoid colectomy
1. Infraumbilical optical port → later enlargement for specimen delivery.

2. RLQ midclavicular line working port.

3. LLQ midclavicular line working port.

4. Additional ports: right side level of umbilicus, suprapubic.

(B2) Sigmoid colectomy
1. Periumbilical hand port → specimen delivery.

2. RLQ midclavicular line optical port.

3. LLQ midclavicular line working port.

4. RLQ working port.

5. Additional ports: suprapubic port.

(C1) Left hemicolectomy (Figure 5–13B)
1. Infraumbilical optical port → enlargement for specimen delivery.

2. RLQ midclavicular line working port.

3. RUQ midclavicular line working port.

4. LLQ midclavicular line working port.

5. Additional ports: right side, level of umbilicus.

(C2) Left hemicolectomy
1. Periumbilical hand port → specimen delivery.

2. RUQ working port.

3. LLQ working port.

4. RLQ working port.

5. Additional ports: suprapubic port.

(C3) Left hemicolectomy
1. Suprapubic Pfannenstiel incision for hand port → specimen delivery.

2. Umbilical optical port.

3. RLQ working port.

4. LLQ working port.

5. Additional ports: RUQ.

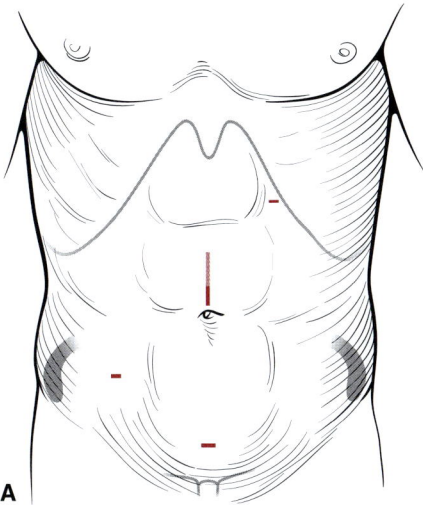

Figure 5–13A. Laparoscopic port placement: right hemicolectomy.

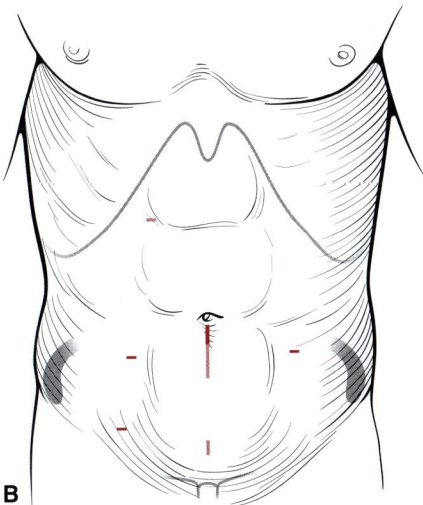

Figure 5–13B. Laparoscopic port placement: left hemicolectomy.

(D1) Subtotal colectomy/proctocolectomy

1. Infraumbilical optical port → later enlargement for specimen delivery.

2. RLQ working port.

3. LLQ working port.

4. RUQ working port.

5. LUQ working port.

(D2) Subtotal colectomy/proctocolectomy

1. Supraumbilical optical port.

2. Right umbilical line working port.

3. Left umbilical line working port.

4. Suprapubic working port → later enlargement for specimen delivery.

(D3) Subtotal colectomy/proctocolectomy

1. Periumbilical hand port → specimen delivery.

2. RUQ working port.

3. LLQ working port.

4. RLQ working port.

5. Additional ports: suprapubic port.

(D4) Subtotal colectomy/proctocolectomy

1. Suprapubic Pfannenstiel incision for hand port → specimen delivery.

2. Umbilical optical port.

3. Right umbilical line working port.

4. Left umbilical line working port.

5. Additional ports: epigastric.

(E) Hartmann reversal (Figure 5–13C)

1. Right umbilical line optical port (away from midline).

2. RUQ midclavicular line working port → free adhesions.

3. RLQ midclavicular line working port → free adhesions.

4. Additional ports: midline (after takedown of adhesions), at colostomy site.

(F) Rectopexy (Figure 5–13D)

1. Infraumbilical optical port.

2. RLQ midclavicular line working port.

3. LLQ midclavicular line working port.

4. Additional ports: suprapubic.

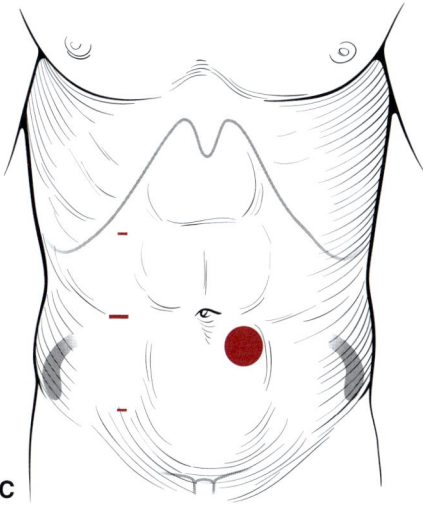

Figure 5–13C. Laparoscopic port placement: laparoscopic Hartman reversal.

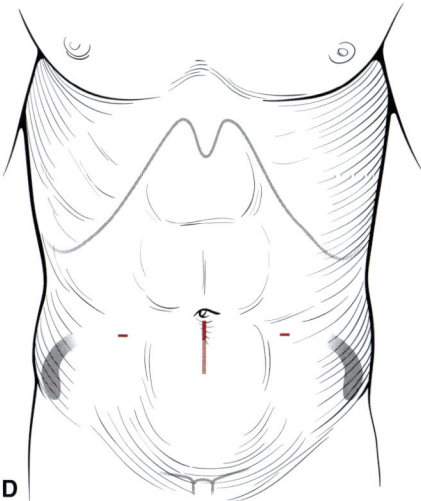

Figure 5–13D. Laparoscopic port placement: laparoscopic rectopexy.

Anatomic Structures at Risk

Epigastric vessels, falciform ligament, bowel, parenchymatous organs, major vessels.

Cross-reference

COLONOSCOPIC STENT PLACEMENT

Principle

Colonoscopic insertion of a self-expandable metallic stent to reopen a LBO, either as a bridge to a definitive resection or as palliation only. Successful decompression converts an emergency situation into a (semi-)elective one and allows for patient recovery, normalization of fluid and electrolyte imbalances, medical tune-up, bowel cleansing, and colonic clearance, and hence reduces the risk that an ostomy will be required.

Setting

Inpatient, endoscope suite or radiology suite (fluoroscopy).

Alternatives

Surgical exploration for LBO.

Indication

- Left-sided colonic obstruction: (1) as bridge to definite surgery, (2) for palliation.
- Right-sided colonic obstruction: only for palliative condition (definitive right-sided resection does not need preceding decompression in order to perform primary enterocolonic anastomosis).

Absolute contraindication: evidence of perforation.

Relative contraindication: low rectal cancer (risk of discomfort or stent end hanging out).

Preparatory Considerations

Resuscitation with rehydration.

Conventional x-rays to rule out perforation.

Limited water-soluble contrast enema (just to level of obstruction, not beyond, otherwise risk of perforation if hyperosmolar contrast causes more fluid to accumulate in distended colon).

Surgical Steps

1. Patient positioning: left lateral decubitus (or supine) position.
2. Insertion of colonoscope and advancement up to distal end of obstruction.
3. Insertion of soft-tipped guidewire through working channel of endoscope: the wire markings should allow for observation of its advancement.

4. Attempting to advance wire through obstruction. These attempts can be fairly aggressive because:

   a. Perforation would typically occur in nondistended and empty part of colon.

   b. Only alternative to stent would be an operation (which at the same time would take care of whatever perforation occurred).

5. Once wire has been placed, endoscope is removed while pushing wire forward to keep it in situ: this step facilitates insertion of actual stent as it has not to be squeezed through biopsy channel.

6. Possible fluoroscopy verification of wire position.

7. Reinsertion of colonoscope to distal end of obstruction.

8. Insertion of stent delivery system over guidewire through lesion: before deployment, correct position in prestenotic colon can again be verified by fluoroscopy while injecting water-soluble radiographic contrast through respective port in delivery system.

9. Careful deployment while keeping distal end of stent about 2 cm distal to obstruction; as long as stent has not been completely deployed, it can be pulled back into sheath.

10. Assessment of deployment success

    a. Successful → immediate decompression of colon with evacuation of gas and liquid stool.

    b. Incomplete → additional stent(s) to be placed through first one (or proceed to surgery).

11. X-ray to rule out perforation.

Anatomic Structures at Risk

Colonic integrity.

Aftercare

Observation for minimum of 24 hours, individualize subsequent workup and plan.

Colonic evaluation: contrast enema vs colonoscopy (after complete decompression and bowel prep).

Plan for definitive surgical care 1–2 weeks after stent placement.

Complications

Unrelieved obstruction, perforation, lost stent, malpositioned/obstructing stent), secondary tumor rupture.

Cross-reference

Operative Techniques

ON-TABLE LAVAGE FOR PRIMARY ANASTOMOSIS IN LBO

Principle

Intraoperative resection of an obstructing segment in the setting of a complete or nearly complete left-sided LBO with washout elimination of the stool (Figure 5–14). This approach avoids an ostomy and therefore is an alternative to two-stage colonic resection (eg, Hartmann resection).

Caveat: while a bowel cleansing is not considered necessary in elective surgery, it may still be desirable under emergency circumstances to eliminate the stool load and decompress the distended colon before effectuating an anastomosis.

Setting

Inpatient, OR procedure.

Alternatives

Colonoscopic stent placement as bridging.

(Sub-)total colectomy with direct enterocolonic anastomosis.

Hartmann-type resection.

Indication

Left-sided colonic obstruction in stable patient.

Absolute contraindication: patient "in extremis," significantly compromised colonic bowel wall.

Caveat: Right-sided colonic obstruction or even descending (or sigmoid) colon obstruction can be addressed with right or extended-right hemicolectomy or a (sub-)total colectomy with primary ileocolonic or ileorectal anastomosis, without bowel prep or preceding colonic decompression.

Preparatory Considerations

Resuscitation with rehydration.

Conventional x-rays to rule out perforation.

Rigid or flexible sigmoidoscopy up to point of obstruction: rule out more distal pathology.

Surgical Steps

1. Patient positioning: modified lithotomy position.
2. Incision and exploration of abdomen to assess extent of disease and rule out secondary pathology.

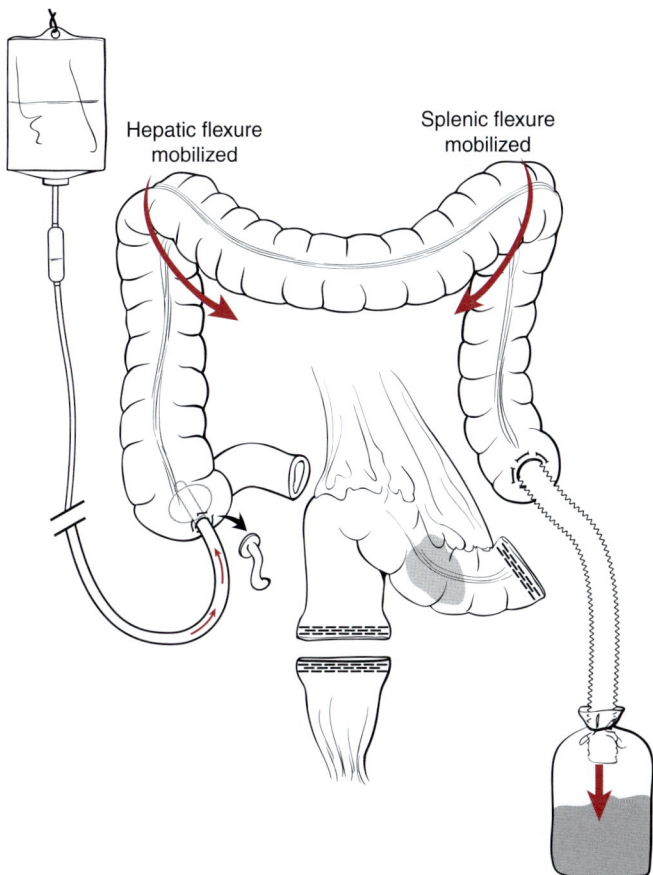

Figure 5–14. On-table lavage for LBO.

3. Isolation and resection of obstructing segment in oncologic technique (see respective topics discussed elsewhere) with adequate vascular ligation and stapling off both proximal and distal ends.

4. Macroscopic assessment of specimen.

5. Assessment of bowel quality and patient stability: primary anastomosis justified or Hartmann-type resection indicated?

6. Logistic preparation for on-table lavage:

   a. Getting a large-diameter tube, eg, corrugated tubing used by anesthesia to connect endotracheal tubing with machine: available sterile or can be soaked in povidone-iodine solution.

   b. Placing intact double plastic bags into trash can next to operating table, secure upper end to edge of trash can to avoid downward traction and disconnection as it fills with fluid.

7. Surgical preparation for on-table lavage:

   a. Massaging colonic content ~10 cm away from distal resection margin and placement of noncrushing bowel clamp; placement of sponges around distal end to minimize uncontrolled spillage.

   b. Opening of distal colon end, insertion of end of corrugated tubing for 3–4 cm and securing it to bowel end with heavy ties around it.

   c. Leading other end of corrugated tubing to bags in trash can and creation of closed system by taping it in securely.

   d. Release of noncrushing bowel clamp → some liquefied stool and gas should start to evacuate through tubing.

   e. Mobilization of both flexures to facilitate massaging colonic content toward tubing.

   f. Appendectomy with placement of two concentric pursestring sutures, insertion of large-diameter Foley catheter, followed by insufflation of catheter balloon.

   g. Connection of Foley catheter to infusion tubing.

8. Pressured infusion of several liters of saline or mixture of saline/povidone-iodine solution into colon until it is completely decompressed and outflow clears.

9. Resection of most distal 5-cm segment of colon and removal from field together with tubing.

10. Staple closure of cecal pole and oversewing of staple line with additional sutures.

11. Continuation of surgery, performing primary anastomosis in the fashion most appropriate for individual patient (stapled, hand-sewn).

Anatomic Structures at Risk

Colonic integrity.

Stool spillage.

Spleen, duodenum (mobilization of flexures).

Aftercare

Fast-track recovery: in absence of nausea or vomiting, oral liquids are started on POD1 and advanced as tolerated.

Complications

Anastomotic leak, prolonged postoperative ileus, sepsis, secondary need for ostomy.

Cross-reference

Operative Techniques

CREATION OF END-ILEOSTOMY OR -COLOSTOMY

Principle

Mobilization of colon or terminal ileum end to adequately reach the abdominal wall, to allow functional maturation. Typically done (1) as part of a discontinuous emergency resection (eg, Hartmann-type resection, total abdominal colectomy), (2) as a definitive procedure (abdominoperineal resection, total proctocolectomy), (3) occasionally for the same reasons as a diverting loop ostomy but with the intent to close off the efferent limb and achieve a complete diversion.

Setting

Inpatient, OR procedure.

Alternatives

End-ileostomy vs Prasad-type ileostomy.

End-colostomy vs Prasad-type colostomy.

Indication

Discontinuous resection: Hartmann-type resection or total abdominal colectomy.

Complete diversion of stool from distal area of concern.

Preparatory Considerations

Elective situation: marking of possible stoma sites, prophylactic antibiotics.

Urgent/emergency: therapeutic antibiotics, resuscitation, stoma site marking if possible (otherwise "educated guess").

Surgical Steps

1. Patient position: supine or modified lithotomy position (depending on surgeon's preference and need to have perineal access).

(A) End-ileostomy (Brooke) with ~3-cm nipple (Figure 5–15A)

2. Mobilization of terminal ileum so that it reaches beyond abdominal wall at planned ostomy site.
3. Excision of skin disk at planned ostomy site: not larger than diameter of small bowel.
4. Dissection of fat and crosswise incision of anterior rectus sheath.

5. Longitudinal splitting of rectus muscle fibers (caveat: epigastric vessels!) and opening of posterior sheath/peritoneum.

6. Width: general 2-finger rule may be too large for ileostomy. Better: as large as necessary, as small as possible (so that loop can be brought through without strangulation), about the diameter of small bowel.

7. Pull-through of bowel and fixation to fascia with three to four seromuscular sutures.

8. For all permanent ostomies: closure of lateral aspect along terminal bowel segment (to avoid internal wrapping of small bowel around that segment), running absorbable suture between bowel and peritoneum.

9. Closure of laparotomy or access ports.

10. Maturing of stoma: avoid stitching through skin because of risk of creating fistulae (particularly in IBD).

   a. Planning of roughly 3-cm symmetric nipple.

   b. Pre-laying of four everting sutures: dermis → base → full-thickness bowel edge.

   c. Gentle traction on all four sutures results in eversion and nipple formation; consecutive tying.

   d. Placement of two to three dermis-bowel edge sutures in between.

11. Appliance.

(B) End colostomy with ~0.3–0.5-cm flat elevation (Figure 5–15B)

2. Mobilization of colon so that it reaches without tension 1–2 cm beyond abdominal wall.

3. Verification that loop reaches planned ostomy site.

4. Excision of skin disk at planned ostomy site: diameter about two fingers wide.

5. Dissection of fat and crosswise incision of anterior rectus sheath.

6. Longitudinal splitting of rectus muscle fibers (caveat: epigastric vessels!) and opening of posterior sheath/peritoneum.

7. Width: general 2-finger rule, but better—as large as necessary, as small as possible (so that loop can be brought through without strangulation).

8. Pull-through of bowel and fixation to fascia with three to four seromuscular sutures.

9. For all permanent ostomies: closure of lateral aspect along terminal bowel segment (to avoid internal wrapping), running absorbable suture between bowel and peritoneum.

10. Closure of laparotomy or access ports.

11. Maturing of stoma: → avoid stitching through skin.

  a. Planning of roughly 0.3–0.5-cm symmetric nipple.

  b. Four slightly everting sutures: dermis → base → full-thickness bowel edge.

  c. Placement of two to three dermis-bowel edge sutures in between.

12. Appliance.

Anatomic Structures at Risk

Mesenteric tears, injury to epigastric vessels, bowel strangulation.

Aftercare

Fast-track recovery: in absence of nausea or vomiting, oral liquids are started on POD1 and advanced as tolerated. Stoma care education.

Complications

Bleeding (surgeon-dependent): eg, traction on mesenteric vessels.

Stoma retraction (obesity), stoma necrosis (insufficient mobilization, strangulation) → stricture (epifascial) or abdominal sepsis (subfascial)

Small bowel wrapping around ostomy-bearing bowel, prolapse, herniation.

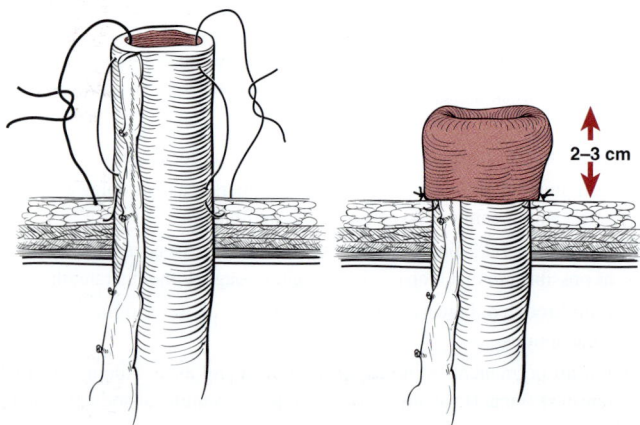

A

Figure 5–15A. Creation of an end-ileostomy.

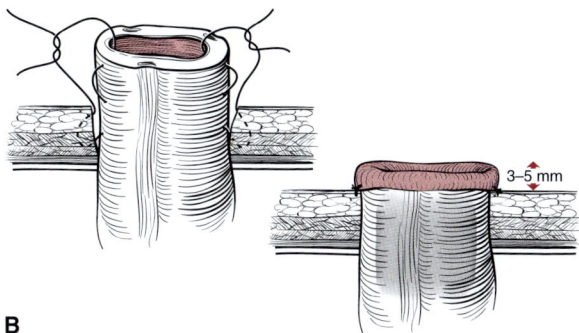

B

Figure 5–15B. Creation of an end-colostomy.

Cross-reference

Operative Techniques

CREATION OF LOOP ILEOSTOMY OR COLOSTOMY *(LAPAROSCOPIC/OPEN)*

Principle

Mobilization of a loop of colon or terminal ileum to adequately reach the abdominal wall, to allow functional maturation. Either done as the last part of a more extensive abdominal surgery (eg, LAR, IPAA) or as a separate independent procedure. A laparoscopic approach generally is suitable for elective circumstances, an open approach as part of a major procedure or for emergency situations with significant bowel distention or expected dense adhesions (eg, after recent exploration, abdominal catastrophe, pelvic sepsis).

Setting

Inpatient, OR procedure.

Alternatives

Ileostomy: preferred stoma if colon empty, no distal obstruction.

Colostomy: preferred in emergency with colon full of stool.

Indication

Diversion of stool from distal area of concern:

- At time of distal surgery, eg, LAR/coloanal, IPAA, etc.
- Independent/elective: fecal diversion to protect distal anastomosis or divert stool from problem area (eg, rectovaginal/-urinary fistula, incontinence, stricture).
- Independent/urgent-emergency: pelvic sepsis from anastomotic leak, perineal wound infection, acute rectovaginal fistula, LBO (eg, in very frail patient).

Preparatory Considerations

Elective: bowel cleansing for all elective cases to avoid stasis of stool, marking of possible stoma sites, prophylactic antibiotics.

Urgent/emergency: therapeutic antibiotics, resuscitation, stoma site marking if possible (otherwise "educated guess").

Surgical Steps

1. Patient position: supine or modified lithotomy position (depending on surgeon's preference and need to have perineal access).

(A) Loop ileostomy with ~3-cm nipple of afferent limb (Figure 5–16)

2. Access:

    a. Indirect access, ie, through laparotomy.

    b. Laparoscopic: (1) midline camera port at some distance from elected stoma sites, (2) one working port through planned stoma site, (3) additional separate working port.

    c. Direct access through planned site: not recommended as opening ends up larger than ideal and carries increased risk of parastomal hernia or stoma prolapse.

3. Open or laparoscopic mobilization of terminal ileum (or in IPAA the most distal small bowel loop proximal to pouch) such that it reaches beyond abdominal wall.

4. Creation of small mesenteric window and placement of Penrose drain.

5. Marking of absolute orientation (eg, one stitch in efferent limb, two stitches in afferent limb).

6. Verification that loop reaches planned ostomy site, adjustment of site if necessary.

7. Excision of skin disk at planned ostomy site: not larger than diameter of small bowel.

8. Dissection of fat and crosswise incision of anterior rectus sheath.

9. Longitudinal splitting of rectus muscle fibers (caveat: epigastric vessels!), opening of posterior sheath/peritoneum.

10. Width: general 2-finger rule may be too large for ileostomy. Better: as large as necessary, as small as possible (so that loop can be brought through without strangulation), about diameter of small bowel.

11. In clean cases: possible wrapping/spraying of loop with antiadhesive (to facilitate later takedown).

12. Pulling through loop with help of Penrose drain, correct orientation/rotation, and possible fixation to fascia with three to four seromuscular sutures.

13. Closure of laparotomy or access ports.

14. Maturing of stoma: avoid stitching through skin—risk of fistulae in IBD.

    a. Planning of roughly 3-cm symmetric nipple.

    b. Transverse incision of efferent limb at skin level, placement of ~3 sutures from dermis to full-thickness efferent bowel edge.

    c. Pre-laying of four everting sutures to afferent limb: dermis → base → full-thickness afferent bowel edge.

    d. Gentle traction on all four sutures with eversion and nipple formation, followed by consecutive tying.

    e. Placement of two to three dermis-bowel edge sutures in between.

15. Appliance.

(B) Loop colostomy

  2. Access:

    a. Indirect access: through laparotomy.

    b. Laparoscopic: (1) midline camera port at some distance from elected stoma sites, (2) one working port through planned stoma site, (3) additional separate working port.

    c. Direct access through planned site: loop transverse colostomy—halfway between midclavicular costal margin and umbilicus; sigmoid colostomy—LLQ.

  3. Open or laparoscopic mobilization of target colon so that it reaches without tension 1–2-cm beyond abdominal wall.

  4. Creation of mesenteric window, placement of Penrose drain.

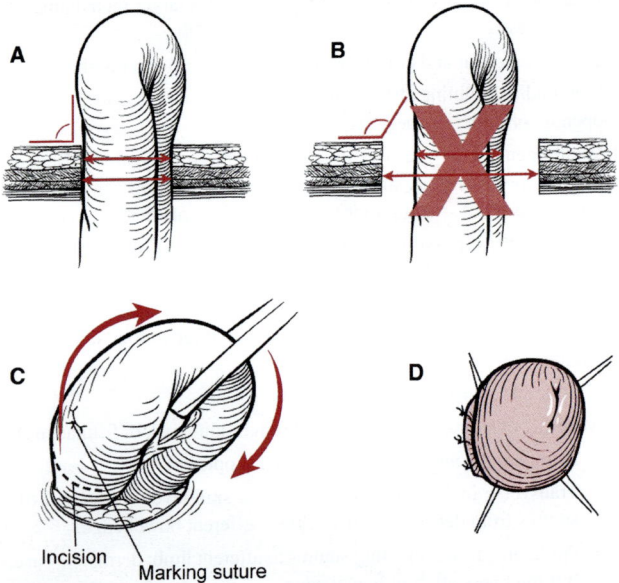

Figure 5–16. Creation of a loop ileostomy.

5. Marking of absolute orientation (eg, one stitch in efferent limb, two stitches in afferent limb).

6. Verification that loop reaches planned ostomy site, further mobilization or adjustment of site if necessary.

7. Excision of skin disk at planned ostomy site: diameter about 2 fingers wide.

8. Dissection of fat and crosswise incision of anterior rectus sheath.

9. Longitudinal splitting of rectus muscle fibers (caveat: epigastric vessels!), opening of posterior sheath/peritoneum.

10. Width: general 2-finger rule, but better—as large as necessary, as small as possible (so that loop can be brought through without strangulation).

11. In clean cases: possible wrapping/spraying of loop with antiadhesive (to facilitate later takedown).

12. Pull-through with help of Penrose drain, correct orientation/rotation.

13. Placement of a colostomy bridge and/or a few seromuscular fixation sutures (3–4) to fascia.

14. Closure of laparotomy or access ports.

15. Maturing of stoma: avoid stitching through skin.

    a. Planning of roughly 0.5-cm symmetric nipple.

    b. Transverse or longitudinal incision of bowel.

    c. Four slightly everting sutures to afferent limb: dermis → base → full-thickness afferent bowel edge.

    d. Placement of two to three dermis-bowel edge sutures in between.

16. Appliance.

Anatomic Structures at Risk

Mesenteric tears, injury to epigastric vessels.

Sigmoid and ileum: ureters.

Aftercare

Fast-track recovery: in absence of nausea or vomiting, oral liquids are started on POD1 and advanced as tolerated. Stoma care education.

Complications

Bleeding (surgeon-dependent): eg, traction on mesenteric vessels.

Stoma retraction (obesity), stoma necrosis (insufficient mobilization, strangulation) → stricture (epifascial) or abdominal sepsis (subfascial).

Small bowel wrapping around ostomy-bearing bowel, prolapse, herniation.

Cross-reference

ILEOSTOMY TAKEDOWN

Principle

Restoration of the intestinal continuity that was interrupted at the level of an ileostomy. The degree of difficulty of such a surgery depends on the extent of adhesions and the actual type of construction of the stoma, in particular whether the two ends to be connected are located in close proximity or not. The more common loop ileostomy is taken down once the distal area of concern (anastomosis, inflammation, etc) has fully recovered. Takedown of an end-ileostomy may involve a more complex surgery with reconnection to a preserved rectum or colon (ileorectostomy), or a completion proctectomy (or proctocolectomy) with ileoanal reconstruction (eg, ulcerative colitis, FAP).

Timing is dependent on general recuperation after first surgery and potential priority need for adjuvant chemotherapy or chemoradiation.

Setting

Inpatient, OR procedure.

Alternatives

Leaving the ileostomy: by choice or if distal problem persists.

Technical variations: laparoscopically assisted, takedown during full laparotomy.

Indication

- Existing loop ileostomy with confirmed integrity of distal anatomy/ reconstruction, > 6 weeks after creation (unless earlier need for reexploration), normalized nutritional status, completely tapered off steroids.
- Existing end-ileostomy with preserved anal sphincter complex and ability to perform reconstruction/reconnection.
- Existing "temporary" loop ileostomy, but unresolvable distal colonic/ pelvic problem → definitive APR with conversion of loop ileostomy into end colostomy.

Preparatory Considerations

Loop ileostomy: appropriate evaluation of distal anatomy of concern; rule out leak or stricture → digital rectal exam, endoscopy, water-soluble contrast enema, or other imaging.

End-ileostomy: appropriate evaluation, discussion about further resection/ reconstruction.

Operative Techniques

Overnight fasting vs low-dose bowel cleansing.

Prophylactic antibiotics.

Stress dose of steroids (eg, IBD patients) if on steroids within last 6 months.

Surgical Steps

1. Patient position: supine or modified lithotomy position (depending on surgeon's preference and need to have perineal access).

(A) Loop ileostomy

2. Limited transverse eye-shaped incision around stoma, tangentially touching mucocutaneous junction at cephalad and caudad border.

3. Division of dermis.

4. Careful dissection through all layers of abdominal wall using sharp Metzenbaum scissors, avoidance of inadvertent injury to bowel segment (excess of traction, cautery injury), otherwise risk of inadvertent enterotomy.

5. Mobilization of bowel through fascia until peritoneal cavity is reached.

6. Completion of dissection all the way around, again with care not to cause inadvertent enterotomies: if this is not adequately and safely possible (10–15% of cases) → midline laparotomy and dissection from inside.

7. Once adequate mobilization of ileostomy-bearing bowel loop achieved: limited division of mesentery to apex of loop.

8. Anastomosis:

   a. Stapled functional end-to-end: creation of enterotomy at base of nipple for insertion of two branches of 75-mm linear stapling device into afferent and efferent limb, device closure and firing without incorporating mesentery → removal of stapler and transverse firing of stapler reload for closure and resection of ileostomy-baring segment at same time; oversewing of stapler line or at least selected areas—stapler edges and cross-points, crotch; closure of mesenteric gap.

   b. Hand-sewn end-to-end: indicated particularly if not adequate length and mobility achieved → excision of ileostomy-baring segment or unfolding of nipple followed by 1- or 2-layered anastomosis.

9. Return of bowel into peritoneal cavity, limited irrigation.

10. Loose approximation of rectus muscle, closure of fascia.

11. Subcuticular closure of skin (alternative: leaving skin open for healing by secondary intention).

(B) End-ileostomy

   2. Laparotomy → careful lysis of intraperitoneal adhesions.

   3. Avoid causing enterotomies, but if they occur → immediate repair to minimize risk of leaving enterotomies unfixed.

   4. Careful takedown of ileostomy: Limited transverse eye-shaped incision at mucocutaneous junction and dissection through all layers of abdominal wall.

   5. Reconnection vs resection/reconstruction:

   a. Ileorectostomy or ileocolostomy: identification of receiving bowel segment → functional end-to-end anastomosis (as described above).

   b. Resection of distal segment (eg, completion proctectomy) → creation of new storage area, ie, IPAA with possible rediverting proximally (ie, loop ileostomy).

   6. Closure of the incision.

   7. Appliance (if another ileostomy was created)

Anatomic Structures at Risk

Enterotomies, mesenteric tears, injury to epigastric vessels.

Aftercare

Fast-track recovery: in absence of nausea or vomiting, oral liquids are started on POD1 and advanced as tolerated.

If loose stool expected → preemptive perianal skin care.

Complications

Bleeding (surgeon-dependent), anastomotic leak 1% (→ abscess and enterocutaneous fistula formation), SBO up to 25%, stricture, unsatisfactory function of anal function, need to recreate another ileostomy, incisional hernia formation. Stoma site infection: ~20%.

Cross-reference

Topic	*Chapter*
"Stomatology"	4 (p 401)
Complications—stoma necrosis	4 (p 468)
Total abdominal colectomy	5 (p 557)
PC/IPAA	5 (p 560)
Creation of loop ileostomy/colostomy	5 (p 596)

Operative Techniques

LOOP COLOSTOMY TAKEDOWN

Principle

Reversal of a temporary loop colostomy once the distal area of concern has recovered. Timing is dependent on general recuperation after first surgery and potential priority need for adjuvant chemotherapy or chemoradiation.

Setting

Inpatient, OR procedure.

Alternatives

Leaving the colostomy: by choice or if distal problem persists.

Technical variations: laparoscopically assisted, takedown during full laparotomy.

Indication

Existing loop colostomy with confirmed integrity of distal anatomy/reconstruction, > 6 weeks after creation (unless earlier need for reexploration), normalized nutritional status.

Preparatory Considerations

Loop colostomy: appropriate evaluation of distal anatomy of concern: rule out leak or stricture → digital rectal exam, endoscopy, water-soluble contrast enema or other imaging.

Full bowel cleansing, possibly an enema into distal limb.

Prophylactic antibiotics.

Surgical Steps

1. Patient position: supine (transverse colostomy) or modified lithotomy position (sigmoid colostomy).
2. Limited transverse eye-shaped incision around stoma, tangentially touching mucocutaneous junction at cephalad and caudad border.
3. Division of dermis.
4. Careful dissection through all layers of abdominal wall using sharp Metzenbaum scissors, avoidance of inadvertent injury to bowel segment (excess of traction, cautery injury), otherwise risk of inadvertent enterotomy.
5. Mobilization of bowel through fascia (and frequently through parastomal hernia sac) until peritoneal cavity is reached.

6. Completion of dissection all the way around, again with care not to cause inadvertent enterotomies: if this is not adequately and safely possible (10–15% of cases) → midline laparotomy and dissection from inside.

7. Once adequate mobilization of colostomy-bearing bowel loop achieved: freshening of wound edge (→ preserving back wall), or complete resection of segment (→completely fresh anastomosis).

8. Anastomosis:

   a. Stapled functional end-to-end: not recommended for large bowel as giant diverticulum is created → potentially relevant functional obstacle (harder stool) + difficult to perform subsequent colonoscopies.

   b. Preserved back wall: 1- or 2-layered transverse closure of bowel.

   c. Freshened bowel edges: 1- or 2-layered end-to-end anastomosis, closure of mesenteric gap.

9. Return of bowel into peritoneal cavity, limited irrigation.

10. Loose approximation of rectus muscle, closure of fascia.

11. Subcuticular closure of skin (alternative: leaving skin open for healing by secondary intention).

Anatomic Structures at Risk

Enterotomies, mesenteric tears, injury to epigastric vessels.

Aftercare

Fast-track recovery: in absence of nausea or vomiting, oral liquids are started on POD1 and advanced as tolerated.

If loose stool expected → preemptive perianal skin care.

Complications

Bleeding (surgeon-dependent), anastomotic leak 3% (→ abscess or enterocutaneous fistula formation), SBO up to 25%, stricture, unsatisfactory function of anal function, need to recreate another colostomy, incisional hernia formation. Stoma site infection: 20–25%.

Cross-reference

Topic	*Chapter*
"Stomatology"	4 (p 401)
Complications—stoma necrosis	4 (p 468)
PC/IPAA	5 (p 560)
Creation of loop ileostomy/colostomy	5 (p 596)
LAR/TME	5 (p 610)

Operative Techniques

HARTMANN REVERSAL
(LAPAROSCOPIC VS OPEN)

Principle

Laparoscopic vs open reversal of a Hartmann-type end-colostomy once the patient has recovered from the acute event that led to the performance of a discontinuous resection (perforation, acute obstruction, etc). The index event often results in significant adhesions (peritonitis), particularly in the midline; nonetheless, a laparoscopic start is usually justifiable.

Timing of the surgery: usually not before 3–6 months after the first surgery, dependent on general recuperation and potential priority need for adjuvant chemotherapy or chemoradiation.

Setting

Inpatient, OR procedure.

Alternatives

Leaving the colostomy: by choice, patient comorbidities, or reconnection impossible (rare).

Completion proctectomy and coloanal anastomosis (with/without temporary ileostomy).

Indication

Existing Hartmann colostomy with confirmed integrity of distal rectal stump, > 3 months after creation, normalized health and nutritional status.

Preparatory Considerations

Full colonic evaluation (barium enema vs colonoscopy), including contrast enema or rectal stump (for assessment of its length and configuration, see Figure 5–17).

Full bowel cleansing.

Enemas into rectal stump + rigid sigmoidoscopy to verify that barium is not impacted.

Prophylactic antibiotics.

Consenting process: making sure that patient understands potential risk that either takedown cannot be completed at all (→ permanent colostomy) or that temporary protection by an ileostomy may again be needed.

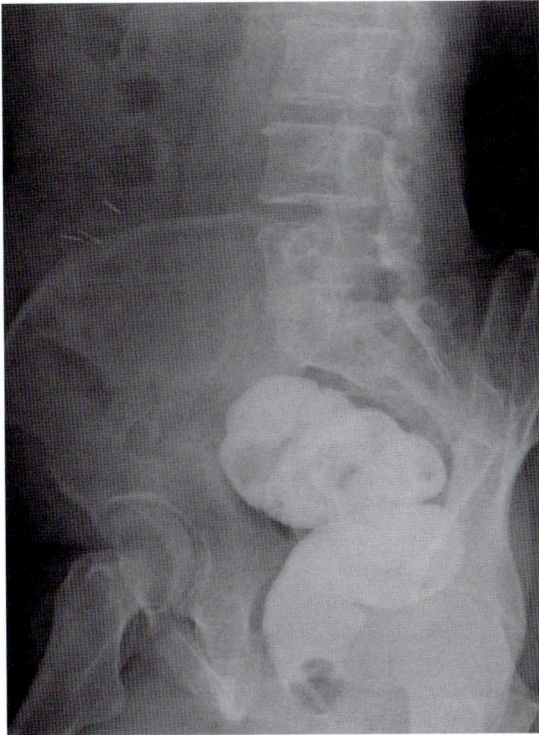

Figure 5–17. Preoperative barium enema of Hartmann pouch.

Surgical Steps

1. Patient position: modified lithotomy position, beanbag, strapped to table, both arms tucked.

2. Access:

   a. Laparoscopic: initial port placement in open port Hasson technique: off midline (eg, right midclavicular line at level of umbilicus). Camera insertion and assessment of density of adhesions: camera lysis until sufficient space developed to insert 2nd/3rd port above and below also on midclavicular line under direct visual control.

   b. Open: midline laparotomy.

3. Takedown of adhesions (ultrasonic shears, scissors, wiping).

4. Target 1: moving small bowel out of pelvis and identification/mobilization of rectal stump.

5. Target 2: identification of ostomy-baring colon, mobilization of splenic flexure.

6. Once that is achieved: limited transverse eye-shaped incision around stoma, tangentially touching mucocutaneous junction at cephalad and caudad border and complete mobilization of stoma-bearing bowel through all layers of abdominal wall (including frequently present hernia sac).

7. Freshening of colonic edge, placement of purse-string suture, insertion of largest possible diameter of circular stapler anvil; bowel dropped back to peritoneal cavity.

8. Stoma site can subsequently either be used as a hand-port, or it is air-sealed by means of axially twisted wound protector or towel clamps.

9. The whole laparoscopic mobilization should clearly advance with time: if adhesions are too dense and no progress is made → conversion to open procedure, eg, through midline laparotomy (see above).

10. Insertion of stapler through anus and deployment of anvil under direct visual control.

11. Completion of anastomosis → testing: submerging anastomosis under water and insufflation of pressured air through sigmoidoscope: air bubbles yes/no?

12. Reevaluation of peritoneal cavity.

13. Port removal and/or closure of abdominal incisions.

14. Stoma site: closure of skin (alternative: leaving skin open for healing by secondary intention).

Anatomic Structures at Risk

Enterotomies, mesenteric tears, injury to epigastric vessels.

Aftercare

Fast-track recovery: in absence of nausea or vomiting, oral liquids are started on POD1 and advanced as tolerated.

Complications

Bleeding (surgeon-dependent), anastomotic leak 3% (→ abscess or enterocutaneous fistula formation), SBO up to 25%, stricture, unsatisfactory anorectal function, need to recreate another colostomy, incisional hernia formation. Stoma site infection: 20–25%.

Cross-reference

Operative Techniques

LOW ANTERIOR RESECTION (LAR)/
TOTAL MESORECTAL EXCISION (TME)

Principle

Oncologic, anatomic, and specimen-oriented resection of the rectum with preservation of an intact mesorectal compartment (Figure 5–18). Benchmark: < 10% local recurrence without adjuvant treatment.

- Two-stage: with temporary ileostomy.
- One-stage: without ileostomy.

Setting

Inpatient, OR procedure.

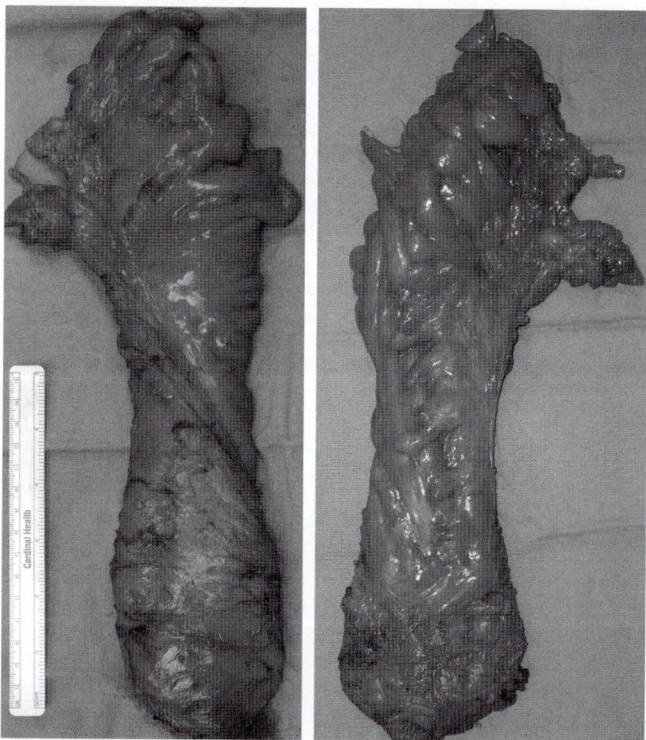

Figure 5–18. TME specimen from front and back showing intact glossy fascial cover.

Alternatives

Partial TME (for tumors in upper rectum).

Abdominoperineal resection.

Coloanal anastomosis, possible intersphincteric dissection.

Pelvic exenteration (advanced primary or recurrent tumor)

Local transanal excision or transanal microsurgery (TEM).

Expectant approach in case of complete clinical response after neoadjuvant chemoradiation. Laparoscopic approach.

Indication

Rectal cancer.

Preparatory Considerations

Full colonic evaluation and histologic documentation.

Rigid sigmoidoscopy to determine level above anal verge.

Staging: ERUS, CT abdomen/pelvis, MRI.

Interdisciplinary management: neoadjuvant chemoradiation (depending on stage, level, preference).

Bowel cleansing (traditional) vs no bowel cleansing (evolving concept).

Ureteral stents for redo cases or extensive disruption of anatomy (eg, inflammation).

Marking of possible stoma sites.

Prophylactic antibiotics.

Surgical Steps

1. Patient position: modified lithotomy position.
2. Laparotomy:
   a. Lower midline: infraumbilical incision sufficient if stomach and splenic flexure can be reached, otherwise extension above umbilicus.
   b. Alternative access: transverse suprapubic (transection of rectus muscle), Pfannenstiel incision (transverse incision to skin and anterior rectus sheath with midline rectus-saving celiotomy).
3. Abdominal exploration: local resectability, secondary pathology (liver/gallbladder, colon, female organs, small bowel), other abnormalities.
4. Installation of abdominal wall retractor (eg, Bookwalter retractor). Insertion of large surgical towel underneath unopened supraumbilical abdominal wall keeps small bowel out of surgical field and allows free access to pelvis.

5. Retrograde dissection from sigmoid toward splenic flexure along white line of Toldt. Opening of retroperitoneum, identification of areolar tissue. Firm pressure against sigmoid mesentery to bluntly reflect retroperitoneal tissues and expose left ureter. Incision of peritoneum continued into pelvis.

6. If needed: complete mobilization of splenic flexure by retraction of distal transverse and proximal descending colon and conjoining the two in stepwise ligation. Avoid splenic tear.

7. Once mobilization is sufficient, serosal incision on right side of mesosigmoid, continuation toward peritoneal reflection

8. Developing avascular plane posterior to superior hemorrhoidal vessels but anterior to hypogastric nerve plexus, caudad continuation leads to avascular plane anterior to Waldeyer fascia.

9. Ligation of vascular stalk (IMA, superior hemorrhoidal) with clamping and transection (ligature, suture ligatures). Before dividing tissue, remote location of ureters to be verified.

10. Stepwise transection of mesosigmoid to proximal point of resection and transection of sigmoid colon with linear stapler.

11. Continuation of nerve-sparing dissection into pelvis under direct visualization, no blunt dissection (avoid presacral veins!).

12. Sharp anterior and lateral dissection all the way to pelvic floor, identification of seminal vesicles (males), careful dissection of rectovaginal plane (females). Anterior or circumferential tumors: dissection with inclusion of Denonvilliers fascia. Posterior tumors: dissection just posterior to fascia to spare autonomic nerve function.

13. (A) Double-stapling technique: transection of distal rectum at puborectalis muscle, ie, ~2–3 cm proximal to dentate line with transverse linear stapler/cutter.

    (B) Hand-sewn technique: Switch to perineal approach, installation of Lone Star retractor, incision of mucosa at dentate line, and mucosectomy up to puborectalis muscle where connection to presacral space is made. Alternatively: intersphincteric dissection by entering at dentate line, accessing intersphincteric groove, and continuing dissection proximally until connection with abdominal dissection.

14. Removal of complete specimen, macroscopic examination (Figure 5–18), frozen section of distal resection margin.

15. Creation of colonic pouch: may be considered in all complete TMEs, but definitely recommended if diameter of proximal colon would not allow insertion of 33-mm stapler anvil:

   a. Colonic J-pouch: folding of distal colon, apical enterotomy, firing of 75-cm linear stapler to create 5–6-cm pouch. Free end of J to be shortened flush to inlet, approximated to afferent limb with a series of interrupted sutures.

   b. Transverse coloplasty: 4-cm longitudinal anterior enterotomy ~3–4 cm proximal to distal resection end. Transverse closure in two layers.

16. (A) Stapled anastomosis: Purse-string suture to distal colon (straight anastomosis, transverse coloplasty), or to apical enterotomy (colonic J-pouch). Insertion of largest possible circular stapler anvil. Insertion of stapler through anus and tension-free anastomosis. Assessment of donuts and digital assessment of anastomosis.

   (B) Hand-sewn anastomosis: Switch to perineal approach, guiding Babcock clamp through anus to grasp end of the bowel or tip of J-pouch and carefully pulling it through → fixation with six seromuscular anchoring stitches, maturing mucosal junction. Removal of retractor.

17. Presacral drains according to surgeon's preference. No need for NGT.

18. For two-stage procedure: creation of loop ileostomy. Excision of skin disk at preoperatively marked site for the ileostomy. Dissection of fat, incision of anterior rectus sheath, splitting of muscle to create gap. Small bowel loop (distal limb marked) wrapped with Seprafilm and carried through abdominal wall.

19. Closure of incision.

20. Maturation of loop ileostomy to 3-cm nipple. Appliance.

Anatomic Structures at Risk

Left ureter, gonadal vessels, hypogastric nerves, fascial planes, presacral vein plexus, vagina.

Aftercare

Fast-track recovery: in absence of nausea or vomiting, oral liquids are started on POD1 and advanced as tolerated. Ileostomy takedown > 6 weeks if clinical/radiologic evidence that anastomosis healed. Takedown postponed if consolidating chemotherapy is given priority: started after 4 weeks.

Complications

Bleeding (surgeon-dependent): presacral veins, inadequate ligature of vascular stalks, splenic tear, gonadal vessels.

Anastomotic leak (5–15%): technical error, tension, inadequate blood supply, poor tissue quality after chemoradiation.

Ureteral injury (0.1–0.2%).

Operative Techniques

Cross-reference

Topic	*Chapter*
Rectal cancer	4 (p 265)
Complications—leak	4 (p 466)
Creation of loop ileostomy	5 (p 596)
APR	5 (p 615)
Transanal excision	5 (p 618)
TEM	5 (p 622)
Chemotherapy protocols—curative intent	6 (p 645)
Radiation therapy	6 (p 654)
Perioperative management—abdominal	7 (p 684)
Fast-track recovery	7 (p 714)

ABDOMINOPERINEAL RESECTION *(APR)*

Principle

Oncologic, anatomic, and specimen-oriented resection of the rectum in TME technique with removal of the anus and creation of a permanent end-colostomy.

Setting

Inpatient, OR procedure.

Alternatives

Sphincter-preserving TME coloanal anastomosis for tumors above puborectalis muscle, possible intersphincteric dissection for lower tumors?

Pelvic exenteration (advanced primary or recurrent tumor).

Local transanal excision.

Expectant approach in case of complete clinical response after neoadjuvant chemoradiation.

Indication

- Rectal cancer at level of puborectalis muscle/sphincter complex.
- Rectal cancer with perirectal fistula.
- Persistent/recurrent anal squamous cell cancer (after Nigro protocol).
- Anal adenocarcinoma (eg, anal glands).

Preparatory Considerations

Full colonic evaluation and histologic documentation.

Digital rectal exam and rigid sigmoidoscopy to determine tumor level.

Staging: ERUS, CT abdomen/pelvis, MRI.

Interdisciplinary management: neoadjuvant chemoradiation (depending on stage, level, preference).

Bowel cleansing (traditional) vs no bowel cleansing (evolving concept).

Ureteral stents for redo cases or extensive disruption of anatomy (eg, inflammation).

Marking of stoma sites.

Prophylactic antibiotics.

Surgical Steps

1. Patient position: modified lithotomy position.

2. Abdominal dissection: in TME technique (see previous discussion).

3. Perineal dissection (separate instrument set, 2-team approach):

   a. Closure of anus using two concentric purse-string sutures with strong suture material.

   b. Marking of planned elliptic incision with pen:

      (1) In women with anterior tumor: extension into vagina, ie, resection of posterior vaginal wall.

      (2) All others: midperineum.

   c. Landmarks of dissection:

      (1) Lateral: ischioanal fossae to ischial tuberosity.

      (2) Posterior: anococcygeal ligament.

      (3) Anterior: transverse perinei muscle (caveat: risk of urethral injury in males).

   d. Connection of perineal with abdominal dissection by entering through anococcygeal ligament.

   e. Loading pelvic floor muscles on finger and slow transection with electrocautery, selective ligation of bleeding vessels.

   f. Once both posterolateral aspects are freed up: posterior delivery of abdominal specimen component and completion of anterior dissection.

4. Removal of complete specimen, macroscopic examination, frozen section of resection margins if any doubts.

5. Closure of perineal defect:

   a. Direct closure: two layers, perineal drains not needed.

   b. Flap closure for larger defect → myocutaneous flap (eg, rectus abdominis muscle).

   c. Internal barrier (eg, omentum patch) and perineal wound left open or covered with wound VAC.

6. Creation of end-colostomy at preoperatively marked site, internal closure of lateral aspect (bowel-abdominal wall) to avoid internal wrapping of bowel around colostomy-bearing segment.

7. Closure of abdominal incision.

8. Maturation of colostomy. Appliance.

Anatomic Structures at Risk

Left ureter, gonadal vessels, hypogastric nerves, fascial planes, presacral vein plexus, vagina, urethra.

Aftercare

Fast-track recovery: in absence of nausea or vomiting, oral liquids are started on POD1 and advanced as tolerated. Consolidating chemotherapy (if needed) started after 4 weeks.

Rare possibility: secondary abdominoperineal reconstruction after APR with pullthrough (perineal colostomy) and placement of artificial bowel sphincter.

Complications

Bleeding (surgeon-dependent): presacral veins, inadequate ligature of vascular stalks, splenic tear, gonadal vessels.

Surgical site infection (perineal wound) in 20% of patients (particularly after neoadjuvant chemoradiation).

Ureteral injury (0.1–0.2%).

Cross-reference

Operative Techniques

TRANSANAL EXCISION *(POLYP, CANCER)*

Principle

Transanal full-thickness excision of circumscribed distal rectal pathology. Ideal for benign pathology; also an option for early-stage rectal cancer, but increased risk of local recurrence even in T1 rectal cancers → important patient selection. Cause for high local recurrence rate (18–30%): risk of positive lymph nodes (for T1 lesion: 7–10%, T2 15–25%), direct implantation of shed cancer cells into the wound closure. Discussion about role of surgery and adjuvant chemoradiation is ongoing.

Caveat: for cancer, the transanal excision should be considered an excisional biopsy until pathologic stage is obtained. T2 → additional treatment, T3 → full oncologic treatment/resection.

Setting

Inpatient (selected outpatient?), OR procedure.

Alternatives

Oncologic resection: low anterior resection (TME), abdominoperineal resection.

TEM.

Indication

Polyp or other pathology (eg, ulcer) in reach of finger:

- No size limit as long as tissue adequate, eg, sufficiently pliable for defect closure.
- Even circumferential lesions acceptable → sleeve excision.

Rectal cancer:

- uT1N0 lesion (invades submucosa).
- < 4 cm largest diameter (less than one-third of circumference).
- Well or moderately differentiated histology.
- No evidence of poor prognostic indicators, eg, lymphatic/vascular invasion.
- Patients not fulfilling above criteria but having significant comorbidities or extensive metastasis but locally highly symptomatic.

Preparatory Considerations

Full colonic evaluation and histologic documentation.

Rigid sigmoidoscopy to determine level above anal verge and exact location on circumference.

Staging: ERUS.

Bowel cleansing: full or two Fleet enemas.

Prophylactic antibiotics.

Surgical Steps

1. Patient positioning: posterior lesion → lithotomy; any other location → prone jackknife position with buttocks taped aside.

2. Pudendal/perianal nerve block with 15–20 cc of local anesthetic in addition to general anesthesia to improve relaxation of anal sphincter muscles.

3. Insertion of Lone Star retractor.

4. Possible placement of holding suture proximal to lesion.

5. Marking of dotted line (electrocautery) around target lesion: 1-cm margin.

6. Incision of mucosa right at lower edge and full-thickness incision into perirectal fat (Figure 5–19).

7. Circumferential dissection and mobilization: avoid traumatizing and fragmentation of specimen.

8. Maintenance of good hemostasis throughout procedure.

9. Continuation until marked area completely excised → maintain orientation of specimen.

10. Placement and needle fixation of specimen onto cork/wax board(Figure 5–19) and absolute orientation as left, right, proximal, distal; in addition inspection of macroscopic margin, permanent fixation (frozen section only if area of uncertainty).

11. Irrigation with dilute povidone-iodine solution.

12. Defect closure with full-thickness suture (interrupted or running).

13. Removal of Lone Star retractor.

Anatomic Structures at Risk

Sphincter complex, rectovaginal septum.

Aftercare

Regular diet as tolerated 6 hours post anesthesia. Maintenance of soft stools (fibers, stool softener, etc).

Assessment of final pathology → possible need for adjuvant treatment vs oncologic resection.

Follow-up (in addition to routine cancer follow-up): ERUS every 3 months (1st year), every 6 months (2nd year), yearly thereafter.

Operative Techniques

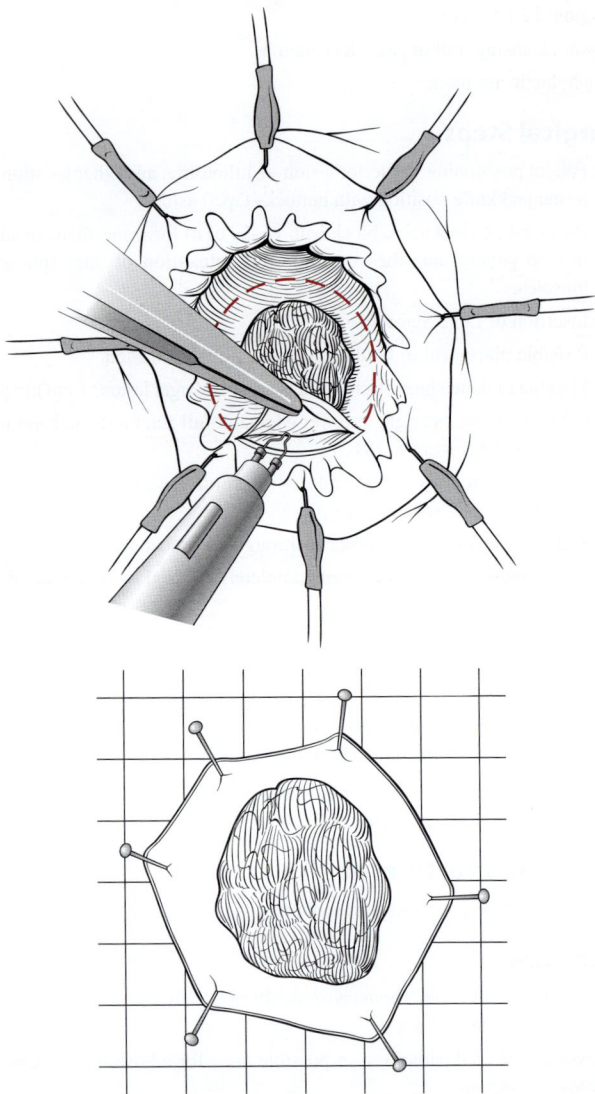

Figure 5–19. Transanal excision of sessile polyp.

Complications

Bleeding (surgeon-dependent).

Infection, abscess/fistula formation.

Anastomotic dehiscence.

Stricture formation.

Formation of rectovaginal fistula → need for colostomy.

Recurrent pathology (cancer, polyp, etc).

Cross-reference

Operative Techniques

TRANSANAL ENDOSCOPIC MICROSURGERY *(TEM)*

Principle

Combination of techniques used for conventional transanal excision with laparoscopic technology and instrumentation: endorectal system to create pneumorectum for optimal exposure and endoscopic magnification for excellent visualization. Indications and contraindications are the same as for conventional transanal excision, except that higher lesions up to 12–14 cm can be targeted. Very low lesions are not amenable and are better treated with a conventional transanal excision.

Setting

Inpatient (selected outpatient?), OR procedure.

Alternatives

Oncologic resection: low anterior resection (TME), abdominoperineal resection.

Conventional transanal excision.

Indication

Polyp or other pathology (eg, ulcer) between 3 and 12(14) cm:

• No absolute size limit (less than hemicircumference) as long as tissue adequate, eg, sufficiently pliable for defect closure.

Rectal cancer:

• uT1N0 lesion (invades submucosa).

• < 4 cm largest diameter (less than one-third of circumference).

• Well or moderately differentiated histology.

• No evidence of poor prognostic indicators, eg, lymphatic/vascular invasion.

• Patients not fulfilling above criteria but having significant comorbidities or extensive metastasis but locally highly symptomatic.

Preparatory Considerations

Full colonic evaluation and histologic documentation.

Rigid sigmoidoscopy: determination of level above anal verge and exact location on circumference are very important for correct patient positioning.

Staging: ERUS.

Bowel cleansing: full bowel cleansing.

Prophylactic antibiotics.

Surgical Steps

1. Patient positioning: the lesion has to be down! ie, posterior lesion → lithotomy; left lesion → left lateral; right lesion → right lateral; anterior lesion → prone jackknife position with legs spread apart (for access).

2. Pudendal/perianal nerve block with 15–20 cc of a local anesthetic in addition to general anesthesia to improve relaxation of anal sphincter muscles.

3. Insertion of 4-cm operating rectoscope/obturator and fixation to supporting arm, insertion of main body with sealing working and gas ports, stereotactic telescope with connection to video system.

4. Exposure of lesion.

5. Using combination instruments (coagulation/suction) and graspers, a dotted line (high-frequency knife, electrocautery) is marked around target lesion: 1-cm margin.

6. Incision of mucosa right at lower edge and full-thickness incision into perirectal fat (caveat: anterior lesions!).

7. Circumferential dissection and mobilization: avoid traumatizing and fragmentation of specimen.

8. Maintenance of good hemostasis throughout procedure.

9. Continuation until marked area completely excised → maintain specimen orientation.

10. Placement and needle fixation of specimen onto cork/wax board and absolute orientation as left, right, proximal, distal; inspection of macroscopic margin, permanent fixation (frozen section only if area of uncertainty).

11. Irrigation with dilute povidone-iodine solution.

12. Defect closure with absorbable full-thickness suture (facilitated by use of preknotted suture and endoscopic suturing device, placement of suture clip at end of suture line).

13. Removal of instruments.

Anatomic Structures at Risk

Sphincter complex (dilation), rectovaginal septum, prostate (hemorrhage).

Aftercare

Regular diet as tolerated 6 hours post anesthesia. Maintenance of soft stools (fibers, stool softener, etc).

Assessment of final pathology → possible need for adjuvant treatment vs oncologic resection.

Follow-up (in addition to routine cancer follow-up): ERUS every 3 months (1st year), every 6 months (2nd year), yearly thereafter.

Complications

Bleeding (surgeon-dependent).

Infection, abscess/fistula formation.

Anastomotic dehiscence (caveat: even without leak there will be extensive retroperitoneal air).

Stricture formation.

Formation of rectovaginal fistula → need for colostomy.

Recurrent pathology (cancer, polyp, etc).

Cross-reference

YORK-MASON APPROACH

Principle

Posterior anoproctotomy, including anal canal and sphincter complex, to expose and gain access to the distal rectum, particularly its anterior aspect (Figure 5–20), with subsequent anatomic reconstruction. Risk of subsequent incontinence is minimal after careful reconstruction, which is facilitated by placement of multiple marking sutures of different colors to corresponding structures on either side. The York-Mason approach provides a wider access to the area than the sphincter-preserving Kraske approach. The target lesion should be palpable on digital rectal exam to qualify for parasacral approach.

Setting

Inpatient, OR procedure.

Alternatives

Abdominal approach: LAR with coloanal anastomosis.

TEM.

Kraske approach (posterior proctotomy without sphincter dissection).

Indication

• Rectourinary (or midlevel rectovaginal) fistula repair.

• Anterior sessile polyp.

Contraindication: proven cancer.

Preparatory Considerations

Full colonic evaluation for all elective cases.

Bowel cleansing mandatory, unless patient already diverted with colostomy.

Prophylactic antibiotics.

Surgical Steps

1. Patient positioning: prone jackknife position with buttocks taped aside.
2. Rectal irrigation with povidone-iodine solution.
3. Marking of planned incision with pen: from posterior anal verge tangentially along tip of coccyx with parasacral extension.
4. Assuring that marking sutures of several different colors are available.
5. Skin incision: maintenance of perfect hemostasis at all times.
6. Longitudinal opening and bilateral suture marking of levator muscles.

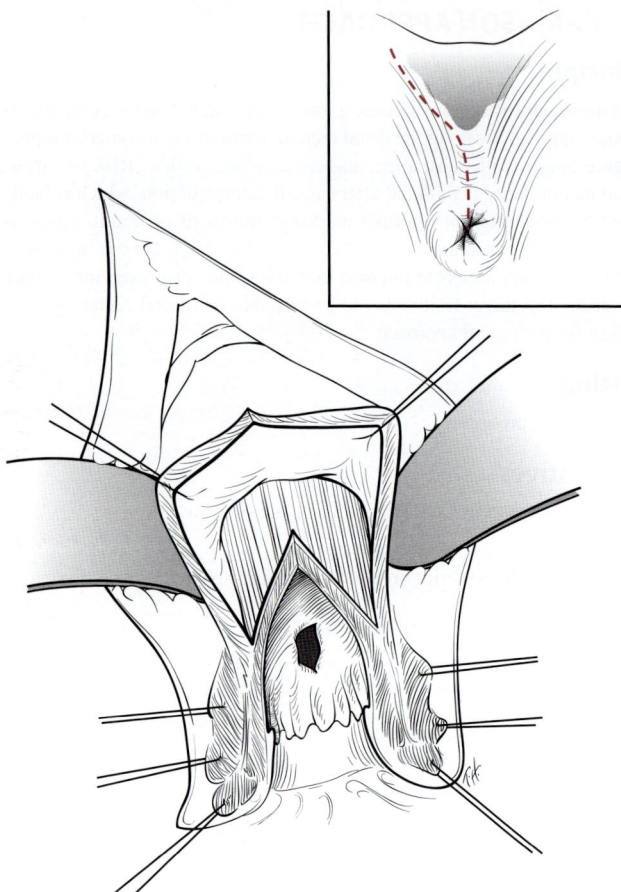

Figure 5–20. York-Mason approach for rectourinary fistula repair.

7. Longitudinal opening of rectum: systematic placement of marking sutures to corresponding structures.
8. Extension of that incision toward anal sphincter complex, marking of external and internal anal sphincter muscle.
9. Marking of anal verge.

10. After complete opening: nice exposure into anterior rectal wall to allow assessment and treatment of the target pathology (eg, layered closure of rectourinary fistula).

11. After completion of target operation → anatomic reconstruction of rectum and anal canal:

  a. Running suture to mucosa (eg, 3-0 Vicryl) up to anal verge marking stitch.

  b. Running seromuscular suture.

  c. Readaptation of internal/external sphincter muscle with three to four interrupted 2-0 or 3-0 Vicryl sutures.

  d. Running closure of levator ani funnel.

  e. Subcuticular closure of incision down to anal verge marking stitch.

Anatomic Structures at Risk

Anal sphincter complex and pelvic floor.

Aftercare

Regular diet as tolerated 6 hours post anesthesia. Wound care dry unless infected.

Complications

Complications of York-Mason access: wound infection, rectocutaneous fistula formation, incontinence to stool/gas.

Complications of target operation: dehiscence, recurrence of tumor/polyp or fistula.

Cross-reference

KRASKE APPROACH
Principle
Parasacral access to the rectum (classical parasacral proctotomy) or the pre-sacral space (extrarectal variation) with or without resection of the coccyx. Similar to York-Mason approach, but preserving anal sphincter complex. Target lesion should be palpable on digital rectal exam to qualify for parasacral approach.

Setting
Inpatient, OR procedure.

Alternatives
Abdominal approach: LAR with coloanal anastomosis.
TEM.
York-Mason approach (posterior anoproctotomy with sphincter dissection).

Indication
• Posterior rectal pathology: sessile polyp.
• Extrarectal/presacral pathology/tumor: possible combined with abdominal approach.
• Anterior rectal pathology (less adequate access): rectourinary (or midlevel rectovaginal) fistula repair, anterior sessile polyp.
Contraindication: proven cancer, lesion not in reach of palpating finger.

Preparatory Considerations
Full colonic evaluation for all elective cases.
Bowel cleansing mandatory, unless patient already diverted with colostomy.
Prophylactic antibiotics.
Consenting patient for possible York-Mason approach with division of sphincter muscle and for possible abdominal exploration and colostomy.

Surgical Steps
1. Patient positioning: prone jackknife position with buttocks taped aside.
2. Rectal irrigation with povidone-iodine solution.
3. Marking of planned incision with pen: posterior to anal sphincter complex, tangentially along tip of coccyx with parasacral extension.

4. Assuring that marking sutures of several different colors are available.

5. Skin incision: maintenance of perfect hemostasis at all times.

6. Longitudinal opening and bilateral suture marking of levator muscles.

(A) Posterior rectal wall pathology

7. Possible coccygectomy if inadequate exposure.

8. Definition of excision under guidance through concomitant digital rectal exam.

9. Transverse incision of rectum with marking sutures to rectal wall part that will be used for closure.

10. Limited transverse vs circumferential sleeve full-thickness excision of rectum.

11. Retrieval of specimen and placement of marking sutures for orientation → frozen section if necessary.

12. Transverse closure of proctotomy in two layers.

13. Running closure of levator ani funnel.

14. Subcuticular closure of skin.

(B) Presacral (extrarectal pathology)

7. Definitive coccygectomy with tumor.

8. En-bloc excision of presacral mass:

  a. Avoiding injury to peritumoral capsule.

  b. Careful hemostasis.

  c. Maintenance of rectal integrity, but avoid wound contamination with rectal exam.

9. Retrieval of specimen and placement of marking sutures for orientation → frozen section if necessary.

10. Running closure of levator ani funnel.

11. Drain placement per surgeon's preference.

12. Subcuticular closure of skin.

(C) Anterior rectal pathology

7. Possible coccygectomy if inadequate exposure.

8. Longitudinal opening of rectum with marking sutures to corresponding structures.

9. After complete opening down to just proximal to sphincter complex to allow exposure into the anterior rectal wall, assessment and treatment of target pathology (see respective discussions).

10. After completion of target operation → anatomic reconstruction of rectum:

   a. Running suture to mucosa (eg, 3-0 Vicryl).

   b. Running seromuscular suture.

   c. Running closure of levator ani funnel.

   d. Subcuticular closure of the incision.

Anatomic Structures at Risk

Anal sphincter complex and pelvic floor, presacral veins.

Aftercare

Unless combined with abdominal approach: regular diet as tolerated 6 hours post anesthesia. Wound care dry unless infected.

Complications

Complications of the Kraske proctotomy: wound infection, rectocutaneous fistula formation, incontinence to stool/gas.

Complications of target operation: bleeding (presacral tumor), need for switch to abdominal approach, recurrent tumor.

Cross-reference

RESECTION OF PRESACRAL TUMOR/LESION

Principle

Depending on the level and size of the presacral lesion and the likelihood of being malignant:

- Lesion below S3 → parasacral access.
- Higher/larger lesion → combined abdominal/transsacral approach.

Goal: to dissect tumor/lesion off the rectum and remove en-bloc with involved coccyx and sacral segments.

Setting

Inpatient, OR procedure.

Conjoined effort with Orthopedic and/or Neurosurgery.

Alternatives

En-bloc resection with LAR and coloanal anastomosis.

Indication

Presacral tumor/lesion.

Preparatory Considerations

Full colonic evaluation for all elective cases.

Bowel cleansing mandatory.

Prophylactic antibiotics.

Counseling/consenting patient: possible sphincter/bladder dysfunction (with/without York-Mason approach), possible colostomy.

Large tumors: ureteral stent placement.

Typed/cross-matched blood products, large-bore access for rapid transfusion if needed.

Surgical Steps

(A) Low tumor/lesion → parasacral approach

1. Patient positioning: prone jackknife position with buttocks taped aside.
2. Rectal irrigation with povidone-iodine solution.
3. Marking of planned incision with pen: posterior to anal sphincter complex, tangentially along tip of coccyx with parasacral extension.
4. Skin incision, maintenance of perfect hemostasis at all times.
5. Longitudinal opening and bilateral suture marking of levator muscles.

6. Coccygectomy.

7. Under traction on resected coccyx (if possible without transanal digital guidance: risk of contamination), dissection of lesion from surrounding structures including rectum; absolutely crucial not to damage integrity of tumor capsule (risk of tumor spillage!) and of rectum (risk of infection/fistula!).

8. Retrieval of specimen, placement of marking sutures for orientation, frozen section if necessary.

9. Running closure of levator ani funnel.

10. Drain placement per surgeon's preference.

11. Subcuticular closure of the skin.

(B) High (above S3) or bulky tumor/lesion → combined abdominal/transsacral approach

1. Patient positioning: supine or modified lithotomy position

2. Rectal irrigation with povidone-iodine solution.

3. Laparotomy.

4. Complete posterior mobilization of rectum down to pelvic floor (if separation not possible → transection of upper rectum and en-bloc resection with coloanal reconstruction).

5. If concern about bleeding: placement of loose vessel loop tourniquets around hypogastric vessels on each side and guided to pelvic floor such that they are reachable from parasacral approach.

6. Placement of sponge behind rectum to serve as protection of rectum during sacral transection.

7. Closure of laparotomy with/without creation of temporary or permanent ostomy.

8. Repositioning to prone jackknife or lateral position.

9. Definitive en-bloc sacrococcygectomy with tumor and its peritumoral capsule.

13. Careful hemostasis, traction on vessel loop-tourniquets if needed.

10. Retrieval of specimen and frozen section if necessary, eg, changing management.

11. Running closure of levator ani funnel, flap closure if needed.

12. Drain placement per surgeon's preference.

13. Subcuticular closure of the skin.

Anatomic Structures at Risk

Rectum, pelvic vasculature, anal sphincter complex, nerve structures.

Aftercare

Fast-track recovery: in absence of nausea or vomiting, oral liquids are started on POD1 and advanced as tolerated. Wound care dry unless infected. Stoma care if ostomy created.

Complications

Bleeding, infection, rectocutaneous fistula formation, incontinence to stool/gas.

Complications of target operation: bleeding (presacral tumor), need for switch to abdominal approach, recurrent tumor.

Cross-reference

Operative Techniques

Chapter 6

Nonsurgical Management

CHEMOPREVENTION OF COLORECTAL CANCER

Principle

Primary cancer prevention: prophylactic measures to intercept tumor development.

Chemoprevention: pharmacologic blocking of intrinsic oncogene- or carcinogen-induced cell proliferation and transformation.

Alternatives

Secondary/tertiary prevention: screening, surveillance.

Indications

- General population at risk.
- High-risk population (eg, status post polypectomy or cancer resection).

Positive Effect Documented

COX inhibitors

Reduced endogenous prostaglandin: COX-2 not elevated in normal colon epithelium, overexpressed in 40–50% of colorectal adenomas, 90% of colorectal cancers.

- Long-term use of ASA: reduction in incidence of colorectal polyps.
- Sulindac: delay of polyp formation and regression of large bowel polyps in FAP.
- Selective COX-2 inhibitors (celecoxib, rofecoxib): same benefits plus presumed less ulcerogenic, but increased cardiac risk.

Calcium (3 g/day)

Decreased incidence of recurrent colorectal adenomata.

Mechanism: intraluminal binding of bile and fatty acids, direct antiproliferative effect in colonic mucosa.

Vitamin D

Decreased incidence of colorectal cancer.

Mechanism: through calcium effect, direct antiproliferative effect of Vitamin D?

Positive Effect Controversial or Awaiting Further Confirmation

- Fiber: benefit is supported by epidemiologic association and "gut feeling" but has not been confirmed by prospective trials.

- Folate.
- Ursodeoxycholic acid.
- Hormone replacement therapy $\rightarrow$ reduction in incidence of colorectal cancer and cancer-specific mortality.
- Selenium.

Positive Effect Not Documented

- Vitamins C and E.
- β-Carotenes.

Cross-reference

Nonsurgical Management

CHEMOTHERAPY—COMMONLY USED DRUGS

Principle

Chemotherapy has evolved as a cornerstone in the treatment of various cancers. There is a large number of known chemotherapy agents overall with a wide range of mechanisms of action, but a limited number of drugs are commonly used in the realm of colorectal surgery patients. Selection of specific drugs, protocol, routes of administration, timing, and duration depend on several patient- and tumor-related factors.

Mechanism of Action Categories

- Antimetabolites: 5-fluorouracil (+ leucovorin), capecitabine, gemcitabine.
- Platin-based alkylating agents: oxaliplatin, carboplatin, cisplatin.
- Topoisomerase inhibitors: irinotecan.
- Targeted immunotherapy (monoclonal antibodies): bevacizumab, cetuximab, panitumumab.
- Cytotoxic/antitumor antibiotics: mitomycin C.
- Tyrosine kinase inhibitors: imatinib, sunitinib.

Specific Drugs

5-Fluorouracil (+ leucovorin)
Antimetabolite (pyrimidine analogue).

Mechanism of action

Intracellular conversion to active metabolites → combined cytotoxic effect from inhibition of thymidylate synthase and incorporation into cellular RNA and DNA.

Leucovorin (LV; folinic acid): increase in cellular levels of reduced folates → modulation of 5-FU.

Protocols

Setting: adjuvant and metastatic colorectal cancer (CRC). 5-FU/LV remains the baseline of current chemotherapy protocols: continuous infusion generally is more effective and better tolerated than bolus administration.

Toxicity and adverse effects

Bone marrow suppression (maximum after 9–14 days), GI toxicity (anorexia, nausea/vomiting, diarrhea, stomatitis = signs of impending toxicity → need to interrupt treatment), dermatologic (reversible maculopapular rash, hand-and-foot syndrome, alopecia, sensitivity to sunlight, hyperpigmentations), neurologic (headache, visual disturbances, cerebellar ataxia).

Dose adjustments

Plasma half-life 10–20 minutes, hepatic catabolism into carbon dioxide and metabolite → urinary excretion. Perioperative discontinuation 3–4 weeks.

Complications

Familial dihydropyrimidine dehydrogenase (DPD) deficiency → risk of severe toxicity.

Capecitabine (Xeloda)

Antimetabolite (pyrimidine analogue).

Mechanism of action

Oral prodrug of 5-FU: intestinal absorption → accumulation in tumor cells → intracellular three-step metabolism to active 5-FU → cytotoxic effect as 5-FU.

Protocols

Setting: adjuvant and metastatic CRC. Dosing convenience: oral administration alone or as part of combination regimens.

Toxicity and adverse effects

Like 5-FU but generally improved tolerance.

Dose adjustments

Renal dysfunction. Perioperative discontinuation 3–4 weeks.

Complications

Familial DPD deficiency → risk of severe toxicity.

Oxaliplatin (Eloxatin)

Platin-based alkylating agent.

Mechanism of action

Exact details unknown: unspecific cytotoxic effect, synergistic with 5-FU.

Protocols

Setting: adjuvant and metastatic CRC. IV administration: FOLFOX4, FOLFOX6, FOLFOX7, CAPEOX, IROX.

Toxicity and adverse effects

Neuropathy (acute/reversible and chronic/irreversible), neutropenia, nausea/vomiting, diarrhea, fatigue. Less ototoxicity and nephrotoxicity than cisplatin and carboplatin.

Nonsurgical Management

Dose adjustments
Half-life 15–30 minutes. Discontinuation 4 weeks before/after elective surgery.

Complications
Febrile neutropenia. Increased toxicity in combination with bolus 5-FU.

Irinotecan (Camptosar, CPT-11)
Topoisomerase I inhibitor.

Mechanism of action
Intracellular conversion into active metabolite SN-38 → inhibition of intracellular topoisomerase-controlled topology/cleavage of supercoiled DNA double helix during transcription/replication → inhibition of DNA relaxation and unwinding necessary for replication and transcription → cell death.

Protocols
Setting: metastatic CRC, not established for adjuvant. FOLFIRI, IFL.

Toxicity and adverse effects
Diarrhea, dehydration, myelosuppression, alopecia.

Dose adjustments
Half-life ~6–12 hours (inactivation by enzyme UGT1A1), but longer lasting biologic effect → discontinuation 4 weeks before/after elective surgery.

Patients with polymorphisms in *UGT1A1* gene → higher effective dose (decreased inactivation) → need for dose reduction.

Complications
Severe diarrhea-induced dehydration, neutropenia.

Bevacizumab (Avastin)
Monoclonal antibody → targeted immunotherapy.

Mechanism of action
Monoclonal antibody against vascular endothelial growth factor (VEGF) → blocking tumor angiogenesis. For adequate tumor response: combination with cytotoxic chemotherapy drug needed (eg, 5-FU).

Protocols
Setting: metastatic CRC, not (yet) established for adjuvant. IV administration every 14 days in combination chemotherapy protocols (with 5-FU/LV, oxaliplatin, irinotecan).

Toxicity and adverse effects
Increased risk of grade 3–4 bleeding, thromboembolism, hypertension. Bowel perforation. Negative impact on anastomotic and wound healing.

Dose adjustments
Half-life ~20 days (range 10–50 days) → discontinuation 4–6 weeks before/after elective surgery.

Complications
GI perforation (1–2%), bleeding 3%, arterial emboli 2–3%, reversible posterior leukoencephalopathy syndrome < 1%.

Cetuximab (Erbitux)
Monoclonal antibody → targeted immunotherapy.

Mechanism of action
Chimeric monoclonal antibody against epidermal growth factor receptor (EGFR): high-affinity binding specifically to extracellular domain of human EGFR → blocks EGF/transforming growth factor-α binding to EGFR, which prevents activation of intracellular tyrosine kinase and EGFR signaling cascade → impaired cell growth and proliferation. Synergistic antitumor activity with conventional anticancer drugs and radiation.

Protocols
Setting: metastatic CRC. Metastatic CRC, combination with irinotecan.

Toxicity and adverse effects
Dermatologic: acne-like rash, xerosis (dry skin), fissures/rhagades.

Dose adjustments
Half-life ~4–5 days → discontinuation 2–3 weeks prior/after elective surgery.

Complications
Severe skin eruptions → pain, superinfection.

Panitumumab (Vectibix)
Monoclonal antibody → targeted immunotherapy.

Mechanism of action
Entirely human monoclonal antibody against EGFR.

Protocols
Setting: metastatic CRC. IV treatment of EGFR-expressing metastatic CRC with disease progression despite conventional chemotherapy.

Imatinib (Gleevec) and Sunitinib
Tyrosine kinase inhibitors → see separate discussion later in chapter.

Mitomycin C
Antitumor antibiotic.

Mechanism of action
Isolated from *Streptomyces caespitosus:* in vivo activation to alkylating agent → binding to DNA with cross-linking → dysfunction resulting in cell-cycle–independent DNA synthesis and transcription.

Protocols
Setting: anal cancer. IV administration.

Toxicity and adverse effects
Myelosuppression, cardiac and pulmonary toxicity, nephrotoxicity.

Dose adjustments
Half-life 15–20 minutes, elimination by hepatic metabolism.

Complications
Myelosuppression (cumulative effect), renal failure and hemolytic uremic syndrome (10%), pulmonary toxicity (40% mortality).

Gemcitabine (Gemzar)
Pyrimidine antimetabolite.

Mechanism of action
Antimetabolite related to cytarabine: intracellular metabolism to active di-/triphosphate nucleosides → S-phase/G1-phase–specific inhibition of DNA synthesis → apoptosis.

Protocols
Setting: metastatic CRC. IV administration.

Toxicity and adverse effects
Myelosuppression, rashes, flulike symptoms, edema, hemolytic uremic syndrome.

Dose adjustments
Half-life 1–10 hours (50% urinary excretion) → discontinuation 4–6 weeks before/after elective surgery.

Cisplatin (Platinol)
Alkylating agent.

Mechanism of action
Exact details unknown: DNA crosslinking resulting in unspecific cytotoxic effect.

Protocols
Alternate protocol to Nigro standard protocol for anal squamous cell cancer.

Toxicity and adverse effects
Dose-dependent cumulative nephrotoxicity, neuro- and ototoxicity, bone marrow suppression.

Dose adjustments
Half-life up to 3 days (!).

Complications
Acute nephrotoxicity. Increased toxicity in combination with radiation therapy.

Raltitrexed (Tomudex)
Antimetabolite.

Mechanism of action
Inhibitor of thymidylate synthase: depletion of cellular thymidine triphosphate (needed for DNA/RNA synthesis) $\rightarrow$ DNA/RNA fragmentation $\rightarrow$ cell death.

Protocols
Setting: metastatic CRC. IV administration.

Toxicity and adverse effects
GI toxicity (nausea, vomiting, anorexia), myelosuppression (neutropenia, anemia, thrombocytopenia), dermatologic, fever, etc.

Dose adjustments
Half-life ~8 days (50% urinary excretion) $\rightarrow$ discontinuation 4–6 weeks before/after elective surgery. Dose reduction for GI or hematologic side effects.

Complications
Life-threatening or fatal combination of leukopenia/thrombocytopenia with GI toxicity.

Experimental drugs (in the pipeline)
- PTK787: multi-inhibitor of vascular endothelial growth factor receptor (VEGFR).
- BAY 43-9006: dual inhibitor of RAF kinase and VEGFR.

Nonsurgical Management

Cross-reference

CHEMOTHERAPY PROTOCOLS—CURATIVE INTENT *(COLORECTAL CANCER)*

Principle

Probability of recurrent cancer 40–50% after "curative" radical resection of stage II and III without residual disease (R0 resection). With better understanding of tumor pathophysiology, availability of different chemotherapy drugs, and more sophisticated protocols, adjuvant or neoadjuvant chemotherapy has secured a role beyond just acceptance, demonstrating superiority over the surgery-only approach for a large number of cancer patients with increased response and survival rates.

Selection of specific drugs, protocol, route of administration, timing, and duration depend on several factors: histopathology, stage, primary and secondary tumor sites, patient performance status, response to treatment, side effects, and performed or planned surgery. Evidence is subject to continuous change or updates as results from trials come in.

Indications

- Colon cancer stage III (pTxN1–2).
- Colon cancer stage IIB (pT4N0), particularly if perforation.
- Colon cancer stage IIA (pT3) with unfavorable features: peritumoral lymphovascular involvement, inadequately sampled nodes, poorly differentiated histology.
- Rectal cancer stage II (u/pT3–4N0) and III (u/pTxN1–2).
- Rectal cancer stage pT2 post transanal local excision.

Summary of Evidence

Stage III colorectal cancer (CRC)

- Postoperative chemotherapy for 6 months is sufficient (no benefit from longer course).
- IV 5-FU/LV is superior to bolus 5-FU/LV.
- Levamisole is not necessary.
- Combination of 5-FU/LV and oxaliplatin is superior to 5-FU/LV alone.
- Capecitabine is similarly effective or even modestly better than IV 5-FU/LV.
- Effectiveness of adjuvant chemotherapy is independent of patient age.
- No documented role in adjuvant setting for the use of irinotecan, cetuximab, or bevacizumab, but subject to ongoing trials.

Stage II CRC
- No documented survival benefit of adjuvant therapy for patients with standard risk stage II disease.
- Chemotherapy in high-risk stage II disease appears logical but remains controversial because of lack of objective validation → needs further studies.

Alternatives

Surgery alone: colon cancer—stage I (pT1–2N0), stage IIA (pT3N0); in medically fit patients routine use of adjuvant chemotherapy is not recommended for stage II colon cancer without poor prognostic indicators.

Radiation alone or radiation + surgery: increasingly unusual approach for GI/anorectal tumors.

Adjuvant Chemotherapy Protocols with Curative Intent

I. Weekly bolus 5-FU + leucovorin (Roswell Park)

Bolus of 5-FU + leucovorin weekly for 6 weeks, 2 weeks of rest → total of three cycles every 8 weeks.

Indication
Standard protocol if oxaliplatin is contraindicated or not tolerated.

Contraindications
Ongoing sepsis, neutropenia, liver failure, kidney failure.

Toxicity and adverse effects
Grade III or IV: diarrhea 40%, stomatitis 1%, neutropenia 4%.

II. Monthly bolus 5-FU + leucovorin (Mayo Clinic)

Bolus of 5-FU + leucovorin on days 1–5, followed by 3 weeks of rest → total of six cycles every 4 weeks.

Indication
Standard protocol if oxaliplatin is contraindicated or not tolerated.

Contraindications
Ongoing sepsis, neutropenia, liver failure, kidney failure.

Toxicity and adverse effects
More toxic than other 5-FU/LV regimens → grade III or IV: diarrhea 13–21%, stomatitis 14–18%, neutropenia 16–55%.

III. Capecitabine (Xeloda)
Capecitabine: two oral doses twice daily for 14 days + 7 days of rest →
total of eight cycles every 3 weeks.

Indication
Alternative/new protocol if oxaliplatin is contraindicated or not tolerated.

Contraindications
Ongoing sepsis, neutropenia, liver failure, kidney failure.

Toxicity and adverse effects
Better tolerated than IV 5-FU/LV regimens.

IV. FOLinic acid + Fluorouracil + OXaliplatin (FOLFOX 4)
Oxaliplatin IV day 1; leucovorin IV days 1 and 2; 5-FU IV bolus, followed by continuous infusion over days 1 and 2 → total of 12 cycles every
14 days.

Indication
Standard intensive chemotherapy of choice if tolerated, particularly for
tumors with aggressive features and younger patients; 18–25% risk reduction compared with bolus 5-FU/LV (78% vs 73% disease-free survival).

Contraindications
Allergic reactions. Preexisting neuropathy.

Toxicity and adverse effects
Neutropenia (> 40%), febrile neutropenia, peripheral neuropathy (grade 3:
12% immediate, 1% persistent long-term).

V. FOLinic acid + Fluorouracil + OXaliplatin (FOLFOX 6)
Oxaliplatin IV day 1; leucovorin IV day 1 only; 5-FU IV bolus, followed by
continuous infusion (higher dose than FOLFOX4) over days 1 and 2 →
total of 12 cycles every 14 days.

Indication
Same as FOLFOX4, but higher dose of oxaliplatin and more convenient for
patient: need for treatment only on day 1 of each cycle.

Contraindications
Allergic reactions. Preexisting neuropathy.

Toxicity and adverse effects
Neutropenia (> 40%), febrile neutropenia, peripheral neuropathy (grade 3:
12% immediate, 1% persistent long-term).

Nonsurgical Management

VI. CAPEcitabine (XELoda) + OXaliplatin (CAPEOX, XELOX)
Oxaliplatin IV day 1; capecitabine PO bid days 1–14 + 7 days of rest →
every 21 days.

Indication
Alternative protocol to FOLFOX with increased dosing convenience.

Contraindications
Ongoing sepsis, neutropenia, liver failure, kidney failure.

Toxicity and adverse effects
Comparable or slightly better toxicity profile than FOLFOX.

Cross-reference

CHEMOTHERAPY PROTOCOLS—METASTATIC COLORECTAL CANCER

Principle

Availability of new drugs, introduction of biologic agents, and refinement of drug combinations and sequences has resulted in improved prospects for patients with metastatic colorectal cancer (CRC), prolonging overall survival from 6 months to currently > 22 months.

Treatment goals in the metastatic setting are:

- Cessation of tumor progression, tumor shrinkage ($\rightarrow$ potential for future resection of metastatic foci).
- Maintenance/improvement of overall quality of life.
- Acceptable profile of adverse effects.
- Prolonged survival.

Presence of limited metastatic disease is still consistent with possibility of resection with curative intent: combination chemotherapy is increasingly established. Route of drug administration: systemic administration (IV/oral) = standard. Regional treatment (hepatic arterial infusion, intraperitoneal chemotherapy) in the majority of situations is of no benefit.

All common regimens of advanced chemotherapy are based on 5-FU/LV (continuous infusion) or its oral prodrug capecitabine (Xeloda) in combination with either oxaliplatin or irinotecan.

Addition of targeted therapies bevacizumab or cetuximab (against vascular endothelial growth factor [VEGF], endothelial growth factor receptor [EGFR]) increases efficacy of chemotherapy with irinotecan and oxaliplatin: $\rightarrow$ FOLFIRI, FOLFOX, or XELOX plus bevacizumab have evolved as similarly effective first-line regimens for metastatic disease with regard to response and progression-free survival. Potentially even better response from combination of irinotecan and oxaliplatin (FOLFOXIRI).

Chemotherapy essentially is continued as maintenance therapy as long as it is tolerated and effective. There is no benefit from a completely chemotherapy-free interval, except interruption of oxaliplatin after 3 months to avoid cumulative toxicity (neuropathy); reintroduction if disease progression under 5-FU/LV. Definition of best modality sequence is subject to ongoing investigations.

Indications

- CRC stage IV.
- Locally recurrent CRC, not amenable to curative resection.

Summary of Evidence

Stage IV (with potential for curative resection):

- Combination of 5-FU/LV with either irinotecan or oxaliplatin superior to 5-FU/LV alone.
- Capecitabine similarly or even modestly more effective than IV 5-FU/LV.
- Bevacizumab or cetuximab added to baseline combination regimen increases treatment response, and prolongs progression-free survival and overall survival.
- Interruption of treatment 4–6 weeks perioperatively.

Stage IV (incurable): same as above, except no benefit from chemotherapy-free interval.

Stage IV (peritoneal carcinomatosis): intraperitoneal chemotherapy may be beneficial after complete macroscopic cytoreduction, otherwise systemic chemotherapy preferable.

Alternatives

Best supportive care.

Chemotherapy Protocols for Metastatic Colorectal Cancer

I. FOLinic acid + Fluorouracil + OXaliplatin (FOLFOX 4) ± bevacizumab

Oxaliplatin IV day 1; leucovorin IV days 1 and 2; 5-FU IV bolus, followed by continuous infusion over days 1 and 2 → cycles repeated every 14 days. Possible addition: bevacizumab IV every 2 weeks.

Indication
Standard intensive chemotherapy regimen for metastatic or recurrent CRC.

Contraindications
Allergic reactions. Preexisting neuropathy. Ongoing sepsis, neutropenia, liver failure, kidney failure.

Toxicity and adverse effects
Neutropenia (> 40%), febrile neutropenia, peripheral neuropathy (grade 3: 12% immediate, 1% persistent long-term).

II. FOLinic acid + Fluorouracil + OXaliplatin (FOLFOX 6) ± bevacizumab

Oxaliplatin IV day 1; leucovorin IV day 1 only; 5-FU IV bolus, followed by continuous infusion (higher dose than FOLFOX4) over days 1 and 2 →

cycles repeated every 14 days. Possible addition: bevacizumab IV every 2 weeks.

Indication
Same as FOLFOX4, but higher dose of oxaliplatin and more convenient to patient: need for treatment only on day 1 of each cycle.

Contraindications
Same as for FOLFOX4.

Toxicity and adverse effects
Essentially similar to FOLFOX4.

III. FOLinic acid + Fluorouracil + OXaliplatin (FOLFOX 7) ± bevacizumab
Oxaliplatin IV day 1; leucovorin IV day 1 only; 5-FU IV bolus, followed by continuous infusion (higher dose than FOLFOX4) over days 1 and 2 → total of six cycles every 14 days.

After that: simple LV/5-FU (without oxaliplatin): LV day 1, 5-FU IV bolus, followed by continuous infusion over days 1 and 2 → 12 cycles every 2 weeks, reintroduction of oxaliplatin if progression of disease. Possible addition: bevacizumab IV every 2 weeks.

Indication
Same as FOLFOX6, but limitation of oxaliplatin duration → maintenance with 5-FU/LV or capecitabine.

Contraindications
Same as for FOLFOX4.

Toxicity and adverse effects
Essentially similar to FOLFOX6, reduced long-term neuropathy.

IV. CAPEcitabine(XELoda) + OXaliplatin (CAPEOX, XELOX) ± bevacizumab
Oxaliplatin IV day 1; capecitabine PO bid days 1–14 + 7 days of rest → cycles repeated every 21 days. Possible addition: bevacizumab IV every 2 weeks.

Indication
Alternative protocol to FOLFOX with increased dosing convenience.

Contraindications
Allergic reactions. Preexisting neuropathy. Ongoing sepsis, neutropenia, liver failure, kidney failure.

Toxicity and adverse effects
Comparable or slightly better toxicity profile than FOLFOX.

V. FOLinic acid + Fluorouracil + IRInotecan (FOLFIRI) ± cetuximab
Irinotecan IV day 1; leucovorin IV day 1; 5-FU IV bolus, followed by continuous infusion over days 1 and 2 → total of 12 cycles every 14 days. Possible combination with cetuximab.

Indication
First-line regimen for metastatic CRC. Alternative to FOLFOX.

Contraindications
Ongoing sepsis, neutropenia, liver failure, kidney failure.

Toxicity and adverse effects
Diarrhea, nausea/vomiting, dehydration.

Bone marrow supression.

Cardiovascular events.

VI. Irinotecan + 5-FU + Leucovorin (IFL, Saltz regimen) ± cetuximab
Irinotecan IV + weekly IV bolus of 5-FU/LV for 4 weeks, followed by 2 weeks of rest → cycles repeated every 6 weeks. Possible combination with cetuximab.

Indication
First-line regimen for metastatic CRC, potential combination with bevacizumab or cetuximab.

Contraindications
Ongoing sepsis, neutropenia, liver failure, kidney failure.

Toxicity and adverse effects
GI syndrome: diarrhea, nausea/vomiting, anorexia, abdominal cramping → severe dehydration, electrolyte imbalances, neutropenia/fever.

Vascular syndrome: acute/fatal myocardial infarction, pulmonary embolus, cerebrovascular accident.

Dose adjustments
Monitoring for signs of impending severe toxicities.

Complications
Increased treatment-induced death rate due to combination of concurrent toxicities (diarrhea, febrile neutropenia, dehydration).

VII. IRinotecan + OXaliplatin (IROX) ± bevacizumab or cetuximab

Oxaliplatin IV, followed by irinotecan IV → every 3 weeks. Possible combination with bevacizumab or cetuximab.

Indication
Protocol in evolution.

Contraindications
Ongoing sepsis, neutropenia, liver failure, kidney failure.

Toxicity and adverse effects
Favorable toxicity profile.

VIII. CAPEcitabine + IRInotecan (CAPEIRI) ± bevacizumab or cetuximab

Irinotecan IV day 1; capecitabine PO bid days 1–14 + 7 days of rest → cycles repeated every 21 days. Possible combination with bevacizumab or cetuximab.

Indication
Second-line protocol.

Contraindications
Ongoing sepsis, neutropenia, liver failure, kidney failure.

Toxicity and adverse effects
Higher rates of severe vomiting, diarrhea, dehydration.

Cross-reference

Nonsurgical Management

RADIATION THERAPY

Principle

Radiotherapy plays an integral part in several standard treatments for anorectal/pelvic and selected extrapelvic malignancies that involve a limited field. In the realm of colorectal surgery, radiation most commonly is done as part of combined multimodality treatment.

Radiation induces direct or indirect (via radicals) ionization damage to biologic molecules (DNA, RNA), which results in single- and/or double-strand DNA breaks: the hit cells react with DNA repair, undergo cell death, or lose their reproductive integrity.

Radiation sensitivity of various tissues is dependent on: type of tissue, cell turnover, oxygenation, anemia (lack of oxygen carriers), and radiation sensitizers (chemotherapy).

Radiation effect in tissues:

• Early effects (within weeks, high cell turnover tissues): tumor shrinkage, skin damage, acute enteropathy, etc.
• Late effects (after months/years): obliterative microangiopathy with neovascularization, interstitial fibrosis, epithelial distortion → nerve injury, renal failure, bowel obstruction or perforation, and fibrosis.

Alternatives

Chemotherapy alone or in combination with surgery.

Surgery alone.

Alternate radiation techniques: intensity-mediated radiation therapy (IMRT), intraoperative radiation therapy (IORT), brachyradiotherapy.

Indications

• Primary rectal cancer stage II and III, selected stage IV: adjuvant vs neoadjuvant setting.
• Recurrent rectal cancer, previously not radiated.
• Anal cancer.
• Selected T4 colon cancers.

Preparatory Considerations

Appropriate imaging and staging.

Radiation planning and calculations: definition of radiation target, radiation dose, fractionation rate, radiation fields and individual technique.

Body marks and limitation of patient and organ movements (eg, through use of body cast) necessary for reproducible targeting of defined radiation field.

Protocols

Rectal cancer

- Standard course: 50.4 Gy radiation therapy (6 weeks) in combination with chemotherapy (see separate discussion).
- Short course: 25 Gy radiation therapy (5 days), followed by surgery 1 week later.

Anal cancer

Radiation therapy (45–59 Gy) in combination with 5-FU and mitomycin C (Nigro protocol) or cisplatin-based chemotherapy.

Toxicity and Adverse Effects

GI (particularly small bowel) toxicity (ie, acute or chronic radiation enteropathy), urinary toxicity, femur head necrosis, increased rate of venous thromboembolism.

Cross-reference

Nonsurgical Management

INTENSITY-MODULATED RADIATION THERAPY *(IMRT)*

Principle

IMRT consists of small radiation beams aimed at a target from many angles and therefore results in a more precise delivery of radiation to the target tissue while sparing surrounding normal and dose-limiting structures.

Three-dimensional (3D) conformal radiation therapy delivery by:

• Inverse treatment planning: CT-image generation for target areas that serve as templates for dose/intensity calculation per each segment. Based on that detailed tissue information, a computer-controlled feedback process calculates needed radiation doses from each angle in order to achieve radiation of just the desired target field.

• During treatment: computer-controlled intensity modulation of the radiation beam on a real-time basis.

Alternatives

Conventional external beam radiation: test radiation to assess effect and distribution to tissue.

Intraoperative radiation therapy: dose-limiting structures kept out of radiation beam.

Brachyradiotherapy: topical placement of radiation probes with relatively short tissue penetrance.

Indications

• Positive radial margins in primary/recurrent rectal cancer.

• Anal cancer.

Preparatory Considerations

Individual body cast is necessary for strict limitation of patient and organ movements.

Intraoperative preventive measures to prevent small bowel from dropping into empty pelvis: eg, omentum flap, etc.

Protocols

Individualized treatment protocol according to tumor location and anatomic structures.

Toxicity and Adverse Effects

GI toxicity 6–10%, urinary toxicity 10%.

Cross-reference

Nonsurgical Management

HIGH-DOSE BRACHYTHERAPY

Principle

Delivery of high-dose of radiation to a limited field and with limited penetration (~1 cm), hence avoiding regional maximal tolerance doses despite previous radiation exposure. Precise placement to areas of concern (positive margins) is achieved by means of afterloading catheters.

Alternatives

Conventional external beam radiation: test radiation to assess effect and distribution to tissue.

Intraoperative radiation therapy; dose-limiting structures kept out of radiation beam.

IMRT.

Indications

Positive radial margins in primary/recurrent rectal cancer or other pelvic malignancy when conventional external beam radiation already performed.

Preparatory Considerations

Intraoperative preventive measures to prevent sensitive structures (eg, small bowel, reconstructed rectum) from direct contact and radiation exposure: eg, placement of omentum flap in between, implantation of absorbable mesh at pelvic entry, etc.

Protocols

Individualized treatment protocol according to tumor location, anatomic structures, type of recurrence, and positive margins: 1600–1800 cGy.

- Intraoperative loading: after completion of resection insertion of afterloading tubes (stabilized with mesh or foldable apparatus). Advantage: empty pelvis, minimized collateral damage. Disadvantage: prolongation of already long surgery.

- Postoperative loading: after completion of resection insertion of afterloading tubes (stabilized with mesh or foldable apparatus) → afterloading 3–5 days after surgery in the radiation oncology facility when patient stabilized and out of the immediate perioperative risk. Advantage: empty pelvis, minimized collateral damage, no need for intraoperative shielding and infrastructure. Disadvantage: potential proximity of sensitive structures, dislocation of tubes.

Toxicity and Adverse Effects

Generally well tolerated, exact number of adverse effects unknown.

Cross-reference

FOLLOW-UP FOR COLORECTAL CANCER

Principle

Even though 70–80% of colorectal cancer (CRC) patients undergo primary treatment with curative intent, 30–50% will develop recurrent/metastatic tumor. More than 80% of recurrences after resection of CRC occur in the first 3 years, whereas the probability after 5 years is much smaller.

The concept of follow-up monitoring is geared to early recognition of recurrent disease at a still-treatable stage to improve survival. The value of intense follow-up remains controversial as improved outcome is not universally documented.

Methods

Clinical evaluation at defined intervals.

Blood work including tumor markers.

Imaging studies (CT, ERUS, PET).

Endoscopy.

Summary of Evidence

- Risk of metachronous cancer: 2–10%.
- Risk of recurrence dependent on primary tumor stage and tumor characteristics, but use of molecular or cellular markers not yet useful as guidance.
- Estimated 30–35% of patients undergoing salvage surgery for recurrent cancer will be cured.
- Benefit of follow-up for stage I cancer limited → colon and rectal surveillance, but no imaging studies.
- Follow-up for stage IV cancer not indicated, reevaluation according to course, treatment, response, progression.
- Intense follow-up for stage II/III CRC indicated as survival benefit suggested: recurrence/metastases occurring at same rate, but detected earlier, therefore increased probability to be addressed with surgery (caveat: lead-time bias).
- Duration of follow-up: not defined (duration, age limit, etc) → rational judgment in consideration of individual's overall life expectancy, comorbidities, risks.

Alternatives

No scheduled follow-up → evaluation if symptomatic.

TABLE 6–1. Suggested Follow-up Schedule for Patients with Stage II/III Colorectal Cancer.

Test Parameter	Months									
	3	6	9	12	18	24	30	36	48	60
History and physical exam	+	+	+	+	+	+	+	+	+	+
CEA	+	+	+	+	+	+	+	+	+	+
Colonoscopy[a]				+		(+)		(+)	(+)	(+)
CT abdomen/pelvis				+		+		+	+	
Rigid sigmoidoscopy and ERUS[b]	+	+	+	+	+	+		+	+	+
CT chest				+		+		+		
PET or PET-CT[c]	?									?
Chest x-ray	●									●
CBC, liver tests, FOBT	●									●

CBC, complete blood count; CEA, carcinoembryonic antigen; CT, computed tomography; FOBT, fecal occult blood test; PET, positron emission tomography.

[a]Frequency of subsequent endoscopies depends on whether and how many lesions are found, and whether there is an underlying hereditary cancer syndrome.

[b]Only for rectal cancer.

[c]Not used as routine test without other suspicion.

Stage-Dependent Follow-up

I. Stage I
Risk of local recurrence or distant metastases < 10%, except after transanal local excision of rectal cancer.

Practical steps
Colonoscopy surveillance: after 3–5 years, higher frequency according to findings and risks. CEA every 3–6 months, clinical follow-up.

Rectal cancer post transanal excision: rigid sigmoidoscopy and ERUS every 3 months (1st year), every 6 months (2nd year), yearly thereafter.

II. Stages II and III
Risk of local recurrence: colon 2%, rectum 10%. Risk of distant metastases: 30–40%.

Practical steps
Scheduled clinical evaluation, scheduled tests (Table 6–1): most weight on clinical evaluation, supplemented by scheduled CEA. Annual CT chest/abdomen/pelvis. Other tests not yet defined. Duration of surveillance not defined. Indication of surveillance in presence of severe comorbidities not defined.

Rectal cancer: Rigid sigmoidoscopy and ERUS every 3 months (1st year), every 6 months (2nd year), yearly thereafter.

III. Stage IV
Unless resection performed with curative intent → no scheduled follow-up for detection of recurrences, but appropriate tests to monitor treatment response or tumor progression or to evaluate symptoms.

Cross-reference

Topic	*Chapter*
Colorectal cancer	4 (pp 252–265)
Rectal cancer	4 (p 265)
Recurrent rectal cancer	4 (p 271)
CEA monitoring for colorectal cancer	6 (p 663)
TNM staging of colorectal cancer	App II (p 740)

CEA MONITORING FOR COLORECTAL CANCER

Principle

Monitoring of CEA in the management of patients with colorectal cancer (CRC) remains controversial. Neither sensitivity nor specificity of CEA is sufficient to be useful as a primary screening tool for detection of early-stage disease. A variety of other diseases may also cause CEA elevation.

The two best indications for CEA monitoring in CRC are (1) as postoperative follow-up in patients who would remain candidates for further treatment and (2) to assess treatment response in patients with metastatic disease. Decision-making process should be comprehensive, ie, not be based on CEA alone, but should incorporate clinical assessment, endoscopic and imaging data.

Methods

- Plasma CEA levels: immunoassay.
- Pathologic specimen: immunohistochemistry and PCR analysis → nearly universal CEA positivity in tumor even if plasma levels normal; search for micrometastases?
- CEA scintigraphy: formerly used to search for hidden disease, no role anymore in era of PET.

Summary of Evidence

- Rectal cancer less likely CEA-positive/-secreting than colon cancer.
- Plasma half-life time of CEA: 4–8 days.
- Other causes of CEA elevation (> 20%):
  – Noncolonic cancers: pancreatic, gastric, lung, breast cancer.
  – Benign conditions: IBD, benign polyps, liver cirrhosis, hepatitis, chronic lung disease, pancreatitis, smoking.
- Value of CEA measurement:
  – Before treatment: minimal/inexistent value for screening, diagnosis, evaluation.
  – Postoperative: valuable for follow-up.
  – Metastatic disease: valuable for monitoring treatment response and disease progression/regression.

Alternatives

Other follow-up tools: history and physical examination, colonoscopy, CT, PET.

Nonsurgical Management

Value of CEA

I. Screening
Disappointing: lack of sensitivity and lack of specificity with > 20% false-positive CEA elevation, eg, in smokers and several benign disorders.

Indication
CEA measurement is not indicated as a screening tool.

Pitfalls
False security; neither supports nor replaces adequate screening tools (colonoscopy, etc).

Data
CEA elevation: < 5% in stage I, < 25% in stage II disease.

II. Symptom evaluation
During evaluation of specific symptoms (ie, bleeding, palpable mass), value of CEA is limited in supporting or ruling out the various differential diagnoses or for guidance of management: lack of specificity as CEA elevation occurs in various other conditions; but CEA > 10–15 is unlikely to be caused by benign disease, and CEA > 20 is highly suspicious for metastatic disease.

Indication
CEA measurement is not indicated as a diagnostic tool, definitive histopathology and imaging studies have absolute preference.

Pitfalls
Negative result cannot provide sufficient certainty to rule out malignancy.

III. Pretreatment (before surgery or chemoradiation)
Value of CEA before surgical resection is limited: information less relevant than pathologic tumor stage, measured value never changes management, prognostic value limited.

Indication
As baseline parameter, expected postoperative normalization (after > 4–6 weeks), persistence suspicious for undetected disease.

Prognostic parameter: CEA < 5 associated with better outcome in colon but not rectal cancer? CEA > 10–15 is unlikely to be caused by benign disease; CEA > 20 is highly suspicious for metastatic disease.

Pitfalls
CEA expression/secretion: rectum is less likely to cause CEA elevation than colon cancer.

IV. Follow-up after treatment with curative intent

Normalization of preoperatively elevated CEA expected within 4–6 weeks after complete surgical resection → early detection of recurrent or metachronous cancer with potentially better chance for successful treatment intervention.

Indication

After complete resection of stage I–III CRC in patients who would again be candidates for surgery (regardless of preoperative CEA level):

- Normal before and after resection: follow every 2–3 months for ≥ 2 years.
- Elevated before, normal after resection: follow every 2–3 months for ≥ 2 years.
- Persistent elevation after resection: evaluation for metastatic or persistent disease, monitoring of treatment response.
- Normal after resection, confirmed rising during follow-up: search for tumor recurrence/metastases.

Pitfalls

CEA level not predictive of resectability of recurrence. Transient CEA elevations caused by liver dysfunction and/or chemotherapy.

Data

CEA and persistent/recurrent disease: sensitivity 50–80%, specificity 90%. CEA rising in > 80% of recurrences. In 50–65% of patients with recurrent disease: CEA rise is seen with/before onset of clinical symptoms. Resectable recurrences: 20% detected through CEA, rest through symptoms or other follow-up techniques.

V. Monitoring of treatment in recurrent/metastatic disease

CEA is a valuable marker for disease response to cancer-specific treatment (chemotherapy, radiation, surgery) in patients with recurrent or metastatic disease. Mandatory complementation with imaging studies (CT, PET).

Indication

Patients with recurrent/metastatic disease undergoing cancer-specific treatment.

Pitfalls

Tumor progression on imaging studies or clinical evidence without concomitant rise of CEA. No correlation of CEA course with survival.

Data

Up to one-third of tumors with progression on imaging studies do not show parallel CEA elevation. CEA elevated in metastatic disease: 80% of liver metastases, 40–50% of other sites.

Nonsurgical Management

Cross-reference

COMBINED MODALITY TREATMENT PROTOCOL—ANAL CANCER

Principle

Combined modality treatment has evolved as the first-line approach to anal cancer involving the anal canal. This is the result of a historical paradigm shift after 1974 from mutilating primary radical surgery (APR) with unsatisfactory survival to highly effective and sphincter-saving chemoradiation (Nigro protocol) as the primary treatment of choice. Radical surgery is reserved as a salvage approach for treatment failures, ie, incomplete response of primary tumor treatment (more likely in large and bulky tumors) or recurrent disease.

Caveat: anal margin cancers (not extending to anal canal) and verrucous Buschke-Lowenstein carcinoma are still primarily treated surgically if negative margins can be obtained.

Indications

Anal squamous cell cancer (involving anal canal).

Summary of Evidence

- Primary chemoradiation: 80–90% complete clinical response, 65–75% 5-year survival.
- 5-year survival after APR alone: 40–70%.
- Cisplatin-based alternative protocols do not result in improved survival but have higher colostomy rate compared with standard mitomycin-based protocols → cisplatin in many centers is only used as a salvage approach or for HIV-positive patients because it is better tolerated.
- Patients with advanced disease at presentation are more likely to have persistent disease after chemoradiation → planning of salvage APR.
- Probability of colostomy 25–40% (persistent/recurrent disease or treatment sequelae).

Alternatives

Surgery alone:

- Anal margin cancers (away from anal canal) → treated like other skin cancers.
- Watchful waiting, possible reexcision, and serial clinical reexaminations:
  - Incidental cancer in condyloma or hemorrhoidectomy specimen.
  - Intraepithelial cancer (carcinoma in-situ): Bowen disease, Paget disease.
- Verrucous carcinoma.

Chemotherapy Protocols with Curative Intent

I. 5-Fluorouracil + mitomycin and radiation 45–59 Gy (Nigro protocol)

- 5-FU infusion on days 1–4, and during last week of radiation therapy.
- Mitomycin C IV on day 1.
- 45–59 Gy in daily doses of 200 cGy → 5 days/week for 5 weeks.
- Radiation evaluated after 45 Gy → if necessary dose escalation by adding further radiation up to 59 Gy.

Indication
Standard protocol for T1–T2 anal cancer.

Contraindications
Ongoing sepsis, neutropenia, liver failure, kidney failure.

Toxicity and adverse effects
Acute toxicity: myelosuppression, cardiac and pulmonary toxicity, nephrotoxicity, anoproctitis, perianal dermatitis, diarrhea. Late toxicity: ulcerations, proctitis, stenosis, impotence.

Dose adjustments
HIV-positive patients (particularly with CD4 < 200 or AIDS): reduced tolerance.

Complications
Myelosuppression (cumulative effect), renal failure and hemolytic uremic syndrome (10%), pulmonary toxicity (40% mortality)

II. 5-Fluorouracil + mitomycin and radiation 55–59 Gy (Nigro protocol)

- 5-FU infusion on days 1–4, and during last week of radiation therapy.
- Mitomycin C IV on day 1.
- 55–59 Gy in daily doses of 200 cGy → 5 days/week for 5 weeks.
- Radiation evaluated after 55 Gy → if necessary dose escalation by adding further radiation up to 59 Gy.

Indication
Standard protocol for T3–T4 anal cancer.

I. 5-Fluorouracil + cisplatin and radiation 45–59 Gy

- 5-FU infusion on days 1–4; cisplatin IV on day 1 → four cycles every 4 weeks.
- After 8 weeks: 45–59 Gy in daily doses of 200 cGy → 5 days/week for 5 weeks.

Indication
Alternate protocol for anal cancer, particularly HIV-positive patients and/or recurrent disease.

Dose adjustments
HIV-positive patients (particularly with CD4 < 200 or AIDS): reduced tolerance.

Complications
No evidence for improved disease-free or overall survival (compared with mitomycin-based standard protocol), but higher risk for colostomy.

Cross-reference

Topic	*Chapter*
Anal cancer	4 (pp 228–230)
LAR/TME	5 (p 610)
APR	5 (p 615)
Tumor staging in TNM system	App II (p 740)

IMATINIB *(GLEEVEC)*

Principle

Imatinib is a specific inhibitor of a selected number of tyrosine kinase enzymes. It is used for treatment of GIST and chronic myelogenous leukemia (CML). GIST: disease control is achieved in 70–85% of patients with unresectable or metastatic disease and is associated with prolonged progression-free survival and overall survival (median 36 months); 90% disease-free survival in adjuvant setting after curative resection of GIST.

Alternatives

Surgery for localized and resectable GIST.

Conventional chemotherapy: notoriously poor results for GIST.

Sunitinib for imatinib-resistant GIST.

Indications

• Unresectable and metastatic GIST.

• CML.

• (Neo-)Adjuvant treatment with surgical resection of GIST?

• Desmoid tumors?

Preparatory Considerations

Risk calculation to assess individual patient's risk of toxicity possible, but often no alternatives to imatinib. Monitoring of CBC, creatinine, and liver parameters.

Protocols

Daily oral administration.

Toxicity and Adverse Effects

Generally very well tolerated.

Side effects include fluid retention and edema (30%), nausea/diarrhea (20%), rash (16–18%), musculoskeletal pain, grade 3 or higher anemia (13%), neutropenia (7%), severe congestive cardiac failure (rare).

Dose Adjustments

Imatinib: hepatic metabolism (half-life 18–20 hours) → still active 1st metabolite (half-life 40 hours) → biliary elimination, only minimal urinary excretion. Dose adjustment for hematologic adverse reactions and hepatotoxicity.

Bleeding risk and potentially higher leak rate, but otherwise no documented negative impact on surgery → discontinuation 1 week prior to elective procedure.

Cross-reference

Topic	*Chapter*
PET	2 (p 126)
GIST	4 (p 283)

MEDICAL MANAGEMENT OF CROHN DISEASE

Principle

Crohn disease is an autoimmune disease of unknown etiology that cannot be cured. Medical management is the treatment of choice unless focal complications mandate a surgical exploration. Nonetheless, key problems often less responsive to nonsurgical management: intestinal fistulae, abscess formation, stricture, etc. Up to 70–80% of patients will require at least one surgical resection. Postsurgical prophylaxis is therefore an additional important aspect.

Indications

- Active intestinal Crohn disease.
- Active perianal Crohn manifestation.
- Maintenance of remission after medical treatment.
- Maintenance of remission after surgical resection.

Medications

Group	Mechanism, Effect	Examples
Aminosalicylates[a]	Unknown, inhibition of proinflammatory cytokines	Sulfasalazine, mesalamine
Steroids, systemic	Multidirectional immunosuppression	Prednisone, prednisolone, hydrocortisone
Steroids, local	Same as above, but locally	Budesonide
Immunosuppressants	Antimetabolites for DNA/RNA synthesis, inhibition of cellular immune response	6-MP, azathioprine (AZA), cyclosporine, methotrexate (MTX)
Anticytokine biologicals	Immunologic elimination of cytokines	Infliximab (Remicade), adalimumab (Humira)
Antibiotics	Suppression of colonic disease activity and secondary problems (abscess, fistulae)	Metronidazole, quinolones

[a]Sulfasalazine = sulfapyridine + 5-ASA → cleavage in colon; mesalamine = 5-ASA + 5-ASA → cleavage level (small bowel, colon) depending on pharmacologic preparation.

Summary of Evidence

Primary medical management

- Steroids: induce remission, no benefit for maintenance, or to prevent recurrence; result in a nine times increased risk for an abscess; response to steroids in 30–80%, steroid dependency in 40%.
- Aminosalicylates: for mild to moderate disease associated with < 40% remission (compared with 15–20% with placebo).
- 6-MP/AZA: induce/maintain remission, prevent recurrence, endoscopic healing with response rate of 70–80%, but long delay of 3–6 months until benefit visible.
- Infliximab: fistula closure in 37–50% temporarily, high probability of recurrence. Concomitant medication with AZA or steroids reduces the risk of antibodies against infliximab → longer effectiveness.
- Cyclosporine: fistula response rate > 80%, fistula closure in > 60% in 1 week, but relapse in > 40% → need for 6-MP or ASA.
- Natalizumab: withdrawn from market because of association with progressive demyelinating leukoencephalopathy, being reintroduced again.

Maintenance of remission

- Steroids: 30–40%.
- 6-MP: in > 80%.
- Mesalamine: data not convincing with no proven benefit over placebo.

Prevention of recurrence after surgical resection

Efficacy: recurrence rates of 6-MP 50% > mesalamine 60% > nothing 70–80%.

Alternatives

Surgery alone: 80% probability that patient will require at least one surgical resection → 50–80% show endoscopic recurrence → 20–30% require 2nd resection.

Watchful waiting: 80% recurrence.

Abdominal fistulae: overall unsatisfactory response to conservative management → remain a surgical target, potentially after preceding priming with immunosuppressants.

Perirectal fistulae: placement of longterm setons.

Treatment Algorithms

I. "Bottom-up" approach

Start with simplest treatment and increase potency if no effect: ie, 5-ASA and/or antibiotics → steroids → 6-MP/AZA → MTX → infliximab vs cyclosporine A.

Efficacy

Endoscopic healing in 20–30%, remission 70–75%, remission with steroid withdrawal 40%.

Pro

Stepwise escalation, reserving powerful biologic agents for later in the game; more cost-effective? Avoidance of known/unknown side effects of biologicals (eg, activation of tuberculosis, lymphoma, encephalopathy).

Con

For Crohn disease (in contrast to ulcerative colitis), there is no safe and effective first-line induction and/or maintenance therapy → increased risk of side effects (eg, abscess, persistent disease, steroid dependency, etc); long delay until 6-MP/AZA takes effect.

II. "Top-down" approach

Start with most potent treatment and go to less potent treatments as disease is suppressed: ie, infliximab + AZA → recurrent infliximab → 6-MP/AZA → steroids.

Efficacy

Endoscopic healing in 75%, remission 70–75%, remission with steroid withdrawal > 75%.

Pro

Rapid and most effective induction suppression of disease activity → prevents hospital admissions, allows return to work, preserves quality of life; 6-MP/AZA may take 3–6 months to show visible effect.

Con

Powerful biologic agents not needed for all patients; once started → needed all the time; very expensive (> $30,000/year); known/unknown side effects of biologicals (eg, activation of tuberculosis, lymphoma, encephalopathy).

Cross-reference

MEDICAL MANAGEMENT OF ULCERATIVE COLITIS

Principle

Ulcerative colitis is an autoimmune disease essentially limited to the large bowel. Medical management is the first-line treatment. Although the disease is surgically curable, only 20–30% of patients will undergo surgical resection.

Indications

- Active ulcerative colitis.
- Maintenance of remission after medical treatment.

Medications

Group	Mechanism, Effect	Examples
Aminosalicylates[a]	Unknown, inhibition of proinflammatory cytokines	Sulfasalazine, mesalamine
Steroids, systemic	Multidirectional immunosuppression	Prednisone, prednisolone, hydrocortisone
Steroids, local	Same as above, but locally	Budesonide
Immunosuppressants	Antimetabolites for DNA/RNA synthesis, inhibition of cellular immune response	6-MP, azathioprine (AZA), cyclosporine, methotrexate (MTX)
Anticytokine biologicals	Immunologic elimination of cytokines	Infliximab (Remicade), adalimumab (Humira)

[a]Sulfasalazine = sulfapyridine + 5-ASA $\rightarrow$ cleavage in colon; mesalamine = 5-ASA + 5-ASA $\rightarrow$ cleavage level (small bowel, colon) depending on pharmacologic preparation.

Summary of Evidence

Primary medical management

- Steroids: induce remission, no benefit for maintenance, or to prevent recurrence.

• Aminosalicylates: induce/maintain remission; for mild to moderate disease, cost-effective.

• 6-MP/AZA: uncertain with regard to induction/maintenance of remission.

• Cyclosporine: last resort in hospitalized patients with severe colitis. Side effects: serious infections, hypertension, renal problems, seizures.

• Infliximab: as of yet not shown to be effective in longterm for refractory colitis.

• Antibiotics: no role in management of ulcerative colitis (except in fulminant episode).

• Specific anti-infectious treatments: flare-up potentially related to superinfection with *C difficile* or CMV → need for respective assessment and initiation of specific treatment; however these pathogens generally indicate poor responsiveness of the ulcerative colitis to nonsurgical management.

• Nutrition: maintained for majority of patients, NPO only for fulminant episode or toxic megacolon.

• TPN: only for severe malnutrition or temporarily as part of treatment of fulminant episode.

Alternatives

Surgery: proctocolectomy with ileal J-pouch anal anastomosis (elective or semi-elective) or total abdominal colectomy with end-ileostomy (emergency).

Treatment Algorithms

I. "Bottom-up" approach

Start with simplest treatment and increase potency if no effect: ie, 5-ASA or budesonide per rectum → 5-ASA per oral → systemic steroids for flare-ups → 6-MP/AZA → cyclosporine? → surgery.

Efficacy

Adequate disease suppression in 70–80% of patients, 30–40% steroid-refractoriness.

Pro

Effective, safe first-line induction and/or maintenance therapy, cost-effective! Avoidance of known/unknown side effects of biologicals (eg, activation of tuberculosis, lymphoma, encephalopathy).

Con

No major considerations.

II. "Top-down" approach
Not currently indicated or defined for ulcerative colitis ($\leftrightarrow$ contrast to Crohn disease).

Cross-reference

Nonsurgical Management

PHYSICAL THERAPY/BIOFEEDBACK TRAINING

Principle

Anorectal dysfunctions commonly have a significant neuromuscular component which may occur as an independent entity or be superimposed on and aggravate a primary morphopathology: loss of muscle strength, muscle discoordination/ dyssynergia, anorectal sensation, spasms, response patterns, etc.

Pelvic floor rehabilitation targets improvement of these baseline components by retraining anorectal sensation, strengthening the residual muscle function, and improving coordination, contraction, and relaxation. In addition, subjective response and coping mechanisms are reinforced. Benefits of this concept include its simplicity, low cost, and absence of any side effects; furthermore, the range of other treatment options is not negatively affected. However, data on efficacy also vary, and subjective and objective outcomes may not correlate.

Indications

- Fecal and urinary incontinence (before/after surgical intervention).
- Pelvic floor dysfunction.
- Functional outlet obstruction (anismus, puborectalis dyssynergia).
- Functional pelvic pain syndromes (levator ani spasm).
- Altered anorectal function, eg, after IPAA, LAR/coloanal.

Summary of Evidence

- Pelvic floor rehabilitation has no side effects (except electrogalvanic stimulation).
- Lack of objective evidence from randomized studies about short-term/long-term efficacy, available studies often with significant methodologic weaknesses.
- Success rates vary for different conditions: 50–80% subjective improvement, but frequently only minimal change to objective parameters. Built-in selection biases: eg, only individuals with improvement complete the training, treatment endpoint when patient is better, etc.
- Patient motivation and smooth interaction with physical therapist strongly correlate with success.

Alternatives

Surgical intervention to improve correctable morphopathology.

Pharmacologic optimization.

Behavioral and habit training.

Rehabilitation Tools

I. Pelvic muscle exercises (Kegel exercises)

Goal: strengthening of muscle contractions.

Protocol: instruction to do extended isotonic/isometric contractions of pelvic floor muscles and quick contract-relax cycles. Timing of exercises to be done independent from bowel activity as well as at the time of bowel activity, eg, conscientious effort to avoid evacuation in the safety of the toilet environment. Intermittent supervision and guidance by physical therapist to instruct independent exercises by patients.

Problems: patients tend to use auxiliary muscles more than actual sphincter complex. Careful supervision and instruction are needed to avoid activation of wrong muscle groups (pseudo-success).

II. Biofeedback training

Goal: re-coordination of pelvic floor muscles.

Protocol: pelvic floor exercises with real-time monitoring and computer-graphic display of the generated effort: guidance through continuous manometry or endorectal or surface EMG probe → patient may see immediate result of activity and learn to coordinate muscles such that desired graphic templates (contraction/relaxation) can be actively reproduced. Weekly sessions of 30 minutes for 9 weeks.

III. Electrogalvanic stimulation

Goal: get spastic (painful) muscle groups into tetany with fatigue and resulting relaxation.

Protocol: insertion of probe and electric pulse delivery at frequency of 80 cycles/second. Incremental voltage starting at 0 with gradual increase and maintenance just below pain threshold for 1 hour.

Problems: lack of documented efficacy, true morphologic cause of pain needs to be ruled out first. Possible side effects from too-high electric stimulation.

Cross-reference

Nonsurgical Management

Perioperative Management

SURGICAL CARE IMPROVEMENT PROJECT
(SCIP)

Overview

Initiative sponsored by several organizations to improve the surgical care and reduce preventable surgical complications (morbidity and mortality). Linked to pay-for-performance quality parameters.

Four major targets for prevention:

• Surgical site infections.
• Venous thromboembolism.
• Cardiac morbidity.
• Respiratory morbidity.

Prevention of Surgical Site Infection

Surgical site infection is responsible for 15% of all nosocomial infections: 2–5% of clean extra-abdominal cases and up to 20% of intra-abdominal cases.

Measures:

• Appropriate selection of prophylactic antibiotics: eg, cephalosporin + metronidazole, ertanpenem, fluorochinolone + metronidazole. Betalactam allergy: fluoroquinolone + metronidazole, clindamycin + fluoroquinolone, clindamycin + aztreonam, etc.
• Prophylactic antibiotics received within 1 hour before surgical incision.
• Prophylactic antibiotics limited to 24 hours (longer duration okay for therapeutic indication).
• Appropriate hair removal for surgical field preparation (clipper, no razor).
• Monitoring and correction of peri-postoperative glucose levels.
• Maintenance of peri-/postoperative normothermia.

Prevention of Venous Thromboembolism

Without appropriate prophylaxis, DVT is a complication in 20–50% of major operations → pulmonary embolism in 10–30%.

Measures:

• Recommended DVT prophylaxis ordered.
• Appropriate DVT prophylaxis initiated within 24 hours before surgery to 24 hours after surgery.

Prevention of Adverse Cardiac Events

Adverse cardiac events (eg, myocardial infarction, sudden cardiac death, congestive heart failure) complicate 2–5% of noncardiac surgeries overall, causing increased mortality rate, length of stay, cost.

Measures:

• Perioperative β-blocker administration if previously required (eg, for angina, hypertension, arrhythmias).

Prevention of Respiratory Complications

Patients on respirator with mechanical ventilation are at increased risk of ventilator-associated pneumonia (10–30%), stress ulcer disease, and GI bleeding.

Suggested (but not yet approved) measures:

• Elevation of head of bed.
• Provision of stress ulcer disease prophylaxis.
• Use of ventilator weaning protocols to reduce duration of mechanical ventilation.

Cross-reference

GENERAL PERIOPERATIVE MANAGEMENT—ABDOMINAL

Overview

Colorectal surgery encompasses an enormously broad spectrum of diseases and conditions through all age and risk groups. Treatment equally varies in a wide range of approaches and is delivered in several different settings (office, OR, endoscopy suite, outpatient/inpatient).

Hence, management is not "one-size-fits-all." Nonetheless, a few principles have evolved that should be considered in the perioperative management of a patient undergoing an abdominal procedure.

Risk Assessment

- < 40 years, no risk factors/symptoms → no specific workup needed.
- > 40 years, no risk factors → ECG, chest x-ray, basic set of lab work.
- Any age, specific risk factors/symptoms → ECG, chest x-ray, basic set of lab work, followed by selective internal medicine or cardiology clearance.
- Pregnancy test in all women of childbearing age.

Bowel Cleansing

- Dependent on surgery and surgeon: see separate discussion in this chapter.
- If mechanical bowel cleansing → monitoring and supplementation of electrolytes and fluid status.

Site Selection (Marking) for Possible Ostomy

Potential need for permanent or temporary ostomy → discussion and pre-operative marking of possible stoma sites (stoma nurse, verification through operating surgeon).

Antibiotic Prophylaxis

See separate discussion in this chapter.

Venous Thromboembolism Prophylaxis

See separate discussion in this chapter.

Management of Medications

- Antihypertensives/β-blockers: should be actively continued.
- Oral antidiabetics: discontinued the day before (fasting period).
- Insulin: reduced dose for fasting and surgery period, ideally titrating drip.

- Steroids: > 20 mg/day of prednisone → give same dose IV (as prednisolone which is 1.25 times more potent that prednisone), < 20 mg/day → dose (as prednisolone) + additional stress dose.
- Past steroids (< 6 months): perioperative steroid stress dose:
- Short boost: 100 mg hydrocortisone IV on call to OR, repeat one dose in evening and next morning, then stop (ie, total of three doses).
- Longer taper: 100 mg hydrocortisone IV twice daily on surgery day (= equivalent to 40 mg prednisone) → switch to oral prednisone and reduce by 10 mg every 5 days down to 20 mg/day, last 20 mg tapered in 5-mg steps every 5–7 days.

Blood Transfusion

Many abdominal colorectal operations do not need a blood transfusion due to bloodless surgical and anesthesiologic technique and a lowered range for blood levels that are still acceptable in a given patient. Minimal blood levels depend on patient age, comorbidities, expected ongoing blood loss, current hemodynamics:

- < 40 years, no risk factors: hematocrit ≥ 25 (or individually even less).
- > 40 years, no risk factors: hematocrit ≥ 28.
- Any age, specific risk factors: hematocrit ≥ 30.
- Preexisting chronic anemia (eg, IBD, renal failure): hematocrit down to 20 acceptable?

Preoperative planning:

- Baseline: type and screen.
- Preexisting anemia, expected blood loss: type and cross.
- Preexisting anemia, bleeding risk, expected high blood loss: type and cross, including fresh frozen plasma, platelets.

Jehovah's witnesses:

- Determine the individual patient's acceptance of cell saver, albumin, fibrin glue, erythropoietin, etc.
- Preexisting anemia: determine whether optimizing blood levels possible, or whether further delay would result in more severe blood loss (eg, active bleeding from tumor, colitis, etc).
- Intraoperative availability of sealing devices, nontraumatic surgical technique; in case of bleeding → rapid packing and damage control.

Pain Management

Crucial to allow for adequate respiratory excursions to avoid atelectasis, pneumonia.

- Epidural analgesia (EDA) at thoracic level (Th6–Th12).
- Patient-controlled anesthesia (PCA).
- On demand: oral analgesics, intramuscular analgesics.

Caveat: postoperative ileus and prerenal borderline kidney function (large fluid shifts) increase risks of ketorolac and other NSAIDs to cause peptic ulcer or acute renal failure.

Foley Catheter

Placement indicated for all abdominal procedures to adequately monitor urine output peri- and postoperatively.

Removal:

- Procedure with pelvic dissection: after 3–5 days.
- Any procedure with EDA in place: continued until 6 hours after discontinuation of EDA.
- Procedure without pelvic dissection, patient stable, no EDA: removal after 1 day or less.
- Procedure without pelvic dissection, but major procedure, comorbidities, or unstable patient: continue until patient stable (eg, large procedure, ICU setting).
- Bladder repair: removal after ~10–14 days (after prior cystogram?).

Ureteral Stents

- Previous history of colorectal or pelvic dissections, ongoing inflammatory process → placement of prophylactic ureteral stents to allow intraoperative identification and protection. Lighted stents for laparoscopy.
- Postoperative management: depending on extent of adjacent dissection or traumatization during surgery removal after 0–2 days.

Nasogastric Tube

- No routine placement.
- Only for symptomatic patient (eg, gastric retention, bowel obstruction) → low intermittent wall suction until output < 200–300 mL/24 hours; limited amount of oral clear fluid intake is okay for patient comfort.
- Removal of NGT: if < 200–300 mL/24 hours; if function is uncertain: transition by intermittent clamping of NGT and checking of residuals every 4–6 hours.

Nutrition

- Fast-track concept → no waiting for passage of gas or stool but feeding on POD1 or as soon as no nausea/vomiting (ie, recovery of upper GI tract function). Caveat: aspiration precautions!

- Inability to have oral intake despite working GI tract (eg, intubated patient) → enteral nutrition.
- > 5 days inability to tolerate enteral nutrition or preexisting malnutrition → TPN. Cycled TPN, if need continued as outpatient.

Mobilization

- Early patient mobilization important: improve lung function, reduce DVT, stimulate GI function, limit decubitus risk.
- Starting no later than first postoperative day, unless patient intubated.
- Bedridden patient: repeated positional changes, soft mattress, physical therapy for prevention of extremity contractures, etc.

Respiratory Care in Nonintubated Patients

- Early patient mobilization and/or frequent positional changes.
- Incentive spirometry.
- Adequate pain control.
- Chest physical therapy.
- Inhaler treatment (bronchodilators, inhaled steroids, acetylcysteine, etc).

Cross-reference

GENERAL PERIOPERATIVE MANAGEMENT— ANORECTAL

Overview

Colorectal surgery encompasses an enormously broad spectrum of diseases and conditions through all age and risk groups. Treatment equally varies in a wide range of approaches and is delivered in several different settings (office, OR, endoscopy suite, outpatient/inpatient). Hence, management is not "one-size-fits-all." Nonetheless, a few principles have evolved that should be considered in the perioperative management of a patient undergoing an anorectal procedure.

Risk Assessment

- < 40 years, no risk factors/symptoms → no specific workup needed.
- > 40 years, no risk factors → ECG, chest x-ray, basic set of lab work.
- Any age, specific risk factors/symptoms → ECG, chest x-ray, basic set of lab work → selective internal medicine or cardiology clearance.
- Pregnancy test in all women of childbearing age.

Bowel Cleansing

- Two Fleet enemas are sufficient for most anorectal procedures.
- Full bowel cleansing for selected indications.
- If mechanical bowel cleansing → monitoring and supplementation of electrolytes and fluid status.

Antibiotic Prophylaxis

See separate discussion in this chapter.

Venous Thromboembolism Prophylaxis

Outpatient procedure: not indicated (except intraoperative intermittent pneumatic compression).

Inpatient procedure: see separate discussion in this chapter.

Management of Medications

- Antihypertensives/β-blockers: should be actively continued.
- Oral antidiabetics: discontinued the day before (fasting period)
- Insulin: reduced dose for fasting and surgery period, ideally titrating drip.
- Steroids: > 20 mg/day of prednisone → same dose IV (as prednisolone), < 20 mg/day → dose (as prednisolone) + additional stress dose.

• Past steroids (< 6 months): perioperative steroid stress dose:
  – Short boost: 100 mg hydrocortisone IV on call to OR, repeat one dose in evening and next morning, then stop.
  – Longer taper: 100 mg hydrocortisone IV twice daily on surgery day (= equivalent to 40 mg prednisone) → switch to oral prednisone and reduce by 10 mg every 5 days down to 20 mg/day, last 20 mg tapered in 5-mg steps every 5–7 days.

Blood Transfusion

Blood transfusion is very unlikely for anorectal surgery.

Pain Management

Combination of NSAID (eg, ketorolac) with opiate generally works well.

Addition of antibiotics (eg, metronidazole), topical nitroglycerine, or topical sucralfate of potential benefit but controversial data.

Foley Catheter

• Routine placement not needed for anorectal procedure as long as anesthesiologist adheres to perioperative fluid restriction (< 500 mL total IV fluids) to avoid bladder distention.
• Selective indications.

Nutrition

Resumption of regular diet as soon as anesthesia has worn off (> 6 hours after end of surgery).

Bowel Management

• Bowel confinement not indicated (except for selected cases).
• Fiber supplementation with adequate fluid intake, stool softener, milk of magnesia (as needed) → soft but formed stool.

Wound Care

• Internal wound (eg, stapled hemorrhoidectomy): no wound care.
• Closed wound: rinsing off after bowel movement, patting dry.
• Open wound: sitz baths 2–3 times, plus after each bowel movement.

Cross-reference

COMORBIDITIES—CARDIAC DISEASE

Overview

Cardiac diseases or surgeries may either precipitate colorectal problems (eg, ischemic colitis) or indirectly interfere with the management of unrelated colorectal diseases. Both the need for colorectal surgeries and the prevalence of cardiac diseases show a parallel increase with age. Adequate cardiac function is a prerequisite for any surgical management. Appropriate risk assessment in view of the urgency and the natural course of the colorectal disease and the cardiac prognosis are relevant in order to adjust the management.

History and background information (eg, risk factors, cardiopulmonary or vascular symptoms and events, previous cardiac evaluations and/or interventions, medications, patient compliance, etc), current physical performance capacity, physical examination, and baseline tests are the basis to assess the need for more thorough cardiac evaluation.

Problems

• Risk assessments reflect a statistical probability and may not predict the individual's outcome.
• Routine placement of pre-/perioperative pulmonary artery catheter is not beneficial, causing potential harm.

Risk Assessment Parameters

• Urgency and extent of colorectal operation: elective vs emergency, abdominal vs anorectal.
• Severity and prognosis of colorectal disease.
• Coexisting morbidity: pulmonary disease, diabetes, peripheral vascular disease, stroke, renal or liver disease, hematologic disorders (anemia, thrombocytosis, etc).
• Nature of cardiac disease:
  – Coronary artery disease (diabetic, nondiabetic).
  – Valvular heart disease (primary vs secondary with biologic or mechanical valve).
  – Arrhythmias and conduction defects.
  – Cardiomyopathy.
  – Post–heart transplantation.

- Assessment of severity and prognosis of cardiac disease and identification of those patients who require cardiologic evaluation:
  - Goldman classification (Table 7–1), and newer modifications (eg, Detsky index).
  - Cardiac risk categories (Table 7–2).
  - Adapted risk stratification for colorectal procedures (Table 7–3).
- Cardiac evaluation and testing:
  - Exercise stress testing: treadmill testing.
  - Ambulatory 24- to 48-hour ECG monitoring.
  - Echocardiography: evaluation of murmurs (diastolic vs systolic vs valvular, etc), congestive heart failure of unknown cause.
  - Dobutamine stress echocardiography.

TABLE 7–1. Goldman Cardiac Risk Index.

Category	Parameters	Points
History	Age > 70 years	5
	Myocardial infarction < 6 months	10
Cardiac exam	Signs of congestive heart failure: S_3 gallop, jugular vein distention	11
	Significant aortic stenosis	3
ECG	Rhythm other than sinus, premature atrial contractions	7
	> 5 premature ventricular contractions per minute	7
General medical conditions	$Po_2 < 60$, $Pco_2 > 50$; K < 3, $HCO_3 < 20$, BUN > 50, creatinine > 3, elevated SGOT, chronic liver disease, bedridden	3
Operation	Emergency surgery	4
	Abdominal or thoracic operation	3

Risk Class	Total Points	Risk of Life-Threatening Complication (%)	Risk of Cardiac Death (%)
I	0–5	0.7	0.2
II	6–12	5	2
III	13–25	11	2
IV	26–53	22	56

TABLE 7–2.   Cardiac Risk Categories.

Category	Conditions
Active cardiac conditions → major clinical risk	Unstable coronary syndromes: angina, acute/recent myocardial infarction (< 1 month) Decompensated heart failure Significant arrhythmias Severe valvular disease

Clinical risk factors
  1–2 → intermediate risk
  ≥3 → major risk
	History of ischemic heart disease
	History of compensated or prior heart failure
	History of cerebrovascular disease
	Diabetes mellitus
	Renal insufficiency

Minor/uncertain predictors	Age > 70 years Abnormal ECG Rhythm other than sinus rhythm Uncontrolled systemic hypertension

– Dipyridamole/adenosine thallium stress test: predictive of postoperative cardiac problems, indicated if functional status cannot be determined otherwise (eg, treadmill).

– Coronary angiogram with/without stenting.

TABLE 7–3.   Adapted Cardiac Risk Stratification for Colorectal Surgical Procedures.

Risk Stratification	Procedure Examples
Major procedures → cardiac risk > 5%	Pelvic exenteration Combined colorectal/liver resection
Intermediate procedures → cardiac risk 1–5%	Average abdominal procedure Major anorectal reconstructions (inpatient)
Simple procedures → cardiac risk < 1%	Endoscopic procedures Average anorectal surgeries (outpatient)

Contraindication to Nonemergency Surgery

Acute ischemic event (< 1 month).

Acute/chronic low output cardiac failure.

Severe comorbidity: pulmonary decompensation, liver failure, renal disease, stroke.

Perioperative Management

Preoperative
- Need for priority cardiac intervention (revascularization, stenting, valve replacement, etc)?
- β-Blockers.
- Management of other medications: continuation of specific cardiac medications (antihypertensives, antiarrhythmics, diuretics, digoxin, etc), but discontinuation of antihypercholesterolemics, aspirin, etc.
- Optimize arterial blood pressure.
- Medical fluid management: diuretics, fluid restriction.
- Patients with need for anticoagulation (eg, mechanical valve) → switch from warfarin to heparin perioperatively.

Intraoperative
- Consideration for epidural anesthesia for preemptive and postoperative pain control to minimize perioperative pain-induced stress.
- Monitoring and correction of coagulopathy: protamine, fresh frozen plasma.
- Monitoring of glucose levels.
- Fluid management: diuretics, fluid restriction.
- Close monitoring of cardiac function: monitoring, continuous transesophageal echocardiography.
- Monitoring whether procedure is tolerated: eg, pneumoperitoneum, steep Trendelenburg position, etc.

Postoperative
- Optimized pain management (avoid pain-induced stress).
- Continuation of β-blockers, resumption of other medications as soon as tolerated.
- Monitoring of glucose levels.
- Anticoagulation maintained with heparin, return to warfarin if no bleeding complication within 5 days.

Cross-reference

COMORBIDITIES—LIVER DISEASE

Overview

Liver diseases may either result in primary colorectal symptoms or indirectly interfere with the management of unrelated colorectal problems. Compensated liver function not only is a prerequisite for steady-state body functions but is absolutely crucial for increased-demand situations in the peri- and postoperative period. Liver dysfunction may result from intrinsic liver diseases (eg, cirrhosis, hepatitis) or secondarily result from extrahepatic problems (eg, metastatic liver replacement, shock liver, etc). Appropriate risk assessment in view of the natural course of the colorectal disease and the liver disease and adjustments to the management are relevant.

History and background information (eg, hepatitis, alcohol abuse, previous evidence of liver dysfunction, cancer load, etc.), stigmata of liver disease on physical exam, and biochemical parameters serve as guidance.

Problems

- Routine liver function tests in patients without risk factors: not recommended, liver parameters do not correlate with chronicity of liver disease.
- Commonly used drugs may accumulate if elimination is primarily through hepatic metabolism.
- Reduced urea and creatinine synthesis → false low serum parameters and overestimation of renal function → better to determine the glomerular filtration rate (GFR) if necessary.
- Portal hypertension:
  - Particularly in conjunction with adhesions from previous surgeries, carries significant risk of intraoperative bleeding.
  - May result in rectal varices (caveat: hemorrhoids are not more common in liver disease patients).
- Risk of perioperative liver decompensation dependent on type of anesthesia (eg, halothane), intraoperative stability, circumstances of the surgery (eg, elective vs emergency), type of surgery, eg, abdominal and cardiothoracic procedures carry a significantly increased risk.
- GI bleeding (pre-/postoperative) may cause decompensation and encephalopathy.

Risk Assessment Parameters

- Urgency and extent of operation: elective vs emergency, abdominal vs anorectal.

- Coexisting morbidity: cardiopulmonary, renal.
- Severity and prognosis of colorectal disease.
- Severity and prognosis of liver disease:
  - Child-Pugh classification (Table 7–4):
    (1) Natural course and life expectancy.
    (2) Mortality of abdominal surgery: Child-Pugh A: 5–10%; Child-Pugh B: 20–40%; Child-Pugh C: 70–80%.
  - MELD score (Table 7–5):
    (1) Predictor of 3-month mortality
    (2) Predictor of surgical mortality: < 10 → surgery okay; 10–15 → surgery with caution; > 15 → surgery contraindicated.
  - Other scores: American Society of Anesthesiologists (ASA) classification, APACHE II score (ICU patients)
  - Tests for synthetic liver function: albumin, factors I (fibrinogen), II (thromboplastin), V, VIII, IX, X, XII, and XIII.
  - Secondary pathologies: thrombocytopenia (hypersplenism), hepatorenal syndrome, encephalopathy, portal hypertension (eg, abdominal and rectal varices).

TABLE 7–4. **Child-Pugh Score and Prognosis for Liver Cirrhosis.**

Measure	1 Point	2 Points	3 Points
Bilirubin (total)			
mg/dL	< 2	2–3	> 3
μmol/L	< 34	34–50	> 50
Serum albumin, g/dL	> 3.5	2.8–3.5	< 2.8
INR	< 1.7	1.7–2.3	> 2.3
Ascites	None	Mild/moderate (suppressed with medication)	Severe (refractory to medications)
Hepatic encephalopathy	None	Grade I–II (mild/moderate)	Grade III–IV (severe)

INR, international normalized ratio.

Score:

5–6 = Child-Pugh A: compensated, expected 1-/2-year survival 100%/85%.

7–9 = Child-Pugh B: severe functional impairment, expected 1-/2-year survival 80%/60%.

10–15 = Child-Pugh C: decompensated, expected 1-/2-year survival 45%/35%.

TABLE 7–5. Calculation of Model for End-stage Liver Disease (MELD) Score.

Measure	1 point
Serum creatinine, mg/dL	$9.57 \times Ln(creatinine)$
Bilirubin (total), g/L	$3.78 \times Ln(total\ bilirubin)$
INR	$11.2 \times Ln(INR)$
Correction factor	6.43
MELD score	SUM

INR; international normalized ratio; Ln, natural logarithm.

Values < 1 are entered as 1; dialysis ≥ twice per week → creatinine entered as 4.

Maximum score: 40 (even if calculated higher).

Contraindication to Nonemergency Surgery

Acute, particularly fulminant hepatitis.

Manifest hepatic failure.

Uncorrectable coagulopathy, severe thrombocytopenia.

Liver cirrhosis Child-Pugh class C, MELD score > 15.

Severe extrahepatic morbidity: cardiopulmonary decompensation, renal disease.

Perioperative Management

Preoperative
- Preemptive TIPS: indicated for portal hypertension, 25% risk of encephalopathy.
- β-Blockers
- Medical management of ascites: diuretics (eg, spironolactone), fluid restriction.
- Correction of coagulopathy: vitamin K, fresh frozen plasma, factor VIIA.
- Consideration of nutritional support.
- Encephalopathy prophylaxis: enteral antibiotics, lactulose.

Intraoperative
- Monitoring and correction of coagulopathy: fresh frozen plasma, factor VIIA, platelet transfusion.
- Placement of a peritoneal overflow drain (to gravity only) even if normally a drain would not be needed.
- Fluid management: medical management of ascites (diuretics, fluid restriction).

- Close monitoring of liver function: prothrombin time, total bilirubin, electrolytes, renal function.

Cross-reference

BOWEL PREPARATION/CLEANSING

Overview

Endoscopy, certain radiologic tests, and some surgical procedures require the absence of fecal matter in the intestines in order to increase the quality and outcome of the intervention or study. Until recently, a full bowel preparation was standard for any colorectal surgery; however, recent data question its benefit and beyond that seem to even suggest a physiologic disadvantage and higher rates of complications.

Disadvantages of unprepped bowels include:

• Inability to palpate lesion of less than obvious size.

• Interference with low anterior stapling procedure.

• Inability to do intraoperative colonoscopy if needed.

• Lack of rational for diverting ileostomy after TME (with reported 5–15% leak rate) if stool column between ileostomy and anastomosis.

At the present time, therefore, "to clean or not to clean" remains a matter of the surgeon's preference and a common rational mind. Different regimens are available to allow patients to choose volume, flavors, and tablets vs liquid.

Caveat: naturopathic colon cleansing for body purification and to promote general well being is not indicated and potentially harmful.

Variations

GoLytely/NuLytely (polyethylene glycol)

• Normal breakfast, clear liquid diet for lunch and dinner.

• 1 gallon of GoLytely PO or via NGT from noon to 6 PM (reduce/increase dose/time depending on pathology and patient constitution).

• Must check and correct serum potassium before surgery.

• Advantage: gold standard. Disadvantage: volume to drink is major challenge for patients → 15% of patients are noncompliant.

Fleet Phospho Soda (caveat: contraindicated for renal failure)

• Normal breakfast, clear liquid diet for lunch and dinner.

• 3 PM: 45 mL Fleet Phospho-soda on ice, followed by > 6 glasses (8 oz) of water or soda between 3 PM and 8 PM.

• 6 PM: 45 mL Fleet Phospho-soda on ice, followed by > 6 glasses (8 oz) of water or soda between 8 PM and midnight.

• Two Fleet enemas (one at a time) in AM and hold each for 3–5 minutes.

• Must check and correct serum potassium before surgery.

• Advantage: lower volume → better compliance. Disadvantage: phosphate accumulation (in kidney failure).

Visicol tablets (40 sodium phosphate tables)
• Normal breakfast, clear liquid diet for lunch and dinner.
• 20 tablets: start at noon; 3 tablets with at least 8 oz of clear liquids, followed by 3 tablets every 15 minutes with clear liquids, last dose only 2 tablets.
• 20 tablets: start 4 hours later; 3 tablets with at least 8 oz of clear liquids, followed by 3 tablets every 15 minutes with clear liquids, last dose only 2 tablets.
• No additional enema or laxative is required.
• Advantage: tablet form (no bad taste) → better compliance? Disadvantage: phosphate accumulation (in kidney failure) visible precipitates.

HalfLytely (bisacodyl + polyethylene glycol)
• Clear liquids but no solid food on the day of cleansing.
• Four bisacodyl tablets → first bowel movement expected in 1–6 hours.
• After bowel movement or maximum of 6 hours: drink HalfLytely solution (2000 mL).
• Advantage: less volume → better compliance.
• Disadvantage: abdominal cramping.

MoviPrep (polyethylene glycol with electrolytes and acorbate/ascorbic acid)
• 2 × 1 L of MoviPrep plus 2 × 500 mL clear liquids PO or via NGT from noon to 6 PM (reduce/increase dose/time depending on pathology and patient constitution).
• Must check and correct serum potassium before surgery.
• Advantage: marketed as low volume prep (in fact only 25% less total fluid), less abdominal cramping because bisacodyl is left out.

Magnesium citrate (caveat: caution in renal failure)
• 1000–2000 mL per 6 hours.
• Advantage: less volume → better compliance; Mg citrate is the only solution with an ability to dissolve barium sulfate precipitates (important for impacted barium).

Mannitol
• Abandoned as bowel prep because sugar leads to bacterial fermentation that results in explosive mixture of hydrogen and methane gas → risk of explosion with use of electrocautery.
• Advantage: none.

Monitoring

- Patient compliance: discussion prior to selection of method.
- All methods invariably result in diarrhea → risk for hypokalemia and other electrolyte imbalances, dehydration, hypotension (elderly patients).
- Prophylactic application of zinc-oxide based barrier cream to perianal skin to reduce irritation.
- Toxic side effects to colonic mucosa: aphthoid lesions particularly in distal large bowel/rectum (caveat: these lesions are not a sign of Crohn disease).

Cross-reference

ANTIBIOTIC PROPHYLAXIS

Overview

Colorectal and anorectal surgery are rarely completely sterile procedures. Antibiotic prophylaxis is considered a crucial component to reduce surgical site infections in patients who do not primarily suffer from an infection. The target is to keep the incidence of wound infections after elective surgery < 10%. The prophylaxis has to be distinguished from therapeutic antibiotic treatment for patients who already have an established infection.

Prophylaxis should be targeted, adequately dosed, and short (< 24 hours) in order to minimize antibiotic side effects and propagation of resistances. Coverage should include both aerobic bacteria (eg, *Staphylococcus, E coli, Klebsiella, Proteus,* etc) and anaerobic bacteria (eg, *Bacteroides fragilis, Clostridia*).

Guidelines

SCIP measures: an appropriate antibiotic must be selected for prophylaxis; it should be started within 60 minutes before incision and ended within 24 hours from the first prophylactic dose. Vancomycin is one of the few exceptions: infusion has to be slow over 1 hour (otherwise risk of "red man" syndrome or hypotension) → start is not restricted to the 60-minute perioperative period. Prophylaxis has to be distinguished from therapeutic antibiotics in the treatment of an infection or severe contamination.

Indication

Clean-contaminated surgeries with expected enteric bacteria:

- Any abdominal colorectal surgery.
- Anal surgery (unless wound primarily left open).
- ERUS-guided anorectal biopsy.
- Endoscopy with polypectomy in immunosuppressed patient.

Clean cases with implant:

- Incisional hernia repair.
- Implantation of central venous access port.

Clean-contaminated case with implant:

- Implantation of ABS.
- Implantation of mesh at time of bowel resection or creation of colostomy.

Endocarditis prophylaxis: see separate discussion in this chapter.

Contraindication

Allergic reactions.

Clean case without implant: generally no need for antibiotic prophylaxis.

Antibiotic treatment in therapeutic intent: → different selection of antibiotics, different duration.

Options

1. Clean-contaminated case:

   a. IV perioperative administration:

      (1) Dual antibiotics: eg, cephalosporin + metronidazole, fluoroquinolone + metronidazole, clindamycin + aminoglycoside, clindamycin + quinolone, clindamycin + aztreonam.

      (2) Triple antibiotics: amoxicillin/clavulanic acid + metronidazole + aminoglycoside.

      (3) Single antibiotic: ertapenem, piperacillin/tazobactam.

   b. Oral prophylaxis (at time of mechanical bowel prep): neomycin + erythromycin, neomycin + metronidazole.

   c. Combination of oral and IV antibiotics (generally no incremental benefit).

2. Clean cases with implant: single dose cephalosporin, vancomycin, etc.

3. Clean-contaminated case with implant: combination prophylaxis, eg, vancomycin + cephalosporin + metronidazole, vancomycin + quinolone + metronidazole, etc.

Monitoring

Quality-control of personal and hospital infection rates and drug resistances.

Cross-reference

Topic	*Chapter*
SCIP measures	7 (p 682)
Perioperative management	7 (pp 684–688)

ENDOCARDITIS PROPHYLAXIS

Overview

Infectious endocarditis is a rare but feared condition that may result from transient bacteremia in high-risk patients.

Basis for 2007 changes in published guidelines:

- No published data convincingly demonstrate efficacy of prophylactic antibiotics in preventing infectious endocarditis associated with bacteremia from invasive procedures.
- Administration of prophylactic antibiotics is (1) not risk-free, and (2) may result in drug-resistant strains.
- Among a multitude of GI bacteria, only enterococci are likely to cause infectious endocarditis.

Revised recommendations (2007):

1. Administration of prophylactic antibiotics solely to prevent endocarditis is not recommended for patients who undergo GI tract procedures, including diagnostic colonoscopy.

2. GI infections may result in intermittent or sustained enterococcal bacteremia → antibiotic regimen to prevent wound infection or sepsis associated with a GI procedure may, in high-risk patients, reasonably include an agent active against enterococci (eg, penicillin, ampicillin, piperacillin, or vancomycin).

3. Skin and soft-tissue infections may result in intermittent or sustained staphylococcal or streptococcal bacteremia → antibiotic regimen for a surgical procedure that involves infected skin or soft tissue may, in high-risk patients, reasonably include an agent active against staphylococci and streptococci (eg, penicillin, cephalosporin; patients with allergy or MRSA → vancomycin or clindamycin).

Guidelines

American Heart Association: revised guidelines 2007.

Indication

Cardiac high-risk conditions:

- Prosthetic cardiac valve or prosthetic material used for cardiac valve repair.
- Previous infectious endocarditis.
- Congenital heart disease:
  - Unrepaired cyanotic congenital heart disease, including palliative shunts and conduits.

- Completely repaired congenital heart defect with prosthetic material or device during the first 6 months after the procedure.
- Repaired congenital heart disease with residual defects at or adjacent to the site of prosthetic patch or device (which inhibit endothelialization).
• Cardiac transplantation recipients who develop cardiac valvulopathy.

Contraindication

Allergic reactions.

Antibiotic treatment in therapeutic intent: different selection of antibiotics, different duration.

Monitoring

Quality-control of personal, hospital, and national infection rates and drug resistances.

Cross-reference

Topic	Chapter
SCIP measures	7 (p 682)
General perioperative management	7 (pp 684–688)
Comorbidities—cardiac disease	7 (p 691)
Antibiotic prophylaxis	7 (p 703)
Prophylaxis of venous thromboembolism	7 (p 707)

PROPHYLAXIS OF VENOUS THROMBOEMBOLISM *(DVT, PE)*

Overview

Thromboembolic events are serious and potentially life-threatening complications even if the majority remain asymptomatic. Surgical trauma with release of procoagulative factors, prolonged intra- and postoperative immobility, and venous stasis contribute to a significant incidence of DVT with or without PE.

Individual risk is dependent on:

• Patient factors: age, habitus (obesity), varicose veins, previous DVT/PE, immobility, smoking, and use of birth control pills.

• Preexisting coagulogenic factors: IBD, malignancy, cancer therapy (radiation, chemotherapy), sepsis, pregnancy, antithrombin III or protein S deficiency, etc.

• Surgery-related factors: type and length of procedure, positioning during procedure, body temperature, etc.

Incidence of venous thromboembolism (VTE):

• Detection with objective test while patient is not necessarily symptomatic: 15–30% after abdominal surgery (without VTE prophylaxis).

• 25–35% of thrombi are located proximally and therefore carry increased risk for PE.

• 10% of hospital deaths are attributable to PE.

Guidelines

ACCP, ASCRS, SCIP: definition of major risk groups for which specific prophylaxis routinely is recommended for all of their respective patients.

• Patients undergoing major general surgical procedures should receive routine VTE prophylaxis:

  – Low-dose unfractionated heparin or low-molecular weight heparin.

  – Mechanical options for individuals with high bleeding risk.

  – Extended prophylaxis for 2–3 weeks after hospital discharge for high-risk patients.

- Patients with no/low risks undergoing minor procedure do not need specific prophylaxis other than early/aggressive mobilization.
- Aspirin alone is not recommended (not sufficient) as VTE prophylaxis for any patient group.
- Placement/removal of epidural catheter should be done when anticoagulant effect is at a minimum (ie, before next scheduled injection). Anticoagulant prophylaxis should be delayed for at least 2 hours after spinal needle insertion or epidural catheter removal.
- Colorectal surgery risk assignment:
  - Low risk: anorectal outpatient surgeries.
  - Low/intermediate risk: anorectal inpatient surgeries, laparoscopic surgeries without additional risk factors.
  - High risk: any abdominal surgery.
  - Highest risk: pelvic surgery for malignancy, particularly after preoperative adjuvant therapy, abdominal surgery in cancer, IBD, morbidly obese patients, patients with history of DVT/PE.
- Management of patients already on long-term anticoagulation/antiplatelet medication:
  - Patients on warfarin: stop warfarin 7 days prior to surgery → switch to therapeutic low-molecular-weight heparin (eg, enoxaparin) → switch to therapeutic IV dose of unfractionated heparin the day before surgery → stop 6 hours prior to surgery and resume 4–6 hours after surgery if no active bleeding.
  - Patients on aspirin or clopidogrel (Plavix): stop 1 week prior to intervention, start 3–5 days postoperatively.
- Documented DVT/PE → therapeutic anticoagulation; if bleeding → Greenfield filter.

Indication

Low risk:	< 40 years, minor surgery, no additional risk factors
Moderate risk:	< 40 years, minor surgery, additional risk factors or 40–60 years, minor surgery, no additional risk factors
High risk:	40–60 years, additional risk factors (prior VTE, cancer, molecular hypercoagulability)
Highest risk:	> 40 years, multiple risk factors (cancer, prior VTE)

Contraindication

Absolute	Relative
Active or significant intraoperative hemorrhage	Thrombocytopenia
History of cerebral hemorrhage	Coagulopathy (INR > 1.5)
Hypersensitivity to heparin	Uncontrolled arterial hypertension
Heparin-induced thrombocytopenia (HIT)	History of cerebral hemorrhage
Warfarin use in 1st trimester of pregnancy	Active intracranial lesions
Epidural catheter	Proliferative retinopathy
Severe head or spinal cord injury < 4 weeks	Bacterial endocarditis
	Jehovah's witness?

Options

- No active measures: → no prophylaxis, early/aggressive mobilization.
- Mechanical measures: graduated compression stockings, intermittent pneumatic compression.
- Pharmacologic measures:
  - Heparin SQ 5000 units every 12 hours up to every 8 hours.
  - Enoxaparin SQ 40 mg qd up to 30 mg bid.
  - Warfarin → target INR 2–3.
- Greenfield filter placement.
- Not adequate for VTE prophylaxis: aspirin, dextran.

Monitoring

All pharmacologic options invariably increase risk of bleeding from surgical site. Increased bleeding may require interruption of DVT prophylaxis, potentially reversal (heparin → protamine, warfarin → fresh frozen plasma).

Thrombocytopenia under heparin treatment (HIT) → stop heparin, start argatroban.

Cross-reference

ANORECTAL ANESTHESIA

Overview

An estimated 10% of anorectal diseases require surgery, the majority of which can be done on an outpatient basis. The anorectal/perineal area is highly innervated and reflexogenic. This implies a need for adequate anesthesia to avoid Brewer-Luckhardt reflex (ie, intense pain, reflex body movements, tachypnea, and laryngeal spasm). Sensation to the distal rectum and anus is conducted through the pudendal nerve (S2–S4 roots).

Effective anesthesia options should achieve:

• Rapid onset and recovery of analgesia and sphincter relaxation.
• Rapid reversibility and ability for quick adjustments during maintenance.
• Low level of intra- or postoperative side effects (local and systemic).
• Low costs.
• Extending postoperative comfort.

Indication

Anorectal problem requiring examination under anesthesia or surgical intervention.

Contraindication

High probability of requiring transabdominal approach.

Inadequate monitoring capabilities.

Options

General anesthesia

• Types:
  – Endotracheal intubation.
  – Laryngeal mask (LMA).
  – Deep intravenous sedation, eg, with propofol (sedative/hypnotic).
• Commonly used drug types: inhalation gases (isoflurance/desflurane, nitric oxide), propofol, muscle relaxants, benzodiazepines, opiates, ketorolac.
• Advantages: complete analgesia and loss of consciousness, muscle relaxation, varying degrees of securing the airways.
• Disadvantage: neurologic, cardiac, and respiratory depression.

Regional anesthesia

- Types:
  - Epidural anesthesia: injection of local anesthetic and/or opioids into epidural or subarachnoid space of spinal canal to achieve complete analgesia in an awake patient.
  - Spinal anesthesia: injection of local anesthetic into spinal canal.
  - Caudal block: avoids transitory neurologic symptoms and postural headache.
- Advantages: preemptive analgesia, avoidance of general anesthesia, minimal postoperative nausea/vomiting, shorter recovery time, no impact on mental/intellectual functions, cost?
- Disadvantages: risk of bleeding in/around spinal canal (particularly with simultaneous DVT prophylaxis), incomplete blockade, prolonged blockade with urinary retention, anxiety related to lower extremity paralysis.

Local (with/without IV sedation): ideal for ambulatory setting

- Types:
  - Complete perianal block with additional relaxation of anal sphincter tone: injection of 5 cc of local anesthetic bilaterally into ischioanal fossae plus ring of SQ injection around anal verge (total 20–30 cc): Figure 7–1.
  - Local sector infiltration: injection just in/around the target area.
  - Local anesthesia with IV sedation/analgesia (propofol, benzodiazepine, opiate).
- Advantages: preemptive analgesia, avoidance of general anesthesia, ease of positioning patient, no postoperative nausea/vomiting, shorter recovery time, no impact on mental/intellectual functions, cost?
- Disadvantages: initial local discomfort, potentially insufficient analgesia and/or relaxation → need for general anesthesia, but patient, eg, in prone jackknife position.

Monitoring

All forms of anesthesia that include more than just local anesthesia need to be performed in an adequate setting with:

- Appropriate monitoring capabilities for patient's heart rate, heart rhythm, blood pressure, respiratory rate, and oxygen saturation.
- Availability of crash cart, antagonistic medications, etc.

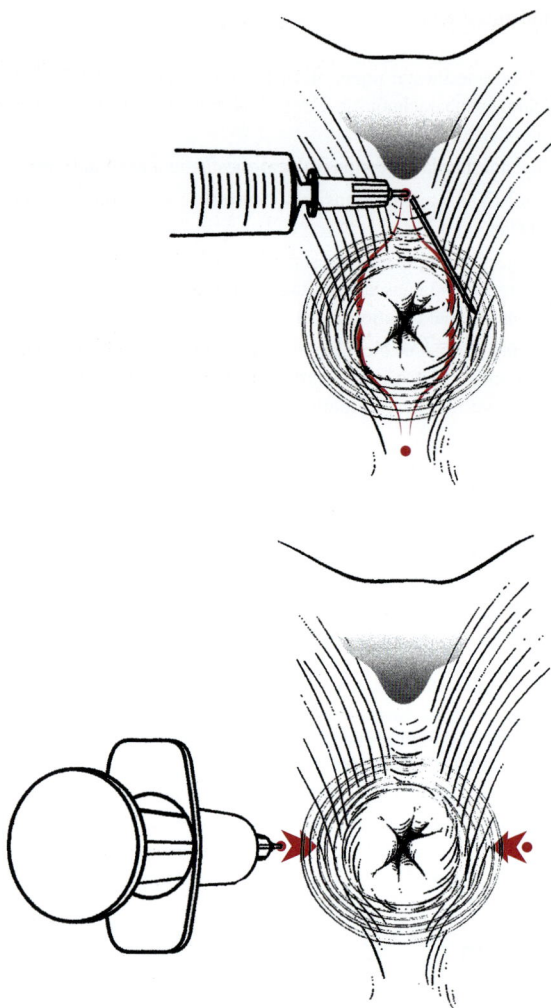

Figure 7–1. Injection of local anesthesia.

Supportive Pain Control Measures

- Ketorolac: effective pain medication (caveat: contraindications/side effects).
- Topical/systemic metronidazole → reduced pain due to reduced inflammation?
- Topical sucralfate to open wound → reduced pain perception, faster wound healing.
- Sitz baths → sphincter relaxation, reduced painful spasms.
- Maintenance of soft stool (rather than bowel confinement).

Cross-reference

Topic	*Chapter*
General perioperative management—anorectal	7 (p 688)

FAST-TRACK RECOVERY

Overview

Fast-track recovery programs aim at an accelerated pace of recuperation after colorectal surgery in a paradigm shift away from traditional approaches with extended physical and bowel resting. The concept consists of a multimodal rehabilitation approach to safely optimize pain management, reduce the patients' surgical stress response, resume early oral nutrition, and support early mobilization.

Compared with traditional peri-/postoperative management after uncomplicated colonic resections, fast-track rehabilitation programs reduce the length of hospital stays and fatigue and allow for earlier resumption of normal activities, without increasing dependence on support after discharge.

Guidelines

Fast-track interventions include:

- Extensive preoperative patient education.
- Reduced preoperative fasting period with carbohydrate loading 2 hours preoperatively.
- Opiate-sparing pain management.
- Preoperative placement of thoracic epidural analgesia for pain management.
- No routine placement of NGT or abdominal drains.
- Maintenance of intraoperative normothermia.
- Forced early mobilization to start ≤ 6 hours postsurgery.
- Forced early resumption of oral diet with energy and protein supplementation.

Indication

Abdominal surgery.

Contraindication

Conservatively managed leak.

Manifest prolonged postoperative ileus.

Patients with individual contraindications to have all measures implemented.

Options

- Absence of complaints of nausea or vomiting on postoperative day 1: start clear liquid diet; subsequently diet advanced as tolerated.
- Supportive measures: use of chewing gums (controversial data)?

Monitoring

Discoordination of upper GI function and lower GI function: $\rightarrow$ 15% of patient will suffer setback and may require readmission to the hospital.

Cross-reference

Medications

Medications

MEDICATIONS FOR ANALGESIA AND SEDATION

Analgesics

Generic Name	Typical Dosage	Trade Name
Acetaminophen/codeine 30 mg	30/300 mg 1–2 tabs PO q 4–6 h	Tylenol #3
Acetaminophen/codeine 60 mg	60/300 mg 1–2 tabs PO q 4–6 h	Tylenol #4
Codeine sulfate	30–60 mg PO tid	Codeine
Fentanyl	25, 50, 75, 100 mcg patch q 72 h	Duragesic Transdermal
Hydrocodone/ acetaminophen	5/325 mg, 5/500 mg, 7.5/750 mg PO q 4–6 h	Vicodin, Norco
Hydromorphone	2–4 mg PO, 0.2–0.6 mg IV	Dilaudid
Ketorolac	15–30 mg IV, 10 mg PO q 6 h (max 5 days)	Toradol
Morphine	10–30 mg PO, 30 mg SR q 8–12 h	MS Contin
Oxycodone	5 mg PO q 4–6 h, 10–40 mg CR q 12 h	OxyContin, Percocet
Propoxyphene napsylate/ acetaminophen	100/650 mg PO q 4 h	Darvocet-N
Tramadol	50–100 mg PO q 4–6 h (max 400 mg/day)	Ultram

NSAIDs

Generic Name	Typical Dosage	Trade Name
Celecoxib	400 mg PO bid	Celebrex
Ibuprofen	200–800 mg PO tid	Advil, Motrin
Sulindac	150 mg PO qd (polyp prophylaxis)	Clinoril

Conscious Sedation

Generic Name	Typical Dosage	Trade Name
Fentanyl	25–50 mcg bolus titration to effect	Sublimaze
Meperidine	25–50 mg bolus titration to effect	Demerol
Midazolam	1–2 mg bolus titration to effect	Versed
Propofol	2–2.5 mg/kg IV, or 40 mg q 10 sec	Diprivan

Antagonists

Generic Name	Typical Dosage	Trade Name
Flumazenil	0.2 mg IV q 1 min (up to five times)	Romazicon
Naloxone	0.4–2 mg IV q 2–3 min (up to 10 mg)	Narcan

MEDICATIONS FOR GI TRACT

Antacids

Generic Name	Typical Dosage	Trade Name
Esomeprazole	20–40 mg PO/IV qd	Nexium
Famotidine	20–40 mg PO qd, 20 mg IV bid	Pepcid
Omeprazole	20–40 mg PO/IV qd	Prilosec
Pantoprazole	40 mg PO/IV qd	Protonix
Rabeprazole	20 mg PO qd	AcipHex
Ranitidine	150 mg PO bid or 300 mg qHs, 50 mg IV tid	Zantac
Sucralfate	1 g PO qid	Carafate

Antidiarrheals

Generic Name	Typical Dosage	Trade Name
Bismuth subsalicylate	2 tabs or 30 mL (534 mg) PO up to 8 doses/day	Pepto-Bismol, Kaopectate
Difenoxin + atropine	2 tabs PO q 6 h (max 8 tabs)	Motofen
Diphenoxylate/atropine	Up to 2 × 2.5/0.025 mg qid	Lomotil
Glycopyrrolate	1–2 mg PO bid–tid	Robinul, Robinul forte
Kaolin-pectin	60–120 mL PO q 3–4 h	Kaopectate
Loperamide	Up to 8 × 1 tab (2 mg)	Imodium
Tincture of opium	5–20 drops qid	Tincture of opium

Bile Acid Binder

Generic Name	Typical Dosage	Trade Name
Cholestyramine	4 g PO bid–qid	Questran

Antiemetics

Generic Name	Typical Dosage	Trade Name
Dolasetron	12.5 mg IV	Anzemet
Droperidol	0.625–2.5 mg IV	Inapsine
Ondansetron	4–8 mg PO/IV tid	Zofran
Prochlorperazine	5–10 mg PO/IV/IM (max 40 mg/day)	Compazine
Promethazine	12.5–25 mg PO/PR/IM	Phenergan

Antispasmodics

Generic Name	Typical Dosage	Trade Name
Hyoscyamine	0.125 mg PO tid	Levsine, Symax

Sphincter-Relaxants

Generic Name	Typical Dosage	Trade Name
Diltiazem 2% ointment	1 fingertip of ointment applied to anus bid	To be compounded
Nifedipine 0.2%	1 fingertip of ointment applied to anus bid	To be compounded
Nitroglycerine 0.2% ointment	1 fingertip of ointment applied to anus bid	To be compounded
Botulinum toxin A	10–20 units bilaterally IM to IAS	Botox

Bowel Prep

Generic Name	Typical Dosage	Trade Name
Magnesium citrate	150–300 mL PO	Magnesium citrate
Neomycin	3 g PO 3–4 doses	Neomycin
Phospho soda enema	Enema 1–2 before procedure	Fleet enema
Phospho soda oral liquid	45 mL PO (8 glasses of water), repeat 3 h later	Fleet
Phospho soda oral tablet	3 tabs q 15 min (20 tabs) × 2	Visicol
Polyethylene glycol with electrolytes	4 L	GoLytely, NuLytely

Medications

Fiber Supplements

Generic Name	Typical Dosage	Trade Name
Methylcellulose	25–30 g/day	Citrucel
Polycarbophil	25–30 g/day	FiberCon
Psyllium	25–30 g/day	Metamucil, Konsyl

IBS

Generic Name	Typical Dosage	Trade Name
Alosetron	Commonly prescribed only by specialists	Lotronex
Dicyclomine	20–40 mg PO qid	Bentyl
Tegaserod	6 mg PO bid	Zelnorm

Laxatives

Generic Name	Typical Dosage	Trade Name
Bisacodyl	10–15 mg PO qd	Correctol, Dulcolax
Castor oil	15–30 mL PO qd	Fleet castor oil, Purge
Lactulose	30–45 mL PO tid–qid	Dulcolax
Lubiprostone	24 mcg bid	Amitiza
Magnesium hydroxide	30–60 mL, 1 tsp to 1 tbsp q 2–4 h	Milk of magnesia
Milk and molasses enema (50:50)	8–10 oz enema	Milk & Molasses enema
Polyethylene glycol	17 g PO in 4–8 oz qd–qid	MiraLax, GlycoLax
Senna	1 tsp granules, 10–15 mL PO	Senokot, Ex-Lax

Stool Softener

Generic Name	Typical Dosage	Trade Name
Docusate calcium	240 mg PO qd	Kaopectate, Surfak
Docusate sodium	100 mg PO bid	Colace

Other Medications

Generic Name	Typical Dosage	Trade Name
Acetylcysteine	600 mg PO bid (prophylaxis contrast nephropathy)	Mucomyst
Botulinum toxin A	10–20 units bilaterally IM into IAS	Botox
Metoclopramide	5–10 mg PO/IV q 6–8 h	Reglan
Neostigmine	2 mg in 100 mL NaCl IV over 2–4 h	Prostigmin
Octreotide	0.125 mcg SQ tid or 20–30 mg IM q month	Sandostatin
Probiotics	1–2 sachets/capsules PO bid	VSL#3
Propantheline	15 mg PO	Pro-Banthine
Simethicone	40–125 mg PO tid	Gas-X

Medications

MEDICATIONS AGAINST VIRAL PATHOGENS

HAART[a]

Generic Name	Trade Name
Abacavir	Ziagen
Amprenavir	Agenerase
Atazanavir	Reyataz, ATV
Combivir lamivudine, zidovudine	Combivir
Darunavir	Prezista
Didanosine	Videx
Efavirenz	Sustiva, EFV
Emtricitabine	Emtriva
Enfuvirtide	Fuzeon
Fosamprenavir	Lexiva
Indinavir	Crixivan
Lamivudine	Epivir, 3TC
Lopinavir-ritonavir	Kaletra
Nelfinavir	Viracept
Nevirapine	Viramune
Ritonavir	Norvir
Saquinavir	Invirase
Stavudine	Zerit, d4T
Tenofovir	Viread, TDF
Tipranavir	Aptivus
Zidovudine	Retrovir, AZT

[a]Commonly prescribed only by specialists.

Other Antivirals

Generic Name	Typical Dosage	Trade Name
Acyclovir	800 mg PO tid	Zovirax
Famciclovir	250 mg PO tid	Famvir
Ganciclovir	5–6 mg/kg IV	Cytovene
Imiquimod	5% cream M/W/F overnight	Aldara
Interferon alfa-2b	4 × 1 million units SQ (after excision of condylomata)	Intron A
Podophyllin	0.5–25% solution	Podocon-25
Valacyclovir	1 g PO bid	Valtrex

MEDICATIONS AGAINST BACTERIAL AND FUNGAL PATHOGENS

Antibiotics

Generic Name	Typical Dosage	Trade Name
Amoxicillin-clavulanate	500/125 mg PO q 8 h, 875 mg PO bid	Augmentin
Azithromycin	1 g PO (one time), 250 mg PO qd (5 days)	Zithromax
Cefazolin	1–2 g IV q 8 h	Ancef
Cefotetan	1–2 g IV q 12 h	Cefotan
Cefoxitin	2 g IV q 12 h	Mefoxitin
Ceftriaxone	125 mg IV	Rocephin
Ciprofloxacin	250–500 mg PO bid (tid)	Cipro
Clindamycin	300 mg PO tid	Cleocin
Doxycycline	100 mg PO bid	Vibramycin
Ertapenem	1 g IV/IM q 24 h	Invanz
Imipenem/cilastin	500 mg IV q 6–8 h	Primaxin
Levofloxacin	500–750 mg PO qd	Levaquin
Metronidazole	250–500 mg PO tid	Flagyl
Metronidazole topical	0.75%	Metronidazole cream
Penicillin G (benzathine penicillin G)	2.4 million units IM (single dose), or 50,000 units/kg IM	Penicillin
Piperacillin/tazobactam	3.375 g IV tid–qid	Zosyn
Rifaximin	200 mg PO tid	Xifaxan
Trimethoprim/ sulfamethoxazole	160/800 mg PO bid	Bactrim
Vancomycin	250–500 mg PO qid (not absorbed) 0.5–1 g IV q 12 h	Vancomycin

Medications

Antifungals

Generic Name	Typical Dosage	Trade Name
Amphotericin B	5 mg/kg IV q 24 h	Abelcet
Caspofungin	50 mg IV q 24 h (loading dose 70 mg IV)	Cancidas
Clotrimazole 1% cream	Topical application bid	Lotrimin
Fluconazole	100–400 mg PO/IV qd	Diflucan
Ketoconazole 2% cream	Topical application bid	Nizoral
Micafungin	150 mg IV qd	Mycamine
Miconazole 2% cream	Topical application bid	Micatin, Monistat
Nystatin	100,000 units/cc	Mycostatin

MEDICATIONS FOR HEMATOLOGIC MANAGEMENT

Anticoagulants

Generic Name	Typical Dosage	Trade Name
Argatroban	Commonly prescribed by specialists or individualized	Argatroban
Enoxaparin	40 mg SQ qd (prophylaxis), 1–1.5 mg/kg (therapeutic) q 12–24 h	Lovenox
Heparin	5000 units SQ bid–tid (prophylaxis), monitored IV dose (therapeutic)	Heparin
Warfarin	Individualized dose (monitoring of INR)	Coumadin

Bone Marrow Stimulant

Generic Name	Typical Dosage	Trade Name
Erythropoietin	40,000 units SQ q week	Procrit

Medications

MEDICATIONS AGAINST TUMOR OR INFLAMMATION

Chemotherapy[a]

Generic Name	Trade Name
5-Fluorouracil	5-FU
Bevacizumab	Avastin
Capecitabine	Xeloda
Cetuximab	Erbitux
Gemcitabine	Gemzar
Imatinib	Gleevec
Irinotecan	Camptosar, CPT-11
Leucovorin (folinic acid)	Leucovorin
Levamisole	Ergamisol
Mitomycin-C	Mitomycin-C
Oxaliplatin	Eloxatin
Panitumumab	Vectibix
Raltitrexed	Tomudex
Sunitinib	Sunitinib

[a]Commonly prescribed only by specialists.

IBD Suppression

Generic Name	Typical Dosage	Trade Name
Adalimumab	Commonly prescribed only by specialists	Humira
Balsalazide	2.25 g (= three 750-mg tabs) PO tid	Colazal
Infliximab	Commonly prescribed only by specialists	Remicade
Mesalamine	800–1600 mg PO tid	Asacol, Pentasa
Mesalamine	800–1600 mg PO tid, 1000 mg supp PR	Canasa
Mesalamine enema	4 g (60 mL) PR overnight	Rowasa
Natalizumab	Commonly prescribed only by specialists	Tysabri
Olsalazine	500 mg PO bid	Dipentum
Sulfasalazine	500–1000 mg PO qid	Azulfidine

Immunosuppressants[a]

Generic Name	Trade Name
Azathioprine	Imuran
Cyclosporine A	Sandimmune
Mercaptopurine (6-MP)	Purinethol
Methotrexate	Methotrexate
Mycophenolate mofetil	CellCept
Tacrolimus (FK506)	Prograf

[a]Commonly prescribed only by specialists.

Steroids, Systemic

Generic Name	Strength Compared to Prednisone	Typical Dosage	Trade Name
Hydrocortisone	0.2×	100 mg IV	Solu-Cortef
Methylprednisolone	1.25×	0.5–1 mg/kg IV	Solu-Medrol
Prednisone	1.0×	5–60 mg PO qd or 0.5 mg/kg	Prednisone

Steroids, Local

Generic Name	Typical Dosage	Trade Name
Budesonide-oral	3–9 mg PO qd	Entocort EC-oral
Budesonide-rectal	2 mg PR qd	Entocort EC-rectal
Hydrocortisone acetate		Analpram 1–2.5%, Cort Enemas, Cort Foam, ProctoCream 1%, ProctoFoam 1%
Hydrocortisone topical	1 supp PR bid–tid	Anusol-HC
Pramoxine	1 supp PR bid + post BM	Anusol, ProctoFoam
Pramoxine + hydrocortisone	1 supp PR bid–tid	ProctoFoam HC

Medications

Appendix II

Diagnostic Guides

SELECTED COLORECTAL REFERENCE VALUES

Tumor Markers

Carcinoembryonic antigen (CEA)

Normal value: < 5.0 ng/mL (smoker).

                     < 2.5 ng/mL (nonsmoker).

Comment: Elevation of CEA in colorectal cancer, but also in a variety of noncolonic cancers (eg, pancreatic, gastric, lung, breast), as well as in benign conditions (eg, IBD, liver cirrhosis, chronic lung disease, pancreatitis). CEA > 20 highly suspicious for metastatic disease. After curative cancer resection, normalization of elevated values expected within 1–2 months.

Prostate-specific antigen (PSA)

Normal value: 0–4 ng/mL.

Comment: Elevation of PSA in prostate cancer, prostatitis, after digital rectal exam.

IBD Markers

Perinuclear antineutrophilic cytoplasmic antibody (pANCA)

Normal value: ≤ 1:8.

Comment: 60–80% positive in ulcerative colitis; 10–25% positive in Crohn colitis.

Anti-*Saccharomyces cerevisiae* antibody (ASCA)

Normal value: ≤ 20.0 units.

Comment: 5–15% positive in ulcerative colitis; 60–80% positive in Crohn colitis.

Celiac Disease Markers

Anti-endomysial IgA

Normal value: < 1:5.

Comment: Sensitivity and specificity for celiac disease > 95% (ie, much better than anti-gliadin IgG).

Anti-transglutaminase IgA

Normal value: < 20 units.

Comment: Positive in celiac disease in > 90% of cases (ie, better than anti-gliadin IgG).

Infectious Diseases

CD4 count

Normal value: 500–1500 cells/μL.

Comment: HIV infection $\rightarrow$ assessment of activity and treatment response with CD4 cell counts and viral load. Critical: < 200 cells/μL.

Plasma HIV-1 RNA monitoring

Normal value: No viral load detectable with appropriate HAART.

Comment: > 100,000 copies/mL $\rightarrow$ sign of drug resistance or disease progression.

Complete Blood Count

White blood cells (WBC)

Normal value: 3.8–10.8 [$\times 10^3$ WBC/mL].

Comment: Marker for acute inflammation.

Hematocrit (Hct)

Normal value: 35–46 [%].

Comment: Assessment of blood levels.

Hemoglobin (Hgb)

Normal value: 12.0–16.0 [g/dL].

Comment: Assessment of blood levels.

Neutrophils relative

Normal value: 42.0–75.0 [%].

Comment: Left-shift/bandemia is a marker for acute inflammation.

Lymphocytes, relative

Normal value: 20.5–51.1 [%].

Comment: Marker for nutritional status.

Blood Chemistry

Creatinine (Cr)

Normal value: 0.5–1.2 mg/dL (SI units: 45–110 μmol/L).

Comment: Serum value dependent on overall muscle volume and kidney function. Elevation does not occur before glomerular filtration rate reduced to 25–40%. IV radiographic contrast to be avoided if creatinine > 2.0 mg/dL.

Diagnostic Guides

Albumin

Normal value: 3.2–5.0 g/dL (SI units: 32–50 g/L).

Comment: Marker for nutritional status and synthetic liver function, < 3.0 → increased risk of postoperative complications.

Prealbumin

Normal value: 20–40 mg/dL (SI units: 200–400 mg/L).

Comment: Marker for nutritional status.

Transferrin

Normal value: 200–300 mg/dL (SI units: 2–3 g/L).

Comment: Marker for nutritional status.

Lactate

Normal value: 4.5–19.8 mg/dL (SI units: 0.5–2.2 mmol/L).

Comment: Elevation suspicious for underperfused/ischemic tissues, false normal possible.

Coagulation

D-dimer (d-dimer)

Normal value: 0.6–1.5 mg/100 mL (SI units: 50–130 µM/L).

Comment: Elevation unspecific through numerous processes (surgery, DVT, etc); high negative predictive value: normal D-dimer → DVT/PE highly unlikely.

INR

Normal value: 0.5–1.4.

Comment: Anticoagulation with warfarin → target range of 2–3.

Bleeding time

Normal value: < 6 minutes.

Comment: Increased with platelet dysfunction (aspirin, von Willebrand disease).

Stool Analysis

Fecal fat

Normal value: 2–6 g/day on 100 g/day fat in diet.

Comment: Increased in pancreatic insufficiency, cystic fibrosis, lipase inhibitor medication.

FOBT (fecal occult blood test)

Normal value:	Negative.
Comment:	Sensitivity: 5 mg hemoglobin in 1 g of stool, false positive and false negative results (eg, vitamin C).

Anophysiology Testing

Pudendal nerve terminal motor latency (PNTML)

Normal value:	< 2.5 ms.
Comment:	Pudendal neuropathy: true elevation (proper test setup), true absence. False pathologic: proper stimulation not achieved. False normal: direct muscle stimulation.

Anal manometry—mean resting pressure

Normal value:	50–100 mm Hg.
Comment:	Relatively reliable as no patient cooperation needed.

Anal manometry—maximal mean squeeze pressure

Normal value:	100–350 mm Hg.
Comment:	Rule of thumb: doubled resting pressure. False low values; patient not cooperating. False normal values: pressure generated by contraction of puborectalis and gluteus muscles.

Anal manometry—high pressure zone (anal canal length)

Normal value:	2–4 cm.
Comment:	Females generally have shorter length of anal canal than males.

Rectoanal inhibitory reflex (RAIR)

Normal value:	Present at 30–60 cc.
Comment:	Absent in Hirschsprung and Chagas disease, megarectum/rectocele, post coloanal or ileoanal (50%); absent for anatomic or technical reasons.

Anorectal sensation—volume at first sensation

Normal value:	10–50 mL.
Comment:	Little value of lower limit as some patients sense the insertion of the probe as such.

Diagnostic Guides

Anorectal sensation—volume at first urge

Normal value:	50–150 mL.
Comment:	Particularly of relevance if no urge felt.

Anorectal sensation—maximum tolerable volume

Normal value:	140–320 mL (females).
	170–440 mL (males).
Comment:	Reduced tolerance: typical finding in IBS. Increased tolerance: rectocele, megarectum, neurological sensory deficiency.

Rectal compliance

Normal value:	2–6 mL/mm Hg.
Comment:	Formula: compliance = Δvolume/Δpressure. Reduced compliance: typical finding in IBS. Increased tolerance: rectocele, megarectum, neurologic sensory deficiency.

Balloon expulsion test

Normal value:	Ability to expel balloon filled with 60–200 mL.
Comment:	If not expelled in left lateral position, recheck when patient sits on toilet.

Balloon retention test

Normal value:	Ability to retain a 100-mL balloon against (minimal to significant) external axial traction of > 0.5 kg.
Comment:	False normal values: pressure generated by contraction of puborectalis and gluteus muscles.

Colonic Transit Time (Sitzmark Study)

Intestinal transit time (baseline reference)

Normal value:	Overall 36–48 hours, stomach 0.5–2 hours, small intestine 1–4 hours, large intestine 30–46 hours.
Comment:	Distinction between upper GI dysfunction and lower GI dysfunction.

Simplified colonic transit test (1-day method)

Normal value: > 80% of all markers eliminated on day 5.

Comment: Three distribution patterns:

(1) < 6 markers left: grossly normal.

(2) diffuse distribution of > 5 markers throughout colon: colonic inertia.

(3) distal accumulation > 5 markers: functional outlet obstruction.

Sequential colonic transit test (3-day method)

Normal value: Segmental transit time: ascending colon: 11.3 hours; descending colon: 11.3 hours; rectosigmoid: 12.4 hours.

Total colonic transit time = 35 hours.

Comment: Pathologic: > 50 markers on day 4, > 70 hours total transit time, > 30 hours segmental transit time.

Defecating Proctogram (Defecography)

Anorectal angle (baseline reference)

Normal value: 90–110 degrees at rest.

Comment: The anorectal angle is the proctographic angle between the midaxial longitudinal axis of the rectum and the anal canal.

AMSTERDAM II CRITERIA FOR HNPCC

Amsterdam II Criteria

A family should be classified as having HNPCC if there is/are:

- One cancer related to colorectal cancer (CRC) or HNPCC in patient ≤ 50 years.
- Two or more generations.
- Three or more relatives with CRC or HNPCC-related cancers with one = first-degree relative of the other two.
- Familial adenomatous polyposis to be excluded!

HNPCC cancers: colorectal, endometrial, gastric, ovarian, ureter or renal, pelvic, biliary tract, small bowel, pancreatic, brain (gliomas), skin cancers (sebaceous adenomas).

Cross-reference

BETHESDA CRITERIA FOR MSI TESTING

Bethesda Criteria (revised 2003, Bethesda II)

Tumors should be tested for microsatellite instability (MSI) in the following situations:

- Colorectal cancer (CRC) in patient < 50 years.
- Presence of synchronous, metachronous colorectal, or other HNPCC-associated tumors, regardless of patient's age.
- CRC in patient < 60 years with histologic features of microsatellite instability (MSI):
  - Crohn-like lymphocytic reaction.
  - Mucinous/signet-ring differentiation.
  - Medullary growth pattern.
- CRC or HNPCC-associated tumor in ≥ 1 first-degree relative, with one cancer at < 50 years of age.
- CRC or HNPCC-associated tumor at any age in 2 first-degree or second-degree relatives.

HNPCC cancers: colorectal, endometrial, gastric, ovarian, ureter or renal, pelvic, biliary tract, small bowel, pancreatic, brain (gliomas), skin cancers (sebaceous adenomas).

Cross-reference

TUMOR STAGING IN TNM SYSTEM

Overview

Most commonly TNM system (other systems abandoned: Dukes, Astler-Coller, etc):

T = primary tumor, N = lymph node involvement, M = distant metastases

Colorectal Cancer

Primary tumor (T)

TX	Primary tumor cannot be assessed
T0	No evidence of primary tumor
Tis	Carcinoma in situ: intraepithelial or invasion of lamina propria
T1	Tumor invades submucosa
T2	Tumor invades muscularis propria
T3	Tumor invades through muscularis propria into subserosa or into nonperitonealized pericolic or perirectal tissues
T4	Tumor perforates visceral peritoneum or directly invades other organs/structures

Regional lymph nodes (N)

NX	Regional lymph nodes could not be assessed
N0	No regional lymph node metastases
N1	Metastasis in 1–3 regional lymph nodes
N2	Metastasis in ≥ 4 regional lymph nodes

Distant metastasis (M)

MX	Distant metastasis could not be assessed
M0	No distant metastasis
M1	Distant metastasis

Extent of resection

RX	Presence of residual tumor cannot be assessed
R0	No residual tumor
R1	Microscopic residual tumor
R2	Macroscopic residual tumor

Modifiers

p	Pathologic assessment
c	Clinical assessment

| u | Ultrasonographic assessment |
| y | Assessment after chemoradiation |

Clinical stage based on most advanced TNM component (bold)

Stage I:	M0 + N0 → T1 or **T2**				
Stage II:	M0 + N0 → T3 or **T4**	IIA	T3	N0	M0
		IIB	T4	N0	M0
Stage III:	M0 → **N+**, any T	IIIA	T1–T2	N1	M0
		IIIB	T3–T4	N1	M0
		IIIC	Any T	N2	M0
Stage IV:	**M1**, any T, any N				

Anal Cancer

Primary tumor (T)

TX	Primary tumor cannot be assessed
T0	No evidence of primary tumor
Tis	Carcinoma in situ
T1	Tumor ≤ 2 cm in greatest dimension
T2	Tumor > 2 cm, but < 5 cm in greatest dimension
T3	Tumor > 5 cm in greatest dimension
T4	Tumor of any size invades adjacent organ(s), eg, vagina, bladder, urethra

Regional lymph nodes (N)

NX	Regional lymph nodes could not be assessed
N0	No regional lymph node metastases
N1	Metastasis in perirectal lymph node(s)
N2	Metastasis in unilateral internal iliac and/or inguinal lymph nodes
N3	Metastasis in perirectal and inguinal lymph nodes and/or bilateral internal iliac and/or inguinal lymph nodes

Distant metastasis (M)

MX	Distant metastasis cannot be assessed
M0	No distant metastasis
M1	Distant metastasis

Diagnostic Guides

Extent of resection

RX	Presence of residual tumor cannot be assessed
R0	No residual tumor
R1	Microscopic residual tumor
R2	Macroscopic residual tumor

Modifiers

p	Pathologic assessment
c	Clinical assessment
u	Ultrasonographic assessment
y	Assessment after chemoradiation

Clinical stage based on most advanced TNM component (bold)

Stage 0:	M0 + N0 → **TIS**	
Stage I:	M0 + N0 → **T1**	
Stage II:	M0 + N0 → T2 or **T3**	
Stage IIIA:	M0 → T1 - **T3** + **N1**	
	M0 + N0 → **T4**	
Stage IIIB:	M0	→ T1 - **T3** + **N2**-3
	M0	→ **T4** + **N1**
Stage IV:	**M1,** any T, any N	

Cross-reference

Topic	*Chapter*
Colorectal cancer	4 (pp 252–280)
Anal cancer	4 (p 230)

FECAL INCONTINENCE SCORING SYSTEMS

(1) Cleveland Clinic Florida Incontinence Score ("Wexner" Score)

Type of Incontinence	Never	Frequency			
		Rarely (< 1/mo)	Sometimes (< 1/wk but ≥ 1/mo)	Usually (< 1/day but ≥ 1/wk)	Always (≥ 1/day)
Solid	0	1	2	3	4
Liquid	0	1	2	3	4
Gas	0	1	2	3	4
Wears pad	0	1	2	3	4
Lifestyle alteration	0	1	2	3	4

DAYS	WEEKS	MONTHS

4	3	2	1

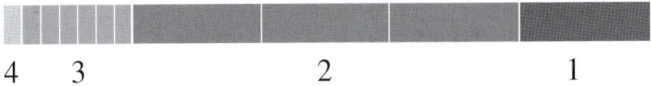

Interpretation
Sum of all parameters: → CCFIS 0 = perfect control, CCFIS 20 = absolute incontinence.

Advantage
• Simplicity and practicality: easy to use and interpret. Most commonly used → comparability.

Disadvantage
• System only based on subjective data input, lack of objective parameters.
• Does not take coping mechanisms into consideration, eg, no accidents if patient always close to bathroom, or "no pad" but change of underwear several times, etc.

(2) Fecal Incontinence Quality of Life Score (FIQL)

	TOTAL	Scale 1. Lifestyle	Scale 2. Coping/ Behavior	Scale 3. Depression/ Self-Perception	Scale 4. Embarrass-ment
Score					
Q1 Subjective report of general health: 1 = excellent → 5 = poor				▓	
Q2 Time quantitation of concerns due to accidental bowel leakage: 1 = most of the time → 4 = never (or N/A)	▓				
a I am afraid to go out		▓			
b I avoid visiting friends		▓			
c I avoid staying overnight away from home		▓			
d It is difficult for me to get out and do things like going to a movie or to church		▓			
e I cut down on how much I eat before I go out		▓			
f Whenever I am away from home, I try to stay near a restroom as much as possible			▓		
g It is important to plan my schedule (daily activities) around my bowel pattern		▓			
h I avoid traveling		▓			
i I worry about not being able to get to the toilet in time			▓		
j I feel I have no control over my bowels			▓		
k I can't hold my bowel movement long enough to get to the bathroom			▓		
l I leak stool without even knowing it					▓
m I try to prevent bowel accidents by staying very near a bathroom			▓		

(Continued)

	TOTAL	Scale 1. Lifestyle	Scale 2. Coping/ Behavior	Scale 3. Depression/ Self-Perception	Scale 4. Embarrass-ment
Score					
Q3 Quantitation of impact of accidental bowel leakage on well-being: 1 = strongly agree → 4 = strongly disagree (or N/A)	■				■
a I feel ashamed	■				■
b I cannot do many of things I want to do		■			
c I worry about bowel accidents			■		■
d I feel depressed				■	
e I worry about others smelling stool on me					■
f I feel like I am not a healthy person				■	
g I enjoy life less				■	
h I have sex less often than I would like to			■		
i I feel different from other people				■	
j The possibility of bowel accidents is always on my mind			■		
k I am afraid to have sex				■	
l I avoid traveling by plane or train		■			
m I avoid going out to eat		■			
n Whenever I go someplace new, I specifically locate where the bathrooms are			■		
Q4 During the past month, have you felt so sad, discouraged, hopeless, or had so many problems that you wondered if anything was worth-while? 1 = extremely so → 6 = not at all.	■			■	

Adapted with permission from Rockwood TH et al: Dis Colon Rectum 2000;43:9–17.

Diagnostic Guides

Interpretation

Psychometric instrument with four separate quality scales for (1) lifestyle, (2) coping/behavior, (3) depression/self perception, (4) embarrassment: higher score → less impact, lower score → more impact of fecal incontinence on quality of life.

Advantage

• Validated patient-reported disease-specific quality-of-life scale for fecal incontinence to assess the direct and very subjective impact of the condition on the patient. Shorter than SF-36 or EORTC-38.

Disadvantage

• System more complex, calculation of scores cumbersome. Question Q3c originally not included in any one of the four scales, best fits in scale 4 (embarassment).

Cross-reference

Topic	*Chapter*
Anophysiology testing	2 (p 78)
Fecal incontinence	4 (p 189)

ABBREVIATIONS (Continued)

UC	Ulcerative colitis
VAC	Vacuum-assisted closure
WBC	White blood cells
XRT	Chemoradiation

Oncological Outcome Parameters

DFS	Disease-free survival
NED	No evidence of disease (cancer follow-up)
ORR	Objective response rate (sum of complete and partial response)
OS	Overall survival
PFS	Progression-free survival
TTP	Time to tumor progression

Organizations

ACCP	American College of Chest Physicians
ACPGBI	Association of Coloproctology of Great Britain and Ireland
ASCRS	American Society of Colon and Rectal Surgeons
ESCP	European Society of Coloproctology
EORTC	European Organization for Research and Treatment of Cancer
ISUCRS	International Society of University Colon and Rectal Surgeons
NCI	National Cancer Institute (USA)
NIH	National Institutes of Health (USA)
SCIP	Surgical Care Improvement Project